Anesthesia

Editor

PAUL J. SCHWARTZ

ORAL AND MAXILLOFACIAL SURGERY CLINICS OF NORTH AMERICA

www.oralmaxsurgery.theclinics.com

Consulting Editor
RICHARD H. HAUG

August 2013 • Volume 25 • Number 3

ELSEVIER

1600 John F. Kennedy Boulevard • Suite 1800 • Philadelphia, Pennsylvania, 19103-2899

http://www.oralmaxsurgery.theclinics.com

ORAL AND MAXILLOFACIAL SURGERY CLINICS OF NORTH AMERICA Volume 25, Number 3
August 2013 ISSN 1042-3699, ISBN-13: 978-0-323-18612-4

Editor: John Vassallo; j.vassallo@elsevier.com
Developmental Editor: Susan Showalter

Oral and Maxillofacial Surgery Clinics of North America (ISSN 1042-3699) is published quarterly by Elsevier Inc., 360 Park Avenue South, New York, NY 10010-1710. Months of issue are February, May, August, and November. Business and Editorial Offices: 1600 John F. Kennedy Blvd., Suite 1800, Philadelphia, PA 19103-2899. Periodicals postage paid at New York, NY and additional mailing offices. Subscription prices are $369.00 per year for US individuals, $543.00 per year for US institutions, $165.00 per year for US students and residents, $431.00 per year for Canadian individuals, $645.00 per year for Canadian institutions, $495.00 per year for international individuals, $645.00 per year for international institutions and $224.00 per year for Canadian and foreign students/residents. To receive student/resident rate, orders must be accompanied by name or affiliated institution, date of term, and the *signature* of program/residency coordinator on institution letterhead. Orders will be billed at individual rate until proof of status is received. Foreign air speed delivery is included in all *Clinics* subscription prices. All prices are subject to change without notice. **POSTMASTER:** Send address changes to *Oral and Maxillofacial Surgery Clinics of North America*, Elsevier Periodicals Customer Service, 11830 Westline Industrial Drive, St. Louis, MO 63146. Tel: 1-800-654-2452 (U.S. and Canada); 314-447-8871 (outside U.S. and Canada). Fax: 314-447-8029. E-mail: journalscustomerservice-usa@elsevier.com (for print support); journalsonlinesupport-usa@elsevier.com (for online support).

Reprints. For copies of 100 or more, of articles in this publication, please contact the Commercial Reprints Department, Elsevier Inc., 360 Park Avenue South, New York, NY 10010-1710. Tel.: 212-633-3812; Fax: 212-462-1935; Email: reprints@elsevier.com.

Oral and Maxillofacial Surgery Clinics of North America is covered in *MEDLINE/PubMed (Index Medicus)*, *Science Citation Index Expanded (SciSearch®)*, *Journal Citation Reports/Science Edition*, and *Current Contents®/Clinical Medicine*.

Printed and bound by CPI Group (UK) Ltd, Croydon, CR0 4YY

Transferred to digital print 2013

Contributors

CONSULTING EDITOR

RICHARD H. HAUG, DDS
Carolinas Center for Oral Health,
Charlotte, North Carolina

EDITOR

PAUL J. SCHWARTZ, DMD
Oral and Maxillofacial Surgeon/Dentist
Anesthesiologist, Private Practice, Southern
Maryland Oral and Maxillofacial Surgery,
Dunkirk, Maryland; Senior Attending and
Director, Ambulatory Anesthesia Education,
Department of Oral and Maxillofacial
Surgery, Medstar Washington Hospital
Center, Washington, DC

AUTHORS

EDWARD C. ADLESIC, DMD
Private Practice, Pittsburgh, Pennsylvania

RAVI AGARWAL, DDS
Assistant Program Director, Department of
Oral and Maxillofacial Surgery, Medstar
Washington Hospital Center, Washington, DC

OSBEL BORGES, DMD
Chief Resident, Department of Oral and
Maxillofacial Surgery, College of Dental
Medicine, Nova Southeastern University,
Fort Lauderdale, Florida

WILLIAM L. CHUNG, DDS, MD
Associate Professor, Department of Oral and
Maxillofacial Surgery, University of Pittsburgh
Medical Center, Pittsburgh, Pennsylvania

DANIEL J. GESEK Jr, DMD
Private Practice, Jacksonville, Florida

JOSEPH A. GIOVANNITTI Jr, DMD
Professor, Department of Dental
Anesthesiology; Director of Anesthesia, Center
for Patients with Special Needs, University of
Pittsburgh School of Dental Medicine,
Pittsburgh, Pennsylvania

ANDREW HERLICH, DMD, MD, FAAP
Professor and Vice-Chair for Faculty
Development, Department of Anesthesiology,
University of Pittsburgh School of Medicine,
Pittsburgh, Pennsylvania

STEVEN I. KALTMAN, DMD, MD
Chair and Professor, Department of Oral and
Maxillofacial Surgery, College of Dental
Medicine, Nova Southeastern University,
Fort Lauderdale, Florida

GEORGE OBEID, DDS
Chairman, Department of Oral and
Maxillofacial Surgery, Medstar Washington
Hospital Center, Washington, DC

**DANIEL L. ORR II, DDS, MS
(anesthesiology), PhD, JD, MD**
Professor and Director, Oral and Maxillofacial
Surgery and Anesthesiology, University of
Nevada Las Vegas School of Dental Medicine;
Clinical Professor of Surgery and
Anesthesiology, University of Nevada School
of Medicine, Las Vegas, Nevada

JAMES C. PHERO, DMD
Professor Emeritus Anesthesiology,
Anesthesiology Department, College of
Medicine, University of Cincinnati Academic
Medical Center, Cincinnati, Ohio

MICHAEL H. PORTER, DDS
Senior Resident, Department of Oral and
Maxillofacial Surgery, Medstar Washington
Hospital Center, Washington, DC

MICHAEL RAGAN, DMD, JD, LLM
Adjunct Professor, Department of Oral and
Maxillofacial Surgery, College of Dental
Medicine, Nova Southeastern University, Fort
Lauderdale, Florida

MORTON B. ROSENBERG, DMD
Professor of Oral and Maxillofacial Surgery;
Head, Division of Anesthesia and Pain Control;
Senior Anesthetist, Tufts Medical Center,
Tufts University School of Dental Medicine;
Associate Professor of Anesthesiology,
Tufts University School of Medicine, Boston,
Massachusetts

PAUL G. SIMS, DDS
Private Practice, Oral and Maxillofacial
Surgery, Butte, Montana

MICHAEL J. STRONCZEK, DDS, MS
Private Practice, Oral and Maxillofacial Surgery
Associates (OMSA), Fort Wayne, Indiana;
Director, Oral and Maxillofacial Surgery
National Insurance Company (OMSNIC),
Rosemont, Illinois

DAVID W. TODD, DMD, MD, FACD
Private Practice, Lakewood, New York

Contents

No legitimate history of anesthesiology can exclude the contributions of American dentistry. Similarly, no history of anesthesiology in dentistry can exclude the contributions of oral and maxillofacial surgery (OMS). Many contributions of OMS to the art and science of anesthesiology have been singular, cutting edge when introduced, have stood the test of time, and have subsequently been universally incorporated into the general discipline. The process continues to this day with regard to the innovations and refinements OMS has proffered to the control of anxiety and pain. This article offers a brief review of some of these gifts.

This article reviews the anesthesia modalities available to the practicing oral and maxillofacial surgeon, including the anesthesia TEAM makeup. If office-based anesthesia is not the best option for the patient, alternative locations are discussed including out-patient surgery centers and hospitals. The American Association of Oral and Maxillofacial Surgeons (AAOMS) has fought long and hard to establish and maintain our ability to provide office-based anesthesia. This is our Standard of Care!

This article discusses the general methods used to assess patients before, during, and after operative procedures, sedation, or general anesthesia by the oral and maxillofacial surgery team. The details about specific disease processes will be discussed in other articles. These methods and modalities are not standards, but are commonly used in offices and clinics in the United States where sedation and anesthesia are provided.

The physical design of an oral and maxillofacial surgeon's office is highly individualized and unique. Every office must incorporate certain essential equipment and features to safely deliver office anesthesia, regardless of the scope of anesthesia services provided. Furthermore, the office design and anesthesia armamentarium must take into account patient safety and comfort. This article discusses the necessary elements, ranging from preanesthesia assessment forms and intraoperative records to office design, anesthesia monitors, and equipment related to the safe and successful administration of office-based anesthesia by oral and maxillofacial surgeons and their staff.

Adult Airway Evaluation in Oral Surgery

James C. Phero, Morton B. Rosenberg, and Joseph A. Giovannitti Jr

Patients with a history of difficult intubation or with conditions associated with difficult airway should be approached with organized primary and secondary plans for airway management. When these potential problems are detected, patient safety may be improved with use of advanced airway management techniques and equipment. Additionally, patient referral for consultation and/or management at facilities where advanced airway management practitioners and equipment are available may be beneficial in some cases.

Management of Allergy and Anaphylaxis During Oral Surgery

Morton B. Rosenberg, James C. Phero, and Joseph A. Giovannitti Jr

Minor and major allergic reactions occur during oral and maxillofacial treatment. Immediate diagnosis and pharmacologic intervention are imperative. Signs and symptoms may be variable. The early administration of epinephrine is critical.

Common Medical Illnesses that Affect Anesthesia and Their Anesthetic Management

Ravi Agarwal, Michael H. Porter, and George Obeid

Patients undergoing an office-based anesthetic require a thorough preoperative evaluation to identify medical illnesses and undertake appropriate investigations or studies. This article addresses common medical illnesses seen in oral surgery offices and provides insight into their anesthetic management, concentrating on open-airway office-based anesthesia.

Pharmacology of Intravenous Sedative/Anesthetic Medications Used in Oral Surgery

Joseph A. Giovannitti Jr

This article provides an overview of historical and current sedative agents available to the dentist anesthetist. The surgeon is given rational choices for sedation and the individualization of drug selection for each patient. Total intravenous anesthesia is becoming increasingly popular for dental sedation because of the availability of ultra–short-acting drugs and computerized infusion technology. Levels of sedation are more easily achieved and maintained, and recovery is enhanced, which gives the operator extreme, moment-to-moment control of the anesthetic experience and improves patient outcomes.

Pharmacology of Local Anesthetics Used in Oral Surgery

Joseph A. Giovannitti Jr, Morton B. Rosenberg, and James C. Phero

This article provides a comprehensive review of the pharmacology of local anesthetics as a class, and provides details of the individual drugs available in dental cartridges. Maximum recommended doses of local anesthetics and vasoconstrictors are presented for healthy adult and pediatric patients, and for patients with cardiovascular system impairments. Various complications and reasons for failure of local anesthesia effectiveness are discussed, and current and future trends in local anesthesia are presented to provide an overview of current research in local anesthesia.

Pediatric Sedation and Anesthesia for the Oral Surgeon

David W. Todd

Even simple oral and maxillofacial surgical procedures can become challenging when the child patient has a high degree of fear and anxiety. This article reviews differences in anatomy and physiology between the adult and pediatric patient, pre-anesthetic assessment, fasting guidelines, and choices of sedation routes, and discusses equipment options for the management of pediatric anesthesia. After reflection on these topics and based on training and experience, oral and maxillofacial surgeons can decide the ages of patients, medical comorbidities, and techniques with which they are comfortable in performing surgery in their offices in a safe and effective manner.

Respiratory anesthetic emergencies are the most common complications encountered during the administration of anesthesia in both the adult and pediatric populations. Regardless of the depth of anesthesia, a thorough review of the patients' health history, including the past medical history, edication list, prior anesthesia history, and complex physical examination, is critical in the promotion of safety in the oral and maxillofacial surgery office. The effective management of respiratory anesthetic emergencies includes both strong didactic and clinical skills.

Perioperative hypertension is a common problem. If hypertension is left untreated in patients at risk, infarctions and stroke are possible. There are limited choices of antihypertensive agents for the office. Aggressive antihypertensive therapy is not indicated because most of the episodes seen in the office are hypertensive urgencies and not emergencies. Hypotension is usually managed by decreasing the depth of anesthesia, intravenous fluids, and then vasopressors, typically ephedrine or phenylephrine. Consider treatment of hypotension whenever the mean arterial pressure decreases less than 60 mm Hg.

Despite the impressive safety of office-based anesthesia, serious emergencies still occur. Early and appropriate treatment is likely to improve outcomes. This article discusses selected emergencies with backgrounds and rationale for emergent treatment.

The safe and efficient use of outpatient surgical anesthesia modalities is a significant part of the training and expertise of the oral and maxillofacial surgeon. Although adverse outcomes are rare, they can have considerable traumatic psychological and professional consequences for the surgeon involved. The goal of this article is to develop guidelines to educate the doctor, the second victim, on how to manage a bad outcome and how to navigate through a difficult and arduous process.

ORAL AND MAXILLOFACIAL SURGERY CLINICS OF NORTH AMERICA

RELATED INTEREST

Anesthesiology Clinics September 2010 (Vol. 28, No. 3)
Current Topics in Anesthesia for Head and Neck Surgery
Joshua H. Atkins, MD, PhD, and Jeff E. Mandel, MD, *Editors*

THE CLINICS ARE NOW AVAILABLE ONLINE!
Access your subscription at:
www.theclinics.com

Preface
Anesthesia

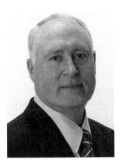

Paul J. Schwartz, DMD
Editor

The majority of surgical treatment rendered by oral and maxillofacial surgeons (OMS) in the United States is completed in an office-based setting. Because of the nature of the surgical procedures we perform and our unique training in the delivery of outpatient anesthesia, our specialty in particular and dentistry in general has historically occupied a unique niche in health care delivery. The ability to provide office-based surgical treatment without pain and anxiety has provided us with an efficient and cost-effective model to serve our diverse patient population. Within this model, the surgeon bears a tremendous responsibility as he/she is expected to make a diagnosis and have the surgical skills and experience to treat the problem, and the medical knowledge to determine if the patient is an acceptable risk to withstand surgery. Perhaps most importantly, the surgeon must rely on his/her training and experience to assess the patient's risk tolerance for office-based anesthesia. The operator/anesthetist anesthesia care team model used by the majority of practicing oral and maxillofacial surgeons in the United States has enjoyed a long history of success in providing individualized patient care with a remarkable record of safety. Our anesthesia care teams must continuously evolve so that we may fortify our position in the health care delivery system, and enable the office-based aspect of our OMS practice to thrive as we continue to make the daily decisions to provide the most efficacious surgical treatment and the safest anesthesia modalities and environment for our patients.

This issue of the *Oral and Maxillofacial Surgery Clinics of North America* is focused on the many challenges embodied within the safe practice of OMS office-based anesthesia. Each of our authors is an OMS or a Dentist Anesthesiologist with a long-standing knowledge and substantial clinical experience of the unique aspects of the OMS office-based anesthesia model. This volume benefits greatly from the quality and diversity of these outstanding contributing authors.

It is my sincere hope that this issue will serve as a valuable reference and resource to the practicing OMS as you face the daily maze of navigating a safe course for your patient.

I would like to extend my gratitude to Dr Richard H. Haug for asking me to serve as editor of this project, and to commend and thank Mr John Vassallo, the series editor, for his obvious expertise and frequent guidance.

Paul J. Schwartz, DMD
Southern Maryland Oral and Maxillofacial Surgery
3150 West Ward Road
Suite 306
Dunkirk, MD 20754, USA

E-mail address:
drpaulschwartz@comcast.net

Oral Maxillofacial Surg Clin N Am 25 (2013) ix
http://dx.doi.org/10.1016/j.coms.2013.04.006
1042-3699/13/$ – see front matter © 2013 Published by Elsevier Inc.

oralmaxsurgery.theclinics.com

The Development of Anesthesiology in Oral and Maxillofacial Surgery

Daniel L. Orr II, DDS, MS (anesthesiology), PhD, JD, MD[a,b]

KEYWORDS

- Anesthesiology • History • Oral and maxillofacial surgery

KEY POINTS

- Oral and Maxillofacial Surgery (OMS) is a specialty because OMS precursors began to incorporate general anesthesia into office-based practices soon after it was discovered by Horace Wells in the 1840's.
- Many contributions of OMS to the art and science of anesthesiology have been singular, cutting edge when introduced, have stood the test of time, and have subsequently been universally incorporated into the general discipline.
- Beginning in the 1970's, the OMS residency anesthesiology educational emphasis began to drift away from the historical one-third or more temporal curricula.
- With the decreased emphasis on dedicated anesthesia training in OMS residencies, recent graduate OMS are providing more sedation and less general anesthesia. OMS should consider reemphasizing anesthesia training in the future in order to preserve the historical team anesthesia model.

No legitimate history of anesthesiology can exclude the contributions of American dentistry. Similarly, no history of anesthesiology in dentistry can exclude the contributions of oral and maxillofacial surgery (OMS). In other words, many contributions of OMS to the art and science of anesthesiology have been singular, cutting edge when introduced, have stood the test of time, and have subsequently been universally incorporated into the general discipline. The process continues to this day with regard to the clinical, management, and other innovations OMS has proffered to the control of anxiety and pain. This article offers a brief review of some of these gifts.

Although dentistry has played a significant role in the development of anesthesiology since it was first discovered (observed and made known) by Horace Wells in December 1844, but for a series of unsuccessful negotiations by Chapin A. Harris, this article on the importance of dentistry in the development of anesthesiology would not be necessary. In fact dentistry itself, at least as administered by those with a DDS or DMD, would not be necessary.

In 1837 Harris approached the University of Maryland Medical College and proposed that the College include in its medical curriculum dental studies.[1] If Harris' plan had been accepted, Maryland Medical College graduates would have been practitioners of dental surgery as physicians. There were no recognized specialties at that time and the only real differing delineation in medical practice was between surgical and nonsurgical practice. However, Harris' logical suggestion to incorporate dentally based procedures into medicine was rejected outright because dentistry was deemed to be a mechanical trade, not rising to the level of a profession. Unwilling to accept defeat, Harris approached the College again in 1838, but with the same result. Resilient in his efforts, Harris in 1839 ultimately organized the first dental school, the Baltimore College of Dental Surgery, which

a University of Nevada Las Vegas School of Dental Medicine, Shadow Lane Campus, 1001 Shadow Lane, MS 7410, Las Vegas, NV 89106-4124, USA; b University of Nevada School of Medicine, Medical Education Building 2040 West Charleston Boulevard, Suite 301, Las Vegas, NV 89102, USA
E-mail address: dlorrii@gmail.com

Oral Maxillofacial Surg Clin N Am 25 (2013) 341–355
http://dx.doi.org/10.1016/j.coms.2013.04.003
1042-3699/13/$ – see front matter © 2013 Elsevier Inc. All rights reserved.

was chartered by Maryland in 1840. The Baltimore College of Dental Surgery established the DDS degree, and in 1867 the Harvard School of Dental Medicine created the DMD (because Harvard preferred a Latin language–based graduation certificate [Dentariae Medicinae Doctorae] and the translation of DDS [Chirurgae Dentium Doctoris] was awkward). Without the creation of the Baltimore College of Dental Surgery, dentists today would likely be physician odontologists or stomatologists.

ANESTHESIA PREQUEL

For millennia man readily understood that the pain from the surgical treatment of physical maladies is often worse than that of simply not treating the condition. Not infrequently, the fear of the pain associated with treatment was such that patients refused treatment altogether, accepting their inevitable fate, often death. Such was the case even if surgical treatment could be predictably successful, simply because patients literally would rather die than submit to the pain associated with surgery.

The Ancients noted that procedures could be completed on unconscious victims, such as those sustaining head trauma, without subjective pain. In short order, therapeutic strangulation to the point of unconsciousness became an option for surgical candidates. Unfortunately, as with any artificial loss of consciousness, complications occasionally occurred. Strangulation, although effective in rendering victims unconscious, also often rendered them dead.

Overdoses of agents, relative to social use, were also used to relieve the pain of surgery. Ethyl alcohol, opiates, and hallucinogens were all used for these purposes from time to time. However, the use of these prescriptions was, sadly, also not predictably safe or effective.

Sensory nerve trunks innervating more peripheral structures could be effectively anesthetized by tourniquets or freezing, which also helped with hemostasis, but these techniques were of limited use. Mesmerism or animal magnetism, hypnosis in modern terms, is effective on some individuals seeking pain relief but, again, is not predictably useful.

It was not until 1799 that Sir Humphrey Davy, the venerable English chemist, noticed that the pain associated with his own erupting third molar was relieved by the inhalation of nitrous oxide. In 1800 he published in *Researches, Chemical and Philosophical*: "As nitrous oxide in its extensive operation appears capable of destroying physical pain, it may probably be used with advantage during surgical operations in which no great effusion of blood takes place."[2] Despite the publication of *Researches*, no practical application of Davy's hypothesis was attempted at this time, and Davy made his name in the course of other chemical pursuits.

The same year *Researches* was published by Davy, future English physician Henry Hill Hickman was born. Hickman's experiments circa 1823 involved in part the partial asphyxiation of animals in glass domes. Hickman confirmed the Ancients' belief that unconscious animals with "animation suspended" could be operated on without reaction to pain. Soon, Hickman added small amounts of carbon dioxide and other agents to the bell chambers, but his use of any more effective agents, such as nitrous oxide, was never documented. Hickman's belief in suspended animation was such that he wrote: "I feel so confident that animation in the human subject could be safely suspended by proper means, carefully employed, that, (although I could not conscientiously recommend a patient to risk his life in the experiment) I certainly should not hesitate a moment to become the subject of it, if I were under the necessity of suffering any long or severe operation."[3] Hickman's suspended animation via asphyxiation found little enthusiasm even after he wrote of his experiments to the Royal Society of London in 1824 (perhaps because Davy was President of the Society that year), and petitioned at least the French courts on the continent.

Many are familiar with Dr Crawford W. Long of Georgia, who successfully administered ether

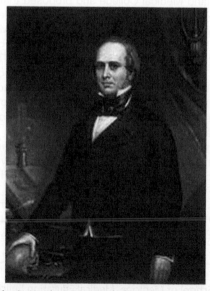

Chapin A. Harris, DDS, MD, believed that dentistry is most properly classified as a profession, an employment requiring advanced education and high ethical standards.

to his patients for straightforward surgical procedures as early as March 1842. However, although Long was one of the first to observe the potential benefits of such an agent he never made his observations known for the benefit of others, thus forgoing the honor of being the discoverer of surgical anesthesia.

In addition, although Long was honored with a United States postage stamp for his early use of ether, medical student William E. Clark actually administered ether to a Miss Hobbie for a dental extraction performed by dentist Elijah Pope in January 1842, predating Long (Yagelia J, personal communication, 2011).

Davy, Hickman, Long, Clark, Pope, and others such as Robert Collier (who mixed opium with rum in 1839) and E.R. Smilie (who combined opium and ether in 1844) all flirted with the potential to be the "greatest benefactor to mankind" for the discovery of anesthesia, but none effectively publicized their observations. That task was accomplished by Horace Wells, DDS.

Horace Wells, DDS

The story of Dr Horace Wells' observation and publication of the beneficial effects of nitrous oxide in surgical operations is well known. Wells attended Professor Gardner Q. Colton's nitrous oxide demonstration in Hartford, Connecticut on December 10, 1844 and noticed frolic participant Samuel Cooley traumatically lacerate his shin without reaction after inhaling nitrous oxide. Wells, a dentist sorely uncomfortable with the pain subjected to his patients by his treatment, was inspired. He was not slow about developing an experiment to test his insight. The very next day, Wells arranged for John M. Riggs, DDS, to

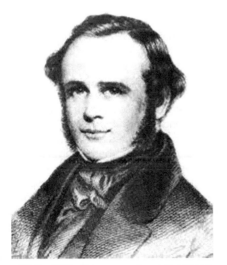

Horace Wells, DDS, discoverer of anesthesiology.

remove Wells' own tooth after receiving nitrous oxide from Colton. Several quotes are attributed to Wells after the successful removal of his tooth by Riggs, but all stress that the operation, and the anesthetic, were a great success. Wells immediately began using nitrous oxide for his own patients. By the time Wells had completed only 12 or 15 procedures in his practice, he had arranged to demonstrate his findings clinically at The Massachusetts General Hospital in the operating room of John C. Warren. On Wells' arrival at the hospital, a patient in need of an amputation was present. However, the patient decided to "die whole" and declined the procedure despite assurances about the likely efficacy of nitrous oxide in relieving his pain. Wells then was allowed to give a lecture to Warren's medical students on his discovery, one of whom determined to have his own troublesome third molar removed at that time with nitrous oxide. Later that day, the student reported that he was completely satisfied and did not recall the extraction. However, while still under the influence of the nitrous oxide he had groaned at the end of the procedure, which led to Wells immediately being hooted out of the ether dome by the student patient's classmates.

Notwithstanding the groan, as time passed the world recognized Wells' singular efforts. In 1864 the American Dental Association (ADA) resolved:

> *...that to Horace Wells, of Hartford, Connecticut, (now deceased) belongs the credit and honor of the introduction of anesthesia in the United States of America, and we do firmly protest against the injustice done to truth and the memory of Dr Horace Wells, in the effort made during a series of years and especially at the last session of Congress, to award the credit to other persons or person.*[4]

In 1872 the American Medical Association resolved "...that the honor of the discovery of practical anesthesia is due to the late Dr Horace Wells, of Connecticut."[5]

Through the years, perhaps culminating in 1944, the centennial anniversary of Wells' discovery, virtually every anesthesia entity has confirmed Wells' primacy as the Father of surgical anesthesia. That year, a year-long worldwide celebration of the event was coordinated by the ADA, which also published a book memorializing the event.[6] Only the American Medical Association (AMA) hedged its prior endorsement, iterating that Wells was "...one of the first..."; the likely reasons for this shift are discussed later.

William Taggert Green Morton, DDS

Dr William T.G. Morton was a member of the inaugural 1840 class of the Baltimore College of Dental Surgery, and subsequently an associate of Wells in Hartford, Connecticut. Virtually everyone in Hartford, including Morton, was familiar with Wells' well-established use of nitrous oxide. On October 16, 1846, Morton repeated Wells' trek to Warren's Massachusetts General Hospital operating room, but to administer a different inhalational agent. Morton arrived at the hospital late because the new inhaler he had ordered was not quite ready. Reportedly, on Morton's arrival Warren pointedly advised: "Doctor, your patient is ready." Morton then administered his "invention" lethion (ether fragranced with perfume), and after a moment boldly counteradvised Warren: "Doctor, *your* patient is ready." The patient, Gilbert Abbot, was successfully anesthetized and, after a neck tumor was quickly removed, Warren announced to the assembled students and faculty in the literal operating-room theater: "Gentlemen, this is no humbug."

Word spread rapidly about Morton's successful demonstration. Lethion was soon disclosed to be ether, and widespread use of the agent immediately followed. Morton, and an opportunistic peripheral contributor, Charles Jackson, also moved quickly, obtaining patent #4848 for lethion on 12 November, 1846. In this case, a conflict between patent law and medical "law" (really the ethical determination to not restrict access to health care innovations, as opposed to other inventions) resulted. After one precedent setting suit, Morton eventually dropped his patent claims to lethion anesthesia, although the process was time consuming over several years. The United States itself played a large role in resolution of the patent rights controversy when, in the Mexican-American War (1846–1848), ether was used liberally and without Morton's permission by the very government that had granted the patent. To his credit, Morton himself later administered 3000 anesthetics gratis during the Civil War.[7]

ADDITIONAL EARLY CONTROVERSIES

In addition to the lingering question about who deserved primacy for the discovery of safe, effective, and reproducible anesthesia, other issues arose almost immediately.

The American Association of Dental Surgeons (AADS) opined that:

> ...every itinerating dentist, who gouges out a tooth or fills a cavity with amalgam...can arm himself with an inhaling apparatus, and a bottle of an anesthetic material, with which he expects to prey on the public...Hence, in all minor operations in surgery, their administration is forbidden; and that their demand in the practice of dental surgery is small...[8]

Then, as today, there seemed to be 3 groups of individuals highly concerned with the practice of anesthesia: (1) doctors who had access to anesthesia, (2) doctors who did not have access to anesthesia, and (3) patients. Interesting dynamics developed within each group.

With regard to doctors who had ready access to the provision of anesthesia, some, such as Wells, stated that anesthesia "should be as free as the air we breathe," seeking first and foremost to provide the gift to the widest patient population possible. Others, such as Morton, by means of his US Patent 4848, sought to significantly restrict the ability of patients to receive anesthesia.

Doctors who did not have ready access to anesthesia, such as the AADS, also generally sought to restrict anesthesia's use by whatever means necessary, including claims that it was uneconomic, unsafe, immoral, hindered healing, and so forth.

Patients, on the other hand, universally wanted more access to anesthesia options, which in part may best explain the incongruous responses of doctors, and others, who saw no need for further anesthesia services. That is, some doctors who had ready access to anesthesia, such as Morton, may have noticed that they had a relative monopoly providing the service, and did not want it to be too easy for other doctors to use the craft. The

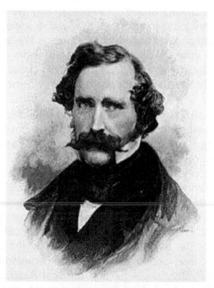

William Taggart Green Morton, DDS, was a student of Wells and introduced the world to the beneficial effects of ether in 1846.

same restraining opinion was held by surgeons who did not have ready access to anesthesia when they noticed their patients leaving in droves, gravitating to others who could provide a pain-free option for their surgeries. It is interesting that much of the same dynamic can be seen even today when one looks at economically competing anesthesia and surgical providers.

Those opining that anesthesia should be limited were not restricted to doctors. Even religionists sought to curb anesthesia, quoting Genesis 3:16 as justification: "Unto the woman he said, I will greatly multiply thy sorrow and thy conception; in sorrow thou shalt bring forth children..."[9] Perhaps ministers noted that members of their flocks seemed to take more comfort in ether or chloroform during times of physical pain than from the words of their religious advisor. Be that as it may, another anesthesia pioneer, James Y. Simpson of Scotland, effectively countered preachers constraining anesthesia by noting not only that in the original Hebrew "sorrow" could also be translated as "labor," but also that God himself apparently approved of anesthesia, as noted during Adam's "deep sleep" for the thoracotomy necessary to create Eve by means of Adam's costae verae (Genesis 2:21).[10] The early debate about the propriety of the use of anesthesia during childbirth diminished greatly when Queen Victoria opted for chloroform during the delivery of her seventh child in 1853.

Nathan Cooley Keep, DDS

Although Simpson is generally rightfully acknowledged as the preeminent pioneer obstetric

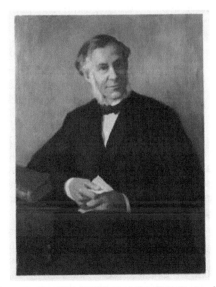

Nathan Cooley Keep, DDS, was the first dean of Harvard School of Dental Medicine and the first to practice obstetric anesthesia in the United States.

anesthesiologist, it should be noted that Nathan Cooley Keep, DDS, later the first dean of the Harvard School of Dental Medicine, was the first in America to provide obstetric anesthesia in 1847, the same year Simpson started the practice in Scotland. In 1867 Dr Keep became the founding dean of the new Harvard School of Dentistry. Keep was also known for his forensic efforts in the sensational Webster/Parkman murder trial, at which he identified a prosthesis he had made for Dr Parkman after Dr Webster had placed it in a furnace along with Parkman's dissected body parts.[11]

First Death

The first death noted in the literature was in 1848 and was that of Hannah Greener, a 15-year-old orphan who passed away during chloroform anesthesia administered by Mr Meggison for surgeon Mr Lloyd, who was addressing an ingrown toenail (unguis incarnatus).[12] The inquest after the incident assigned no legal blame to either Meggison or Lloyd. Later analyses of the cause were mixed, with Mr Sibson opining that the etiology was "paralysis of the heart," the French Academy of Medicine publishing "asphyxia alone," and the AMA stating it was due to "overdosage." For decades, early clinicians vigorously argued between a cardiovascular and pulmonary cause of death under anesthesia.

First Sexual Assault Claims

In 1847 a Parisian dentist was convicted of sexual assault on 2 girls. In 1854, United States dentist Stephen T. Beale was convicted and sentenced to 4.5 years in prison after a highly publicized trial in Philadelphia. However, the sentence was immediately overturned,[13] and the legal principle that the accusation of an anesthetized patient needs the corroboration from a noncompromised witness was established. Even today, an important function of OMS anesthesia team members is as objective witnesses to events as they actually occur, particularly when patients' memories are compromised by drugs or psychological reactions.[14]

Samuel Stockton White, DDS

Dr S.S. White, perhaps best known to OMS for carbide burs, was also the first to commercially render N_2O into liquid form in 1881 by means of hand-pump compression. Before this innovation, those administering N_2O had to produce the gas themselves for patient use, stored and delivered via large rubber bags. The SS White Company

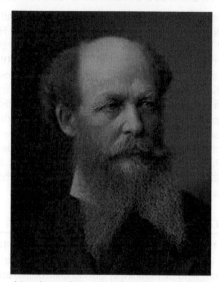

Samuel Stockon White, DDS, founder and underwriter of the *Journal of the American Dental Association* precursor *Dental Cosmos*, liquefied nitrous oxide for clinical use.

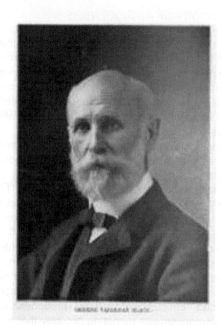

Greene Vardeman Black, DDS, father of modern dentistry, founding dean of Northwestern School of Dentistry, and general anesthesia educator.

was also a leading manufacturer of early anesthesia machines and equipment. White's efforts also facilitated Thomas Crapper's (of plumbed toilet fame) creation of an N_2O hyperbaric chamber.[15]

Alfred Coleman, DDS

Dr Ralph Waters, founding director of the first anesthesiology residency in the United States, is widely acknowledged as being the first to use CO_2 absorption clinically in 1919. However, the *British Medical Journal* published that Dr Coleman reported it was possible to save some of the products of respiration for further use as early as 1868. Coleman also described his invention of a CO_2 absorber that allowed N_2O to be reused, naming the device, in true dental entrepreneurial fashion, The Economizer.[16] Coleman was later named the first dental fellow of the Royal College of Surgeons.

Greene Vardiman Black, DDS

Dr G.V. Black, the father of Modern Dentistry and the founding dean of the Northwestern University School of Dentistry, developed the carious lesion classification system ubiquitously used by dentists to this day. Black also lectured on the "Introduction of Bromide of Ethyl as an Anesthetic for Dental Purposes or Any Very Short Operation" in 1883.[17]

Ferdinand Hasbrouck, DDS

When President Grover Cleveland was diagnosed with an intraoral tumor in 1893, the President's

surgeons chose Dr Hasbrouck as his dental surgeon and anesthesiologist. The operation was performed in secret on the yacht *Oneida* in the Long Island, New York Sound. Hasbrouck, as an operator anesthetist, induced President Cleveland with 100% N_2O and extracted teeth from the corpus of the tumor. As President Cleveland recovered from the N_2O, Hasbrouck began the administration of ether for the remainder of the procedure as performed by a team of surgeons. This incident was kept secret from the American public for decades.[18]

Statistically, it is not surprising that the President's anesthesiologist was Dr. Hasbrouck because dentistry was the qualitative and quantitative leader in the provision of anesthesia at this time. For instance, at Presbyterian Hospital in New York, 1,714 total anesthetics were administered in 1911. There were only a few hundred medical anesthesia providers in the country. On the other hand, "signs on dental offices everywhere proclaimed" the availability of general anesthesia for tooth extraction.[19] Many dentists administered thousands of anesthetics annually in their own offices.

Charles Teeter, DDS

In 1902, Dr Charles Teeter introduced the first anesthesia machine capable of delivering N_2O/O_2, ether, and chloroform. The gasses could be warmed, rebreathed, and administered under

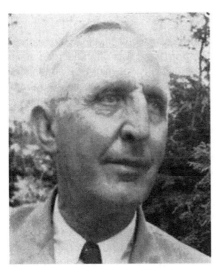

Charles Teeter, DDS, President of both the American Society of Anesthesiologists and the International Anesthesia Research Society. (*From* ADSA. Available at: adsahome.org. Accessed May 1, 2013.)

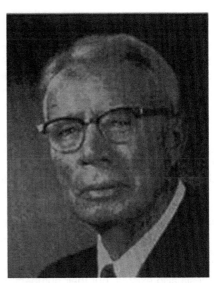

Jay A. Heidbrink, DDS, was an exemplary entrepreneurial exodontist/pre-OMS specialty educator and inventor. The preeminent anesthesia award of the American Dental Society of Anesthesiology is named in his honor. (*From* ADSA. Available at: adsahome. org. Accessed May 1, 2013.)

positive pressure. Later Teeter added mercury columns to observe the flow of inhalational agents. He also designed the first nasopharyngeal tubes for clinical use. Teeter was well accepted by his medical colleagues, publishing in the *Journal of the American Medical Association*[20,21] and speaking at the AMA annual meeting several times about anesthesia. Teeter was elected President of both the International Anesthesia Research Society and the American Society of Anesthesiologists (ASA).

Jay A. Heidbrink, DDS

Dr Heidbrink successfully modified the Teeter machine into a "rather complicated" unit. The Heidbrink innovation and others were ultimately purchased by the Ohio Chemical Company, a leading manufacturer of anesthesia machines for decades. Heidbrink was the first to color code anesthesia gas tanks, and invented the pin index safety system. An exodontist before the formalization of OMS as a specialty, Heidbrink owned a practice in Minnesota that employed 3 dentist anesthesiologists. Heidbrink would transition room to room, operating as the dentist anesthesiologists would sequentially induce and recover patients with 100% N_2O. The American Dental Society of Anesthesiology (ADSA) Heidbrink Award is named after him.

Edgar Randolph Rudolph Parker, DDS

Dr Edgar R.R. Painless Parker was a highly successful, though controversial, dental entrepreneur

in California at the beginning of the twentieth century. Parker legally supplemented his name with Painless after the California State Board of Dental Examiners opined that his prior use of "painless" in promoting his dental practice was unethical. Unethical or not, the patients flocked to Parker's offices, enabling him to gross US$3 million in that era. Parker was at least relatively truthful in his use of "painless" because he was an early advocate of the routine use of local anesthesia, formulating his own solution dubbed "Hydrocaine."[22] The routine use of local anesthesia in dentistry did not come to fruition until the 1930s.[23]

1920 TO 1940: ORAL AND MAXILLOFACIAL SURGERY PREQUEL

1920 to 1940 were the years immediately preceding the formalization of OMS. Since the days of Wells and Morton, an insightful number of dentists had used general and local anesthetics in dentistry as they became available. The use of general agents was always controversial, as it also was in medicine, because of the less favorable patient risk/benefit analysis that existed or was perceived to exist for many decades. The success of Painless Parker in ushering in the increased acceptance of using local anesthetic resulted in dentistry gravitating toward that mode of pain relief. However, a core of dentists committed to the use of general anesthesia successfully persisted. This group, including early exodontists from Wells and Morton to Hasbrouck in the 1800s and followed by Teeter, Heidbrink, and many others, were the precursors of today's specialty practitioners of OMS. Without question, what set OMS pioneers apart from the rest of dentistry was their use of general anesthesia.

In 1918 the American Society of Exodontists (ASE) was formed, and in 1921 the ASE renamed itself the American Society of Oral Surgeons and Exodontists (ASOSE).[24] The group's literature and annual meeting presentations from the 1920s and 1930s were dominated by the topic of inhalation general anesthesia, but also included talks about intravenous agents such as sodium thiopental as a cutting-edge presentation in 1934. Non-ASOSE dentists who used general anesthesia also existed, but their numbers began to be dwarfed by the ASOSE members in terms of both practitioners and anesthetics delivered. In large part this was because OMS exodontia operations are of short duration compared with dental restorations, which require a much longer and more labor-intensive general anesthetic. During this era, dentists were the most prolific providers of general anesthesia not only in dentistry, but in all the health professions, largely secondary to the outpatient office-based niche.

The American Board of Oral Surgery was established in 1940, and for decades Board candidates spent nearly equivalent amounts of time studying subject matter relating to surgery and anesthesiology.

Harry Seldon, DDS

The list of major contributors to anesthesia in the specialty at this time is impressive, but this chapter focuses on Dr Harry Seldon as a prototypical exemplar of the surgeon anesthesiologist from this era. In 1918 Seldon graduated from New York University College of Dentistry, and went on to publish several highly successful editions of *Practical Anesthesia for Dental and Oral Surgery—Local and General* in the 1930s, 1940s, and 1950s. He was the Director of Dentistry at the New York Metropolitan Hospital and Chief of Anesthesia of the New York University. He was elected President of the ASOS in 1956, and the Center for OMS at the Israeli Government Hospital in Haifa is named after him. Seldon's texts present a wonderful retrospective history of the advancements in anesthesiology and surgery during these years.

1940S

This decade was significant in that anesthesiology changed from what was often deemed an insignificant afterthought that might be administered by technicians during surgery to an area that began to be embraced as essential by dentistry, medicine, veterinary medicine, and nursing.

The remarkable growth of anesthesiology in the 1940s was brought on by 2 major factors. First, it was the decade that recognized the 100th anniversary of the discovery of anesthesia, even as it was still a somewhat controversial question. A US postage stamp was issued in recognition of Crawford W. Long in 1942, the centennial of his first use of ether. Long did not make known his observation of ether's effectiveness until years later, so cannot be acknowledged as the discoverer of the art.

The ADA, recognizing since 1864 that Horace Wells was the first to observe and make known the benefits of general anesthesia, planned a centennial celebration for its annual meeting in 1944. However, the ADA's plans were truncated by restrictions on travel secondary to World War II. The ADA ultimately issued a book[25] acknowledging Wells' efforts with testimonials from virtually every dental association and developed country in the world.

In 1944 Paramount Pictures released a feature-length movie titled "The Great Moment" based on Rene Fulop-Miller's *Triumph Over Pain* (1940) and starring Joel McCrea as Morton.

The second factor influencing the remarkable recognition of anesthesia was World War II itself. In fact, wars did much to promote the art during the previous century. Morton provided 3000 anesthetics during the Civil War.[7] The American Association of Nurse Anesthetists traces its founding to the same conflict. However, World War II was the first time that the military formally planned for the provision of anesthesia during surgery. For instance, the Pitt Brigade, led by Leonard Monheim, DDS, was just one dental unit that was dedicated to providing anesthesia for wartime surgical procedures. Other dentists such as Milton Jaffe were also leaders in these groups of dentist anesthesia providers.[26] Heidbrink's anesthesia mask was modified for aviation use and more than 1 million such masks were produced for aviators.

In 1945, the ASA underwent its fifth and final name change after being initially formed in 1905. The American Board of Anesthesiology was formed in 1941, 1 year after the American Board of Oral and Maxillofacial Surgery (ABOMS).

Also in this decade, Leonard Monheim published "A, B, and C" preanesthesia risk categories while Harry Archer offered "1, 2, and 3" risk classifications. In 1963 the ASA first produced its Physical Status Classification, of which later versions are ubiquitous today.

Adrian Orr Hubbell, DDS

Adrian Orr Hubbell graduated from the University of Southern California School of Dentistry in 1937 and subsequently trained as a resident in oral surgery and anesthesiology at the Mayo Clinic through 1939. The Mayo Clinic was the second anesthesiology residency, established by John Lundy, MD, following Wisconsin's program Chaired by Ralph Waters, MD.

While at the Mayo Clinic, Hubbell was introduced to the new intravenous short-acting barbiturate sodium thiopental. Contrary to all the current conventional wisdom, Hubbell determined that thiopental would be a valuable drug for office-based OMS procedures and immediately began to use it at his private practice in Long Beach, California after successful completion of his dual residency training. During the course of his career, Hubbell administered more than 300,000 thiopental anesthetics without mortality. Hubbell demonstrated his preoperative diagnostic acumen, evidenced by the fact that 3 patients he admitted for inpatient anesthetics succumbed during the hospital procedures.

Hubbell published his findings extensively in the dental and medical literature,[27–34] and also

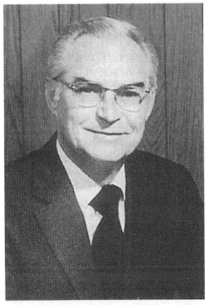

Adrian Orr Hubbell, DDS, intravenous office-based outpatient anesthesia pioneer. (*From* American Association of Oral and Maxillofacial Surgeons. The building of a specialty: oral and maxillofacial surgery in the United States. J Oral Maxillofac Surg 1989; 47(10 Suppl 2):1–271.)

obtained US Patent #2,471,623 for An Apparatus for Handling Fluids.[35] Popularly known as the "Hubbell Bubble," the device featured a hand-held rubber bulb by which incremental doses of thiopental could be conveniently dosed. Later versions were modified so that dosing could be accomplished by a knee or foot bulb. Similar to earlier N_2O/O_2 practitioners, Hubbell used thiopental as his single agent, usually omitting even local anesthesia.

In the early 1950s, Hubbell and Harold Krogh, another early Mayo Clinic OMS/anesthesia resident, offered their successful thiopental techniques as nationwide continuing education to the OMS community, thus establishing the basis of the preferred intravenous techniques used by many OMS to this day. Hubbell was the first to publish the term "team anesthesia" to describe the office-based, outpatient general anesthesia experience developed by OMS.[36]

1950S

The decade started with the momentous decision of the ASA to rescind unrestricted membership for dentists, which included dentist anesthesiologists and many OMS.[37] The ADSA was then established by and for former ASA dentist members and others who realized that dentistry needed a platform from which to address anesthesia issues.

As an interesting aside, in 1953 the AMA attempted to define Oral Surgery and produced a document the ADA found to be inaccurate and objectionable. The Board of Trustees of the AMA subsequently rescinded the document.[38] The AMA's 2009 Scope of Practice Data Series comments on OMS are nothing new...but have not been rescinded to date.[39]

1960S

In 1960 The American Association of Oral and Maxillofacial Surgeons (AAOMS) (American Society of Oral Surgeons [ASOS]) Committee on Graduate Training issued the document "Essentials of an Adequate Training Program in Oral Surgery." The document stressed the primacy of anesthesia training in OMS residencies, which were 3 years' duration at that time, by iterating: "Ideally, training in anesthesia should extend throughout a twelve-month period. Such a schedule of study allows for the other 2 years to be devoted exclusively to the various aspects of clinical oral surgery." In addition to the ideal 12 consecutive months of operating room–based anesthesia, OMS residents were generally immersed in OMS office-based team general anesthesia paradigms such as the Hubbell Los Angeles County/University of Southern

California/Medical Center (LAC/USC/MC) intravenous thiopental paradigm and OMS Morgan Allison's Ohio State University intubated inhalational model.

Although most of the anesthetics provided by OMS in the 1960s were general anesthetics, sedative techniques were present. Niles Jorgensen, DDS, at Loma Linda University, had developed the popular "Jorgensen Technique" of intravenous pentobarbital, meperidine, and scopolamine. Harry Langa, DDS, in New York, advocated the "relative anesthesia" technique, which was a shift from N_2O/O_2 general anesthesia to N_2O/O_2 sedation. Milton Jaffe, DDS, reported his use of intravenous ether for sedation, an effective technique familiar to the author.[40,41] Diazepam was made available by Hoffmann-La Roche in 1963.

In 1967 the ADSA initiated its Fellowship Examination process, open to any dentist who had a minimum of 1 year of operating room–based anesthesia residency training.

The Southern California Society of Oral and Maxillofacial Surgeons

In 1967, the Southern California Society of Oral and Maxillofacial Surgeons (SCSOMS) began voluntary in-office anesthesia evaluations as a society.

Southern California OMS leaders, such as John "Jack" Lytle, DDS, MD, who trained at LAC/USC/MC in the 1950s and 1960s, were purists of the "Hubbell School," although thiopental had been largely replaced by methohexital. The LAC/USC/MC

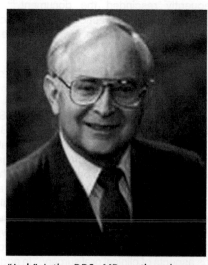

John "Jack" Lytle, DDS, MD, authored many early OMS anesthesia safety articles in the professional literature. (*From* American Association of Oral and Maxillofacial Surgeons. The building of a specialty: oral and maxillofacial surgery in the United States. J Oral Maxillofac Surg 1989;47(10 Suppl 2):1–271.)

technique typically used 8 to 14 mL of a 1% solution. Patients generally became apneic, but the initiation of the surgery as the last of the methohexital was entering the vein stimulated ventilation. No monitors were attached to the patient, so skin and mucosal color were used to determine the level of oxygenation.[42]

Harry Seldin, DDS, had reported about OMS office anesthesia safety beginning in the 1950s.[43,44] Lytle magnified the early reporting efforts of Seldin on morbidity and mortality, beginning a series of publications about anesthesia in OMS offices in 1974.[45–47] Similar studies are now regularly published to this day. Over the years, the OMS-coordinated team paradigms have seen the incidence of mortality reported initially by Seldin as 1 in 66,000 decrease to less than 1 in 720,000, a safety record second to none for any surgical procedure in any venue.

1970S

That the AAOMS (ASOS) was supportive of the rapidly spreading concept of state component in-office evaluations was demonstrated by the publication of the ASOS *Office Anesthesia Manual*, cost $4.50 prepaid, in 1976. The eighth edition of this resource was published in 2012.

In 1977 the prescient SCSOMS initiated its OMS Anesthesia Assistant Courses, which are still ongoing and are scheduled to be presented in large part online in 2013. The AAOMS Oral and Maxillofacial Anesthesia Assistant Program started in 1986 and evolved into the Dental Anesthesia Assistant Certification Examination (DANCE) in 2009.

The 1970s saw the AAOMS residency educational emphasis begin to change markedly with regard to anesthesia rotations. Even as single degree programs increased to 4 years and dual degree programs to 6 years, operating room–dedicated anesthesia experiences were reduced to 6 months. The additional years of training were composed of medical school and/or rotations with emphasis on internal medicine. This change came about in an effort to prepare OMS to effectively represent the specialty in hospitals when competitor physicians questioned the OMS's ability to complete adequate history and physical (H&P) examinations and hospital admissions overall. ABOMS applicants of this era might never be asked a question about teeth, but could fully expect queries about ectopic tubal pregnancies or be asked to listen to and diagnose heart sounds.

During this decade the author was a dentist anesthesiology resident at the University of Utah Medical Center Department of Anesthesiology,

1 of more than 150 programs that had produced dentist anesthesiologists up to that time.[40] Not a few OMS at this time completed 2 years in anesthesiology, 1 year as a dedicated anesthesia resident and an additional year during OMS residency training. This training gave OMS a cadre of individuals with training and insight into both anesthesiology and OMS, doctors who were valuable to the profession clinically, academically, in research, and politically.

In 1976 the ASA introduced the resident's written examination as the first step in becoming board certified in anesthesiology. Dental residents at the University of Utah were enrolled for the test, and one first-year dental resident achieved the second highest score in the program on the examination, competing against more than 30 other first, second, and third (research) year physician residents. The University of Utah and other medical anesthesiology programs petitioned the ASA to allow dentists to continue on the track to ASA board certification. These requests were refused by the ASA, in a decision reminiscent of the 1950 determination to rescind full unrestricted dentist anesthesiologist membership in the ASA.[37]

During the author's residency, the ADA Council on Judicial Procedures determined that dentist residents in anesthesiology residencies were in parallel situations to those in Commission on Accreditation (CODA) accredited residencies (W. Elliott Dunn. Secretary, Council on Judicial Procedures, Constitution and Bylaws, American Dental Association. personal communication, 1976). Dental anesthesiology residencies ultimately became CODA accredited in 2005.

In early 1976 the opening of Utah's first outpatient surgical center was announced to university anesthesia residents at rounds. It was explained that this was a facility where patients could be admitted in the morning, receive an anesthetic for a surgical procedure, and return home on the same day! The anesthesia faculty discussed in an animated fashion whether this new model was safe and questioned if it would even survive. One of the dental residents then commented that dentistry had been doing the same thing for 100 years (actually since December 1844), out of private dental offices in fact, causing consternation for the physician anesthesiologists in the room. There is no question that dentistry, and specifically OMS, in large part helped to develop the outpatient anesthesia paradigm that grew rapidly after Hubbell's contributions. That medicine finally began to adopt part of this model in the 1970s is telling. Only recently has medicine begun to investigate the second component of the dental model, namely providing outpatient services outside the operating room.[48]

One final note about the author's anesthesia residency experiences is somewhat humorous and relates to differences in dental/medical training. For students learning anesthesia in dental schools, training usually involves student-on-student practice, particularly with local anesthesia. This model has been criticized, but has been the status quo in dentistry since the day dentistry adopted the use of local anesthesia.[49] One evening, preparing for the next day's case load, 2 of Utah's dental residents determined to administer an interscalene brachial plexus block for an upper extremity procedure. Part of the dentists' late evening preparation involved intentionally eliciting digital paresthesia while practicing needle placement for the block on each other in classic dental-school fashion. When discussing the proposed upper extremity case anesthetic the next morning with the faculty, it was difficult to determine who was more incredulous, the speechless faculty when advised of the practice session, or the dental students who could not fathom the faculty's shock at the resident's dental-school mode clinical practice session.

1980S

Although the basic OMS office-based team anesthesia paradigm has remained essentially the same for decades, it has progressed in terms of monitoring, that is, from skin color in the early 1970s to end-tidal CO_2 today. The drugs used have changed too, from sodium thiopental to sodium methohexital to propofol for typical Hubbell-type short general anesthesia cases.

With the decreased emphasis on dedicated anesthesia training in OMS residencies, many more recent graduate OMS have moved to drugs that can be classified as more of a sedative than a general anesthetic. From the early days of the Jorgensen technique, the introduction of diazepam produced a significant number of diazepam/meperidine OMS sedation providers. The introduction of midazolam, which is shorter acting than diazepam, in 1986 produced a logical midazolam/fentanyl sedation combination that is popular to this day.

Ketamine is commonly used today, largely because OMS clinicians who realized early on that one could avoid the infamous emergence deliria by a marked reduction of the Physician Desk Reference (PDR) suggested dosage, which was originally designed for longer-duration general anesthesia. The PDR-advised doses of more than 1 mg/lb were reduced to less than 1 mg/kg, and were found to be effective for dental office-based procedures.[50]

Tony Protopappas, DDS

Not everything related to dental anesthesia that emanated from Southern California was positive. The 1980s also saw the beginnings of media sensationalization of dental office–related morbidity and mortality. This continuing trend of disproportionate media scrutiny, relative to surgical center–based or hospital-based anesthetic complications, started in 1983 when Orange County dentist Tony Protopappas was prosecuted for second-degree murder for mishandling anesthesia for 3 patients who died under his care. Protopappas was sentenced to life in prison, but was paroled in August 2011.[51] This case helped voluntary societal SCSOMS office examinations evolve into nationwide state board regulated general anesthesia permits for all dentists.

Popular Media Assaults

The American Broadcasting Company (ABC) aired a 2-part exposé on dental anesthesia in 1983. The ratings-driven cyclical media assault on dental anesthesia has continued, and occasionally OMS paradigms are specifically mentioned. Fortunately, dental/OMS office–based anesthesia has flourished in the United States, in part because the ADA have a well-trained cadre of dentist anesthesiologist spokespersons who effectively defend dental anesthesia, including the OMS model, when dealing with the media.

Poswillo Report

In other areas of the world, for instance in Great Britain since 2002, dentists have lost the legal ability to provide general anesthesia in their offices. The National Health Service, after evaluation of the 1990s Poswillo Report, opined that the only safe place to administer general anesthesia was in a hospital. Historically, millions of general anesthetics were safely administered in dental offices in Great Britain annually, as is the case now in the United States. A mere 8 dental-office mortalities from 1996 to 1999 precipitated the Report. OMS David Poswillo's committee recommended that dentists needed to receive standardized postgraduate training (other than that received in dental school). The recommendation was impossible to implement because there was no formalized residency or specialty training in dental anesthesiology in Great Britain.[52] Poswillo passed away in June 2003 in London.

OMS Political Shift

OMS support was fundamental to the formation of the ADSA in 1953. The first issue of the *ADSA*

Newsletter mentioned, 3 times in the first 3 paragraphs, the advisability of establishing a specialty in anesthesiology in dentistry.[53] In 1979, AAOMS President Bill Wallace openly supported a specialty of anesthesiology in dentistry. Partially in response to the trends seen in Great Britain, in 1980 OMS Tom Quinn recommended anew that the ADSA pursue ADA specialty status for anesthesiology. In 1982 the American Dental Board of Anesthesiology (ADBA) formed, and original Board members included preeminent OMS such as President Dan Laskin, Robert Campbell, and Frank McCarthy. Progress to the specialty application continued, and in 1986 the ADBA proposed that ADSA Fellows, including all dentist anesthesiologists and OMS practitioners, would be grandfathered as anesthesia specialists. However, in 1988 the AAOMS Board determined to not continue to support the specialty application, stating in part that a specialty was not in the best interest of OMS.[54] AAOMS then sent a missive to all AAOMS members of the ADSA encouraging them to oppose the specialty effort for reasons such as: "…may greatly affect the anesthesia practice of OMS…could potentially have a detrimental affect [sic] in a court of law."[55]

1990S

This decade saw 3 anesthesiology specialty applications, sponsored by The American Society of Dentist Anesthesiologists (ASDA), successfully advance through the ADA specialty application structure to the last ADA arbiter, the House of Delegates. Each application, in 1994, 1997, and 1999, failed to be approved by the House of Delegates. In each case organized OMS, via AAOMS, led the fight against the application.

Historically, there were more than 150 anesthesia residencies that had allowed dentist residents through the decades. In June 1990 the ASA was advised about the numbers of dentist anesthesiologists that had been trained in medical residencies through the years. The ASA then contacted the Accreditation Council for Graduate Medical Education (ACGME) and opined that residencies that deigned to train dentists should not be accredited. The ACGME then contacted all accredited anesthesiology residencies and iterated that if dentists continued to be rostered, programs might lose accreditation. Almost overnight, all but a handful of medical residencies determined to no longer admit dentists for training. The AAOMS, however, was able to negotiate continued rotations on anesthesiology services for OMS residents.

In October 1991, the ADSA voted to discontinue its funding support for a specialty of anesthesiology in dentistry.[53]

2000S

In 2000, the AAOMS published its first *USA Today* supplement. Covered topics included the broad scope of all OMS, including a section on anesthesiology.

Also in 2000, the AAOMS initiated the Office Anesthesia Study, which was to evaluate 4 areas: (1) characterization of the types of anesthesia used; (2) variations in the types of anesthesia based on ASA status, OMS training, the surgical procedures, and the facility used; (3) associated complication rates; and (4) patients' views about the anesthesia experience. The overall purpose of the study was to protect the OMS niche from those who would attack it. The results of the study were published in the *Journal of Oral and Maxillofacial Surgery*.

In 2001 Laerdal introduced SimMan, which was first used in an ADSA course in 2002. Beginning in 2005, the AAOMS annual meeting developed continuing education course options for attendees, enabling certification in Advanced Cardiac Life Support and Pediatric Advanced Life Support.

The CODA approved accreditation for dental anesthesiology residency training in 2005. The numbers of 3-year anesthesiology programs available to dentists is now increasing annually.

In 2008 at the annual meeting of the American College of Legal Medicine (ACLM), a professional society comprising dentist and physician attorneys, a paper was presented stating: "In addition, anesthesia is sometimes being administered by the surgeon himself/herself even though it is *far safer* to employ an anesthesiologist or other adequately trained health care professional to manage anesthesia and sedation." This article's author responded with concern to the disingenuous posture of the ACLM paper with regard to anesthesiology in dentistry. To date, the subject has not been broached again at the ACLM.

In 2012 the AAOMS released the eighth edition of the *Office Anesthesia Evaluation Manual*. In addition, all AAOMS members had to now successfully complete an in-office anesthesia evaluation as a prerequisite for membership.

ABC's most recent media exposé on dental anesthesia, "Death, Greed, at the Dentist, American Children at Risk," was aired in July 2012.[56] The ADA continues to reach out to anesthesiology-trained dentist spokespersons to defend in the media all modes of anesthesia in dentistry, including OMS. These ADA voices are able to point to an overall safety record second to none in any venue, and continue to be effective.

The most important issue considered at the October 2012 ADA Annual Meeting was the anesthesia specialty application, the fourth in 20 years and fifth overall. Once again, after vetting and approval of the application by the ADA's Council on Dental Education and Licensure, Committee on Recognition of Specialties and Interest Areas in General Dentistry, and the Board of Trustees, the House of Delegates voted against the application. As with the anesthesia specialty efforts in the 1990s, organized OMS, after leading the opposition to the application, once again applauded its defeat as the result most optimal for dentistry and OMS. OMS once again established itself as the only ADA-recognized specialty with a significant emphasis on advanced pain control. Shortly after the 2012 ADA vote against the anesthesiology specialty application, the ASDA removed language from its founding documents that specifically supported the traditional OMS anesthesia model.

THE FUTURE OF ANESTHESIOLOGY IN OMS

Just as dentistry began to be accepted as a profession only after Wells introduced anesthesiology to the world, so OMS became a specialty primarily because a group of pioneer exodontists set themselves apart from their dental colleagues by embracing general anesthesia.

The modern OMS anesthesia model inspired by surgeons such as Hubbell in the 1930s must be diligently and judiciously enhanced both clinically and politically by today's OMS anesthesia educators, researchers, and private practitioners. Continued progression in the art and science of OMS office-based team anesthesia will do much to preserve OMS's anesthesia heritage and ensure its future preservation.

REFERENCES

1. DeFord WH. Lectures on general anaesthetics in dentistry. Pittsburgh: Smith & Son; 1912.
2. Davy H. Researches, chemical and philosophical, chiefly concerning nitrous oxide or dephlogisticated nitrous air and its respiration. 1st edition. Bristol: Biggs and Cottle; 1800.
3. Raper HR. Man against pain, the epic of anesthesia. New York: Prentice-Hall; 1945.
4. American Dental Association. Transactions of the Fourth Annual Meeting. Niagara Falls, July 26, 1864.
5. American Medical Association. Transactions of the Twenty-First Annual Meeting. Washington, DC, May 3, 1870.

6. American Dental Association. Horace Wells Dentist, father of surgical anesthesia, Proceedings of Centenary Commemorations of Wells' Discovery in 1844. Hartford, 1948.

7. Morton EW. The discovery of anaesthesia. McClure's Magazine 1896;VII:4.

8. American Society of Dental Surgeons. Resolutions adopted at Eighth Annual Meeting. Am J Dent Sci 1848;9:1.

9. Bible (Authorized King James version). Salt Lake City (UT): The Church of Jesus Christ of Latter Day Saints; 1979.

10. Simpson JY. Anesthesia, or the employment of chloroform and ether in surgery, midwifery, etc. Philadelphia: Lindsay & Blakiston; 1849.

11. Christian AG, Christian JA. The 1850 Webster/Parkman trial: Dr. keep's forensic evidence. J Hist Dent 2003;51(1):5–12.

12. Section on legal medicine, fatal application of chloroform. Edinburgh Medical and Surgical Journal 1848;69:498.

13. Strickland RA, Butterworth JF. Sexual dreaming during anesthesia: early case histories (1849-1888) of the phenomenon. Anesthesiology 2007; 106(6):1232–6.

14. Orr DL. Conversion phenomena secondary to outpatient general anesthetic. J Oral Maxillofac Surg 1985;43:817–9.

15. Wynbrandt J. The excruciating history of dentistry. New York: St. Martins's Press; 1998.

16. Rogers TA. Odontological Society of Great Britain, reports of societies. Br Med J 1881;31.

17. Black GV. Introduction of the bromide of ethyl as an anesthetic for dental purposes or any very short operation. The Annual Journal of the Illinois State Dental Society, Ohio State Journal of Dental Science 1883;67–70.

18. Algeo M. The president is a sick man. Chicago: Chicago Review Press, Inc; 2011.

19. Volpitto PP, Vandam LD. The genesis of contemporary American Anesthesiology. Springfield, IL: Charles C Thomas; 1982.

20. Teeter CK. 13,000 administrations of nitrous oxid with oxygen as an anesthetic. JAMA 1909;53:448.

21. Teeter CK. The limitations of nitrous oxid with oxygen as a general anesthetic. JAMA 1849;59:1912.

22. Donovan R, Whitney D. Painless Parker. Collier's Magazine 1952;5:12.

23. Driscoll EJ. Jorgensen Memorial Lecture. American Dental Society of Anesthesiology Newsletter 1977; 9(3):27.

24. MacIntosh RB, Kelly JP. The American Board of Oral and Maxillofacial Surgery, a history. Chicago: American Board of Oral and Maxillofacial Surgery; 2010.

25. American Dental Association. Horace Wells, dentist, father of surgical anesthesia, centenary commemorations, case. Hartford (CT): Lockwood and Brainard; 1844.

26. Diaz JH. Calling all anesthetists to service in World War II. Anesthesiology 2002;96:3.

27. Hubbell AO, Adams RC. Intravenous anesthesia for dental surgery with sodium ethyl (l-methylbutyl) thiobarbituric acid. J Am Dent Assoc 1940;27:1186–91.

28. Hubbell AO. Intravenous anesthesia in the dental office with sodium ethyl (l-methylbutyl) thiobarbituric acid. J Am Dent Assoc 1941;28:1039–43.

29. Hubbell AO. Pentothal sodium anesthesia for dental surgery in office practice and control of recovery time. Anesthesiology 1943;4:174–80.

30. Hubbell AO. Laryngospasm in oral surgery. J Oral Surg 1954;12:286–92.

31. Hubbell AO. Methohexital sodium anesthesia for oral surgery. J Oral Surg Anesth Hosp Dent Serv 1960;18:295–8.

32. Hubbell AO, Krogh HW. Management of intravenous anesthesia to control recovery time. Oral Surg Oral Med Oral Pathol 1956;9:403–10.

33. Hubbell AO. Laryngeal stethoscope to monitor the respiratory exchange. J Oral Surg 1958;16:20–1.

34. Hubbell AO. Brevital sodium and pentothal sodium, a clinical comparison. Oral Surg Oral Med Oral Pathol 1963;16:426–31.

35. Hubbell AO, Apparatus for handling fluids. US Patent 2,471,623. 1949.

36. Hubbell AO. On general anesthesia. Anesth Prog 1968;15:316–9.

37. American Society of Anesthesiologists. Newsletter 1951;5:15.

38. Lynch DF. Are you interested in the definition of oral surgery? Anesth Prog 1957;4:6.

39. American Medical Association. AMA scope of practice data series, oral and maxillofacial surgeons. Chicago: September 2009.

40. Jaffe M. The evolution of ambulatory anesthesiology in dentistry. Anesth Prog 1980;27:76–84.

41. Orr DL. The history of anesthesiology in dentistry, AAOMS Annual Meeting. San Diego, September 11, 2012.

42. Lytle JJ. Intravenous sedation in a teaching environment, SCOA Proceedings. Southern California: SCOA; 2012.

43. Seldin HM. The safety of anesthesia in the dental office. Oral Surg Oral Med Oral Pathol 1955;13:199.

44. Seldin HM, Recant BS. The safety of anesthesia in the dental office. J Oral Surg 1955;13:199.

45. Lytle JJ. Anesthesia morbidity and mortality survey of the Southern California Society of Oral Surgeons. J Oral Surg 1974;32:739–44.

46. Lytle JJ, Stamper ES. Report of the 1988 anesthesia survey of the Southern California Society of Oral and Maxillofacial Surgeons. J Oral Maxillofac Surg 1989;47:834.

47. Lytle JJ. Anesthesia morbidity and mortality in the oral surgery office. Oral Maxillofac Clin North Am 1992;5:759.

48. Gross WL, Gold B. Anesthesia outside the operating room. Anesthesiol Clin 2009;27:1.

49. Rosenberg MR, Orr DL. Student-to-student local anesthesia injections in dental education: moral, ethical, and legal issues. J Dent Educ 2009;73:127–32.

50. Orr DL. Reduction of ketamine induced emergence phenomena. J Oral Maxillofac Surg 1983;41:1.

51. Welborn L. Former dentist who killed three people paroled, Orange County Register. 2011. Available at: http://www.ocregister.com/articles/protopappas-310503-pfeiffer-prison.html. Accessed November 14, 2012.

52. Laurance J. Dentists to stop giving general anesthetic, The Independent, 2000. Available at: http://www.independent.co.uk/life-style/health-and-families/health-news/dentists-to-stop-giving–general-anaesthetic-706184.html#. Accessed November 14, 2012.

53. Kinney WB, American Dental Society of Anesthesiology Newsletter, April 1954, 1:1.

54. AAOMS, Report to the American Association of Oral and Maxillofacial Surgeons Board of Trustees and committees, 1988. September 29-October 3, 1998.

55. Letter to the AAOMS members of the ADSA. December 29, 1989.

56. ABC, death, greed at the dentist: American children at risk. Available at: http://abcnews.go.com/Blotter/death-greed-dentist-american-children-risk/story?id=16763109. Accessed November 14, 2012.

Determining the Appropriate Oral Surgery Anesthesia Modality, Setting, and Team

Michael J. Stronczek, DDS, MS[a,b],*

KEYWORDS

- Local anesthesia and nitrous oxide • Minimal sedation (anxiolysis) • Moderate sedation
- Deep sedation • General anesthesia

KEY POINTS

- Most oral surgery procedures can be accomplished using local anesthesia.
- When providing minimal sedation, the American Dental Association and the American Association of Oral and Maxillofacial Surgeons (AAOMS) mandate that at least one additional assistant trained in basic life support be present in the room to assist the treating surgeon.
- As of January 1, 2014, the AAOMS has mandated the use of carbon dioxide monitoring (capnography) for any procedure considered to be at the level of moderate sedation to general anesthesia.
- When potential triggers of malignant hyperthermia, like the halogenated agents (sevoflurane) and succinylcholine, are used, the surgeon must have dantrolene immediately available to manage a malignant hyperthermia emergency.

INTRODUCTION

Most surgical treatment rendered by oral and maxillofacial surgeons (OMFS) in the United States is completed in a clinical setting. What makes our specialty unique is the training received in the delivery of anesthesia. The ability to provide office-based surgical treatment without pain and anxiety has provided us with a great deal of freedom and an appropriate amount of responsibility. The oral surgery model is complex. The surgeon is expected to make a diagnosis, have the surgical skills and experience to treat the problem, and the medical knowledge to determine if patients are fit to withstand surgery. Finally, the surgeon and patients must agree on the best anesthesia modality. The operator/anesthetist model used in every oral surgeon's office has given us a great advantage in the provision of individualized patient care.

PATIENT ASSESSMENT

As a surgeon, it is valuable to have a consistent protocol for every patient. The initial focus is on the patient's chief complaint. Listen carefully to patients and get an accurate history. Continue the investigation with a comprehensive examination of the maxillofacial region to establish the correct diagnosis. Treatment options can then be discussed, and a specific course of action can be determined. Once the surgical procedure has been chosen, the type of anesthesia and the location of the procedure must be determined.

a Private Practice, Oral and Maxillofacial Surgery Associates (OMSA), 10008 Dupont Circle Court, Fort Wayne, IN 46825, USA; b Oral and Maxillofacial Surgery National Insurance Company (OMSNIC), 6133 North River Road, Suite 650, Rosemont, IL 60018, USA
* Private Practice, Oral and Maxillofacial Surgery Associates (OMSA), 10008 Dupont Circle Court, Fort Wayne, IN 46825.
E-mail address: Michael.stronczek@omsnic.com

Oral Maxillofacial Surg Clin N Am 25 (2013) 357–366
http://dx.doi.org/10.1016/j.coms.2013.03.008

Before any procedure, patients must be evaluated to determine their fitness to undergo the proposed surgery and anesthesia. This process begins at the initial office visit. There are 3 essential steps necessary to complete a physical evaluation:

1. Medical history questionnaire
2. Physical examination
3. Open discussion with patients about their medical history

The surgeon is obligated to carefully review the patient history, ask appropriate questions, and fill any unanswered gaps. This process can be tedious and time consuming, but it must be done with meticulous precision. If patients cannot answer specific questions, then the surgeon is obligated to find the answers. These questions might be answered by consulting the family physician or a specialist. It is important that the surgeon explain the patient's diagnosis, planned treatment, and anesthesia choice with the consultant so they can provide focused information and recommendations.

Patients' social and family history is also important. Smoking and drinking in moderation has little effect on our anesthesia delivery, but any of these habits in excess can severely affect the anesthesia and surgical outcome. Patients must be questioned about drug use, especially street drugs, like cocaine, if the surgeon is suspicious. Finally, questioning patients about family complications during anesthesia can provide valuable information that can be used to determine how and where patients' treatment will be provided.

The surgeon must have a complete list of each patient's medications, including herbal remedies. Asking patients why they take a specific medication provides the surgeon with targeted information regarding their medical status. It is difficult to understand the pharmacology of every medication, the potential side effects, and how anesthetic drugs will react in this environment. Fortunately, there are excellent resources that can be accessed online in real time to provide this information.

The surgeon must have a complete list of patients' drug and food allergies. This information is essential knowledge that directs the anesthesia care as well as the prescribing of medication to strictly avoid patient-specific allergens. Knowing the specific response to an allergen helps the surgeon determine patients' level of reactivity.

Once the review of systems and patient history has been completed, a physical assessment must be done. Several key observations and questions provide the surgeon with the information necessary to choose the appropriate anesthesia modality. These observations and questions include the following:

1. Height and weight, including body mass index (BMI) if indicated
2. Initial vital signs, including electrocardiogram (EKG) reading if indicated
3. Oral range of motion, jaw size, neck size, and range of motion
4. Mallampati classification
5. Cardiovascular and respiratory reserve (Metabolic Equivalent of Task [METS])

The examination can be completed very quickly. In some patients, this process will expose significant risks, including poor cardiovascular reserve, a difficult airway, poor intravenous (IV) access, and a multitude of other problems. When the examination process is complete, the OMFS should have the knowledge to give patients an American Society of Anesthesiologists' (ASA) classification and decide on an appropriate anesthesia modality. The ASA classification system is highlighted here:

ASA Physical Status Classification System

1. A normal healthy patient
2. A patient with mild systemic disease
3. A patient with severe systemic disease
4. A patient with severe systemic disease that is a constant threat to life
5. A moribund patient who is not expected to survive without the operation
6. A declared brain-dead patient whose organs are being removed for donor purposes

Traditionally, oral surgeons have limited anesthesia delivery to patients who are classified as an ASA 1 or 2. With changes in reimbursement and a population that is older, frequently obese, and surviving with multiple comorbidities, the surgeon is now challenged to treat patients who are classified as an ASA 3 and even 4 at times. The decision to treat then becomes more complicated. Every surgeon must understand their limits based on training, experience, confidence, and ability.

LOCAL ANESTHESIA

The American Dental Association (ADA) defines local anesthesia as "the elimination of sensation, especially pain, in one part of the body by the topical application or regional injection of a drug."[1] The use of local anesthesia is the foundation of pain control in dentistry. It is safe if used correctly and in appropriate doses. It is critical that the surgeon understand the pharmacology of the local anesthesia and the maximum dose allowed per patient. This understanding is especially important in children.

Most oral surgery procedures can be accomplished using local anesthesia. This treatment option is practical and cost-effective. This modality assumes patients can handle the stress of the surgery and tolerate the needle. Topical anesthetics can be helpful to decrease the pain of the injection. A preoperative medical assessment is necessary even for patients treated with local anesthesia. Although rare, there are true allergies to local anesthetic solutions. More frequently, patients are intolerant of the vasoconstrictor drugs like epinephrine, especially those with cardiovascular disease. The surgeon must weigh the risk of using epinephrine against the need to provide profound local anesthesia. Local anesthesia can be deadly, leading to central nervous system depression and even death if overdosed; this is especially true in children who do not tolerate an overdose well.

LOCAL ANESTHESIA WITH NITROUS OXIDE

Nitrous oxide can be used in conjunction with local anesthesia and provide an effective sedative and analgesic effect for many patients. States have specific guidelines as to who can start and supervise the use of nitrous oxide. Be aware of your specific state guidelines. The ADA specifies that you must have a scavenger system to pull off the residual nitrous oxide gases.

There are few disadvantages to using nitrous oxide inhalation. As long as nitrous is accompanied by at least 20% oxygen, it is a safe anesthetic agent. Nitrous is not a potent anesthetic; unfortunately, there will be a percentage of patients who will not achieve the desired effect. This situation is most commonly seen in disruptive children and adults. If the child or adult cannot or will not breath through their nose, the effects of the drug cannot be achieved.

There are no true contraindications to the use of nitrous oxide in combination with adequate O_2 delivery. Nitrous is not, however, an innocuous agent. Chronic exposure to low levels of nitrous oxide has been associated with an increased risk of spontaneous abortion, fetal deformities, and other congenital health concerns. Chronic exposure to high levels of nitrous oxide has been linked to severe sensory neuropathies. This occurrence has been found in overdosing of nitrous and is usually associated with addictive individuals who have direct access to nitrous oxide gas.

MINIMAL SEDATION

The ADA defines minimal sedation (anxiolysis) as "a minimally depressed level of consciousness, produced by a pharmacologic method that retains the patient's ability to independently and continuously maintain an airway and respond normally to tactile stimulation and verbal command. Ventilatory and cardiovascular functions should be unaffected."[2] This definition is supported by the American Association of Oral and Maxillofacial Surgeons' (AAOMS) Parameters of Care.

The ADA is very specific about the dose of drug used to produce minimal sedation. According to the guidelines, a single enteral drug can be given at a dose not to exceed the maximum recommended dose. This dose is the dose adult patients can take for prescribed and unmonitored home use. The ADA further states that "if nitrous oxide is used in conjunction with a single sedative agent, levels of anesthesia deeper then minimal sedation can be reached, so patient's must be appropriately monitored."[2]

In the cooperative adult population, oral sedation may be useful in oral surgery. This article is not about specific drugs or doses, but the benzodiazepines are the workhorse of this technique. Patients can be maintained in a comfortable, sedated state and, in combination with nitrous oxide, have little recall of the procedure. Profound local anesthesia is essential. These drugs have a margin of safety that allow patients to maintain their airway, respond to position changes, and swallow when surgical irrigation is used. Patients must understand that some recall of the procedure is likely. Unfortunately, the oral sedative drugs can be unpredictable based on the gastric absorption and peak effect of the drug. Triazolam (Halcion) is the most commonly used drug because of its short half-life (1.5–5.5 hours) and the fact that it has no active metabolites. Peak plasma levels are seen at 1.5 hours after oral administration, although this can vary. Typically, these patients will have minimal residual drowsiness.

Patients occasionally ask for medication to calm their anxiety before arriving at the office. The cooperative adult can be given a dose of triazolam or diazepam (Valium) to promote stress-free rest the night before surgery. A single dose is then taken 1 hour before surgery. Nitrous oxide can then be used to assist with the delivery of local anesthesia or the placement of an IV to allow drug titration. The team should expect an accentuated response to titrated medication if oral sedatives have been given. These patients must have a responsible escort to drive them home.

When providing minimal sedation, the ADA and the AAOMS mandate that at least one additional assistant trained in basic life support be present in the room to assist the treating surgeon. The ability to provide positive pressure oxygen must be immediately available in the case of an airway emergency. The oxygen and nitrous delivery system must have a fail-safe system to prevent the delivery of less then 30% oxygen.

The ADA recommends the use of pulse oximetry, although it is not mandated for minimal sedation. The AAOMS recommends the use of pulse oximetry during all sedation procedures. The blood pressure and heart rate must be evaluated preoperatively, postoperatively, and intraoperatively as needed. An appropriate sedation record that includes the names of all drugs given and the listed vital signs taken for the procedure is mandated.

Pediatric patients are a more complex problem. Pediatric dentists have used a myriad of drugs to sedate children, some with better results than others. For the oral surgeon, oral versed is the most commonly used medication for enteral sedation. Unfortunately, the clinical effect of oral versed can be unpredictable. The child must be cooperative enough to drink the medication. Rectal and nasal versed can also be used based on the tolerance of the surgeon, the parents, and the child. The child's response to the initial dose may not provide the level of sedation necessary to complete the procedure with local anesthesia and nitrous oxide. Children frequently do not react appropriately to the sedative feeling and may require IV placement to deepen the level of anesthesia via drug titration. Using the initial medication to allow venipuncture seems to be the modality chosen by most oral surgeons, allowing the child to be titrated to moderate or deeper sedation.

MODERATE SEDATION

Moderate sedation is defined as "a drug-induced depression of consciousness during which patients respond purposefully to verbal commands, either alone or accompanied by light tactile stimulation. No interventions are required to maintain a patent airway, and spontaneous ventilation is adequate. Cardiovascular function is usually maintained."[1] The ADA specifically recommends that the drugs used in the delivery of moderate sedation must carry a margin of safety that would render the unintended loss of consciousness unlikely.

The benefit of moderate sedation is the use of drug titration, most commonly provided by a parenteral route. The ability to give incremental doses of any drug allows you to control the level of sedation. It is essential that the surgeon understand the pharmacology of each drug used and allow the full effect of the drug to occur before administering more medication.

The ADA mandates that at least one additional trained individual must be present in the room during the delivery of moderate sedation. The regulations recommend that the surgeon remain in the room and recover patients until they reach a level of minimal sedation. A trained assistant can then recover patients until discharge.

Monitoring guidelines for moderate sedation include the mandated use of pulse oximetry. The ADA's guidelines recommend the continuous use of an EKG monitor for patients with cardiovascular disease. The AAOMS' *Parameters of Care* and the Office Anesthesia Evaluation Program are more stringent regarding the use of an EKG. The guidelines clearly state the benefits of continuous EKG monitoring of all sedated patients. The blood pressure should be continuously monitored and recorded at appropriate intervals. A time-oriented record must be maintained during the procedure that includes the vital signs at regular intervals as well as all drugs given, including local anesthesia.

Alert to all Oral Surgeons!

As of January 1, 2014, the AAOMS has mandated the use of carbon dioxide (CO_2) monitoring (capnography) for any procedure considered to be at the level of moderate sedation to general anesthesia. This decision stems from the collaborative relationship the AAOMS has developed with the ASA. It is clear through research that capnography provides the earliest evidence of respiratory distress or failure. Early diagnosis leads to early treatment. Capnography will allow surgeons to respond to airway concerns expeditiously. The AAOMS intends to continually improve the safety of anesthesia delivery. As of January 1, 2014, capnography will be the standard of care.

Practically speaking, moderate sedation is very effective in the oral surgery office. Most surgeons refer to this modality as IV sedation. The Oral and Maxillofacial Surgery National Insurance Company's (OMSNIC) data for the past 12 years show that oral surgeons use IV sedation approximately 27% of the time in their day-to-day activities. The ability to titrate patients to an appropriate level of sedation and maintain this level with incremental dosing is predictable. Profound local anesthesia to prevent pain during the surgical procedure is essential to allow the smooth delivery of moderate sedation. This technique is ideal for almost any procedure completed in the outpatient setting. Patients must understand the limitations of this technique, realizing they may have some recall of the procedure if sedation is the anesthesia end point.

The value of mild to moderate sedation cannot be understated for patients with a difficult airway. Oral surgeons are faced daily with a population of patients who have a compromised airway. Whether from obesity, obstructive sleep apnea, poor head and neck mobility, jaw size, or a combination, these patients are at a high risk for airway complications. The surgeon is obligated to explain the risks the difficult airway creates. Deeper levels of anesthesia require that the surgeon be able to maintain or reestablish the airway in the case of respiratory distress. Keeping patients light allows the airway to be maintained spontaneously while allowing patients to respond to direct commands. This ability for the patient to respond to direct commands is the patient's lifeline. The OMSNIC's data clearly show that the difficult airway is a primary factor in many death cases in the oral surgeons office. Choosing this modality takes discipline and understanding on both the surgeon and the patients' part. If sedation is not acceptable to patients, and the surgeon is uncomfortable providing a deeper plane of anesthesia, another location, like the hospital or outpatient surgery center, should be considered.

Children are a unique part of every day oral surgery, occasionally becoming disruptive. Some tolerate local anesthesia with or without nitrous oxide very well. Other children cannot be managed in this fashion and require some level of sedation. Moderate sedation requires the child to tolerate the placement of an IV for titration. Most children handle this well if they understand what is going to happen. Nitrous oxide can be very helpful for the venipuncture. Some surgeons use combination preparations of lidocaine and prilocaine cream to prevent the pain of venipuncture. EMLA (Eutectic Mixture of Local Anesthetics) is the trade name of the preparation marketed by APP Pharmaceuticals. Some surgeons will choose an oral sedative like versed to assist with patient management. The advantage of having good IV access to allow titration of the medication is paramount.

Our population is aging. People are living longer, and many people have significant medical comorbidities. They are educated and desire comprehensive treatment. Age has significant physiologic effects on the body, so the elderly may have a unique and sometimes abnormal response to anesthesia drugs. Sedation must be undertaken with care, allowing the full effect of each small incremental dose to reach its peak effect before giving more. The elderly metabolize drugs differently and are prone to more rapid cardiovascular and respiratory depression. Proceed slowly with elderly patients.

Every oral surgeon has a list of preferred anesthetic medications. Most medications are drugs that were studied and used during residency training. The drugs most commonly used in oral and maxillofacial surgery for moderate sedation are fentanyl as a narcotic and versed for its amnesic and sedative effects. Regardless of the surgeon's choice of medication, the slow titration of each drug and the use of profound local anesthesia are the key elements in the delivery of moderate sedation.

DEEP SEDATION

By definition, the ADA describes deep sedation as "a drug-induced depression of consciousness during which patients cannot be easily aroused, but respond purposefully following repeated or painful stimulation. The patient's ability to independently maintain ventilatory function may be impaired, and the patient may require assistance in maintaining a patent airway. Cardiovascular function is usually maintained during deep sedation."[2]

Deep sedation is the workhorse anesthetic technique in most oral and maxillofacial surgery offices. According to the OMSNIC's statistics from 2000 to 2011, the average surgeon provides approximately 670 anesthetics every year, with 73% of these being either deep sedation or general anesthesia. This technique is ideal for most short-duration procedures, including wisdom teeth removal and placement of dental implants. Because of the depth of anesthesia, the team concept of anesthesia delivery that has been pioneered in oral surgery is a must. The oral surgery operator/anesthetist model has been challenged on multiple occasions, yet our record of safety is unmatched.

Every patient should be appropriately evaluated medically and given an ASA classification before deep sedation. Patients who are classified as an ASA 1 and 2 are considered to be of minimal risk. The AAOMS' *Parameters of Care* discusses the treatment of patients classified as an ASA 3 and 4 and recommend a physician or medical specialist consultation before treatment if clinically indicated. It is important to recognize that the higher the ASA classification, the higher the BMI, and the higher the Mallampati scale, the more risk we incur when the patient is under deep sedation.

The anesthesia team for deep sedation must consist of at least 3 individuals. This guideline is clearly spelled out in the ADA's guidelines and supported by the AAOMS' *Parameters of Care*. The OMFS must be current in advanced cardiovascular life support training. At least 2 other individuals who are current in basic life support must be in the treatment room at all times. Using the operator/anesthetist model, one of the assistants must be designated for patient monitoring.

The AAOMS has developed a staff certification training program called Dental Anesthesia Assistant National Certification Examination (DANCE). This 2-part program consists of 36 hours of self-study material with associated quizzes followed by a computer-based competency examination. The program must be completed over a 6-month time period. This is an amazing program further preparing your team members for their day-to-day activities and for anesthesia emergencies. The AAOMS is also strongly suggesting that the surgeon and team take part in simulation training (Sim-Man [Laerdal, Wappingers Falls, NY, USA]) or in office emergency training on a regular basis.

In some states, registered nurses and licensed practical nurses can legally place IVs and presedate patients under the doctor's supervision. Regardless, the designated assistant or nurse is given the responsibility of monitoring patients and maintaining the airway. This individual is responsible for maintaining a time-accurate record of the anesthetic, including periodic monitoring of vital signs. Hiring nurses is an additional employee expense, but the comfort of having highly trained individuals to assist with patient management and emergency care cannot be overlooked. Nurses who have had intensive care unit (ICU) experience provide a unique skill set, including airway management and IV placement, that can be critical in an emergency situation.

During the delivery of deep sedation, the following monitors are mandated by the ADA:

- Oxygenation must be continuously monitored using a pulse oximeter.
- **End tidal CO_2 was previously mandated for intubated patients only. As of January 1, 2014, CO_2 monitoring will be mandated in all patients from moderate sedation to general anesthesia.**
- EKG must be used to evaluate the heart rate and rhythm.
- Continuous blood pressure monitoring must be used.
- The ability to take patients' temperature must be available, especially when using agents that could trigger malignant hyperthermia (MH).

The monitoring technology we use today is unbelievable, and yet patient monitoring is much more than watching numbers on a screen. The doctor and the assistants must be acutely aware of patients. Teach the team to watch the patients' respiratory pattern, the color of the skin, the color of the blood, and feel for a pulse as needed. Monitors cannot provide us with this information. A precordial stethoscope is an extremely valuable tool used to auscultate the patients' respirations and heart rhythm and rate. This technique may seem like old-school technology, but in children especially, this is a great monitoring technique.

In the case of an emergency during deep sedation, the OMFS must have the following equipment available for appropriate resuscitation:

- The ability to provide positive pressure oxygen must be available.
- The anesthesia equipment must have a fail-safe system that will not allow less then 30% oxygen delivery.
- A scavenging system must be available if nitrous oxide or halogenated gasses are used.
- The ability to place an IV must be available.
- The equipment to provide a patent airway must be immediately available for both children and adults. The use of the laryngeal mask airway (LMA) is now included in the airway management algorithm and has become mainstream in the management of the difficult airway.
- Medications necessary for resuscitation and a defibrillator must be immediately available. Most offices have moved toward using an automatic external defibrillator (AED) rather than the traditional defibrillator. Dosing guidelines for emergency medication should be immediately available for both children and adults.

Because of the deeper level of sedation delivered, the recovery of patients after surgery becomes more labor intensive. The ADA and AAOMS recommend the following guidelines:

- Oxygen and suction must be immediately available if a separate recovery area is used. Practices may have different means of recovery, including using the treatment room for the recovery process. Regardless, appropriately trained assistants must have direct contact with recovering patients. A recovery checklist like the Modified Aldrete Scale is useful to document the patients' fitness to leave the office.

Deep sedation is likely the most common form of anesthesia provided in the OMFS office. Most oral surgery procedures are short in duration (<30 minutes), so deep sedation provides patients with the satisfaction of excellent pain control, amnesia of the surgical event, and a comfortable arousal usually with minimal side effects. With a skilled team providing the anesthesia, the risks are very low for patients classified as an ASA 1 and 2. Again, the risk becomes greater as the ASA level increases and the depth of anesthesia increases. The surgeon must be comfortable with the choice of anesthesia and understand potential limitations.

Deep sedation of the small child is a more complex subject. The ADA defines the child as someone aged 12 years or younger. The ADA's guidelines clearly support the use of the American Academy of Pediatrics/American Academy of Pediatric Dentists' guidelines for the management of pediatric patients during and after sedation for diagnostic and therapeutic procedures. Practically speaking, each surgeon must determine their ability to manage the anesthesia needs of children. Based on their training, experience, and comfort level in providing advanced anesthesia techniques, the appropriate decision can be made as to the modality and location of the anesthesia. Children are less tolerant of moderate sedation, so frequently we are forced to deepen the level of anesthesia for control purposes. The surgeon must be acutely aware of the anatomic (airway) and physiologic differences in children. Children also decompensate quickly, so the team must respond rapidly to every emergency. Some OMFS are simply not comfortable with the risk of treating children. In that situation, taking the child to an outpatient surgery center or local hospital is a better option.

In the cooperative child, the use of nitrous oxide can be extremely valuable to assist in the placement of an IV. EMLA cream can also be stocked in the office and used for comfortable venipuncture. If a sedative is desired before deep sedation, oral versed is still the drug of choice. These children must be directly monitored to watch for potential respiratory depression, so providing this medication at home under parent supervision is not recommended.

Deep sedation in patients with a difficult airway is a significant concern. Looking at the OMSNIC's data for the past 12 years, it is clear that airway compromise can be the beginning of the end. We see patients daily who have complex medical problems and airways that are suspect at best. The deeper the anesthesia, the more likely an airway event will occur. It is essential that the surgeon can recover or reestablish an airway quickly and efficiently. The presurgical evaluation can give you clues as to the patients' airway status; but in the end, it is the training and skill level of the surgeon that will be tested. The difficult airway patient might best be treated with a lighter form of sedation, or by securing the patient's airway with endotracheal intubation at an outpatient surgery center depending on the length and complexity of the surgical procedure.

GENERAL ANESTHESIA

The ADA defines general anesthesia as "a drug-induced loss of consciousness during which patients are not arousable, even by painful stimulation. The ability to independently maintain ventilatory function is often impaired. Patients often require assistance in maintaining a patent airway, and positive pressure ventilation may be required because of depressed spontaneous ventilation or drug induced depression of neuromuscular function. Cardiovascular function may be impaired."[5]

Deep sedation and general anesthesia are closely linked in the continuum of anesthesia. Clinically they are almost identical. Both techniques require that the surgeon have the skill and knowledge to manage the patient's airway, maintain cardiovascular stability, and be able to resuscitate patients in case of an emergency. For this reason, the delivery of deep sedation/general anesthesia is restricted to only those dentists who have completed an oral and maxillofacial surgery residency or a dental anesthesia residency.

The ADA's guidelines for the facility, training, team, and emergency response is identical to the guidelines for deep sedation. Because the depth of general anesthesia places patients in a more compromised state, the OMFS and the team must be well trained in airway management and emergency care. The AAOMS' *Parameters of Care* (2012) and the *Office Anesthesia Evaluation Manual* clearly specify everything from the team makeup to the room size. It is recommended that the emergency medications and algorithms be meticulously organized. Drug doses and emergency airway equipment specific for both children and adults must be immediately available. These documents are an excellent resource for the surgeon and staff and can be accessed on the AAOMS' Web site at aaoms.org.

General anesthesia can take on many forms in the OMFS office. For the surgeon who is comfortable with children and less cooperative adults, mask ventilation anesthesia is a reliable technique. Since the development of sevoflurane, the use of mask anesthesia induction for short procedures in children, adults, and even patients with special needs has become more predictable. In longer procedures, a mask induction can be followed with IV placement and transition into a parenteral technique, or an endotracheal tube or LMA can be placed. The rapid onset, favorable aroma, and relative lack of cardiac ectopy seen in sevoflurane when used in conjunction with local anesthesia make this a reliable and relatively safe technique. The surgeon must be comfortable and experienced in this procedure to make it a viable and predictable modality.

Some surgeons are comfortable with the use of intramuscular ketamine for the uncooperative child or adult. Ketamine given at a dose of 2 to 4 mg/kg will create a cooperative patient in several minutes, allowing venipuncture and further titration of medication. The airway must be evaluated carefully based on the patient's response to the medication, but typically ketamine supports the cardiovascular and respiratory parameters. Postoperative hallucinations, especially in the absence of benzodiazepines, can complicate the recovery period.

The LMA is emerging as a viable option in the outpatient setting. The ability to place this airway blindly without the need for paralytic agents is advantageous. As the LMA has matured, different versions of this airway, like the flexible LMA, allow placement and improved vision of the surgical field. These patients can be maintained with an inhalation agent or a parenteral (propofol) pump titrated to allow for spontaneous ventilation. In the case of an emergency, the airway is already in position. The LMA does not protect the airway from emesis and aspiration. Once again, the surgeon must feel comfortable and confident with this specific technique.

Intubated general anesthesia is still used in the modern OMFS practice, although it seems to be less popular. The surgeon must have the skill, training, and confidence to be able to place the endotracheal tube both orally and nasally. This technique is superb for procedures that require unimpeded access to the mouth and oropharynx, like osteotomies and advanced dentoalveolar procedures. The doctor and team must protect and maintain the patients' airway and cardiovascular status. Intubated anesthesia is more complex and stressful, especially during induction and arousal. The surgeon who uses this technique in the operator/anesthetist fashion must be absolutely confidant with their own abilities and the ability of their team. When performed in the office, the assumption is that patients will be discharged to home, so the length, complexity, and postoperative needs of patients must be taken into consideration before using this technique.

When potential triggers of MH like the halogenated agents (sevoflurane) and succinylcholine are used, the surgeon must have dantrolene immediately available to manage an MH emergency.

Some surgeons choose to use the services of a certified nurse anesthetist or a medical or dental anesthesiologist to provide general anesthesia and even moderate and deep sedation in their office. This choice depends on the training, skill level, and comfort of the oral surgeon as well as the complexity of the procedures completed in the office setting. Obviously, this team choice has both professional and economic concerns that must be discussed with patients.

OUTPATIENT SURGERY AND ANESTHESIA

It is appropriate to take certain patients to an outpatient surgery center for both surgical and anesthesia services. Factors affecting this decision include

- Patient health status: ASA 3 or higher
- Difficult airway
- Complexity of the surgical procedure
- Management problems (children/patients with special needs)
- Length of surgery
- Surgeon preference

Every surgical procedure is unique in its own way. More importantly, every patient has unique needs based on their health, size, and level of cooperation. Occasionally the simplest of procedures cannot and should not be completed in the office. The benefit of the outpatient facility is the anesthesiologist or certified registered nurse anesthetist who will manage your patients' anesthesia needs, which allows the surgeon to focus on the surgery at hand without the stress of also providing the anesthesia.

Young children are occasionally very difficult to manage in the office setting. Every surgeon has a comfort level with children. If the surgeon is not comfortable with a specific child in the office, then an outpatient surgery center is an appropriate setting, depending on the health of the child and the complexity of the surgical procedure. Most of these procedures are of short duration and minimal complexity and do not require a hospital stay. Most anesthesiologists are very willing to use a mask induction to breath a child down for tooth extraction without intubating or placing an LMA, similar to the technique used in the oral surgeons office.

Patients with special needs may at times be best managed at an outpatient facility, depending on their level of cooperation and health status. The complexity and length of the surgical procedure must also be taken into consideration. If patients are unable to cooperate for the surgery or for the anesthesia, an outpatient setting is a good option, assuming the patients will not need overnight hospital care.

The surgeon should communicate directly with the anesthesiologist to determine the best airway and anesthesia technique regardless of the facility. This information is usually determined by the anatomic requirements of the procedure and the surgeons need for access.

HOSPITAL-BASED ANESTHESIA

Not every procedure can or should be handled in the office. Some patients do not belong in an outpatient center either. Taking patients to the hospital is usually based on several factors:

- Patient diagnosis
- Complexity and length of the procedure
- Patient health
- Need for comprehensive hospital services, including extended admission
- Need for critical care
- Patient is already in the hospital

Orthognathic surgery, cancer surgery, severe maxillofacial infections, temporomandibular joint surgery and cleft and craniofacial surgery require a level of surgical skill and a depth of anesthesia that may necessitate hospital admission. Typically these procedures require careful planning and coordination with our medical colleagues. The surgeon must have an anesthesia plan and clearly communicate it with the anesthesiologist. This plan includes the choice of an airway (nasal verse oral endotracheal intubation), patient positioning, and specific needs like relative hypotension when bleeding is expected.

Intubated anesthesia is still the standard of care, although the LMA is being used more frequently for shorter cases, especially with children. Occasionally a surgical airway will be necessary for long-term hospital care. Placing a tracheostomy requires precise coordination with the anesthesiologist and an experienced surgeon. In most intubated cases, patients are extubated before leaving the surgical suite and anesthesia services end when the anesthesiologist transfers the patients to the postanesthesia care unit. Occasionally it is appropriate to leave the endotracheal tube in place for several days to allow swelling to resolve or to allow patients to be completely awake before extubation. Orthognathic surgery for patients with severe obstructive sleep apnea and severe maxillofacial infections are cases when extended intubation is appropriate. Anesthesia will assist with the ICU transfer and coordinate care with the intensivist before signing off from patients.

Cases completed in the hospital have the benefit of postanesthesia care and good medical/surgical treatment as the patients begin to recover. In the case of a complication or mishap, the patients and surgeon have direct access to all services provided by the hospital, including immediate anesthesia. Depending on the specific geographic area, some hospitals will have more goods and services available to your patients.

Children who need surgery and overnight hospital care will require general anesthesia. Consultation with the anesthesia staff should be considered if the child presents unique medical or anatomic challenges that might affect the delivery of anesthesia. If intubation is necessary, this plan should be coordinated with the anesthesiologist, specifying the type of airway and anesthesia needed to best accomplish the surgery.

Depending on the size of your community, anesthesia will be provided either by a board certified anesthesiologist or a certified nurse anesthetist who is supervised by the anesthesia staff. Regardless of your provider, open communication is the key to excellent anesthesia care.

CHOOSING THE CORRECT MODALITY

Anesthesia delivery for the control of anxiety and pain has a rich history in dentistry. Our forefather's tested the waters, pushed the limits, and perfected the techniques of the anesthesia delivery we use today. Oral surgery is the most painful specialty in dentistry. Fortunately, we have the gift of anesthesia to provide patients with pain-free care in a safe environment. The operator/anesthetist model that is the standard of care for oral surgeons throughout the United States has stood the test of time. Many of our medical colleagues are copying our model as they are forced to manage more patients in an outpatient setting. Our safety record is second to none.

This article is about anesthesia options and the different modalities available to the OMFS. It is not a comprehensive review of the techniques and drugs. Every surgeon brings a unique skill set to the delivery of anesthesia. The guidelines are clearly spelled out by the AAOMS and the ADA. In the end, the choice of anesthesia modality, team, and location is left to the surgeon and the patients.

REFERENCES

1. American Dental Association (ADA). Guidelines for teaching pain control and sedation to dentists and dental students. (As adopted by the October 2007 ADA House of Delegates). Available at: http://www.ada.org.
2. American Dental Association (ADA). Guidelines for the use of sedation and general anesthesia by general dentists. (As adopted by the October 2007 ADA House of Delegates). Available at: http://www.ada.org.

FURTHER READINGS

American Association of Oral and Maxillofacial Surgeons (AAOMS). Parameters of care: clinical guidelines for oral and maxillofacial surgery (AAOMS ParCare 2012), anesthesia in outpatient facilities. Available at: http://www.aaoms.org.php.

American Association of Oral and Maxillofacial Surgeons (AAOMS). Office anesthesia evaluation manual. 8th edition. Available at: http://www.aaoms.org.

American Academy of Pediatric Dentists (AAPD). Guidelines for monitoring and management of pediatric patients during and after sedation for diagnostic and therapeutic procedures: an update. Available at: http://www.aapd.org/media/policies.asp.

American Society of Anesthesiologists (ASA). Practice guidelines for sedation and analgesia by non-anesthesiologists. Available at: http://www.asahq.org.

American Society of Anesthesiologists (ASA). Guidelines for office-based anesthesia. (Approved by the ASA House of Delegates on October 13, 1999 and last affirmed on October 21, 2009). Available at: http://asahq.org.

American Society of Anesthesiologists (ASA). Continuum of depth of sedation: definition of general anesthesia and levels of sedation/analgesia. (Approved by the ASA House of Delegates on October 13, 1999 and amended on October 21, 2009). Available at: http://asahq.org.

American Society of Anesthesiologists (ASA). Standards for basic anesthetic monitoring. (Approved by the ASA House of Delegates on October 21, 1986 and last amended on October 20, 2010 with an effective date of July 1, 2011). Available at: http://asahq.org.

Malamed SF. Sedation: a guide to patient management. 4th edition. Saint Louis (MO): Mosby; 2003.

Roizen MF, Fleisher LA. Essence of anesthesia practice. (PA): W.B. Saunders; 1997.

Preoperative, Intraoperative, and Postoperative Anesthesia Assessment and Monitoring in Oral Surgery

Paul G. Sims, DDS

KEYWORDS

- Preoperative evaluation • Medical history • Physical examination • Monitoring • Discharge

KEY POINTS

- Preoperative history and physical examination are critical before anesthesia is induced.
- An evaluation of the airway for potential obstruction is essential.
- Laboratory testing and radiographic studies need to be customized to the clinical situation.
- Physiologic monitoring must be done throughout anesthetic administration.
- Postoperative monitoring is critical.
- Discharge criteria and standards must be used.

PREOPERATIVE EVALUATION

The statement is often made, "do not operate on a stranger". The same statement also is applied to providing anesthesia services. Many offices require elective surgery patients to visit the office for a preoperative consultation and evaluation, which allows a detailed medical and dental history and appropriate physical examination. An anesthesia history should also be obtained as well as a description of the benefits and risks of the proposed procedure, allowing a comprehensive and appropriate surgical consent to be obtained. Preoperative medication alterations can be discussed, postoperative medications can be prescribed, and nothing by mouth (NPO) status can be addressed. Postoperative instructions can be presented and discussed with the patient and family.

A thorough discussion of the patient's symptoms and a limited or complete physical examination is necessary to establish a diagnosis. Once this diagnosis is decided upon, a discussion about the various modalities to treat the problem must occur. This discussion must be done to arrive at an Informed Consent. The practitioner must have various consent forms that are available for each type of procedure. There are many sources to obtain informed consent forms that are available to the practitioners that have been customized for the various surgical and anesthesia procedures.

Offices with experienced screening staff can obtain much of the pertinent information necessary to allow surgery and anesthesia to be performed without a separate preoperative consultation. The scheduling can be done on American Society of Anesthesiologists 1 and stable 2 patients. Many times emergency patients are treated in this manner. A drawback to this type of practice is there may be times that surgeries have to be postponed and rescheduled when information obtained compromises patient safety.

In the past routine adjunctive testing was done on all patients preoperatively. This practice has changed and only appropriate studies are ordered. Appropriate radiographic studies must be

The author has nothing to disclose.
Private Practice, Oral and Maxillofacial Surgery, 775 West Gold, Butte, MT 59701, USA
E-mail address: pgsims@ddsmt.com

Oral Maxillofacial Surg Clin N Am 25 (2013) 367–371
http://dx.doi.org/10.1016/j.coms.2013.03.007

ordered and diagnosed when appropriate. These studies include the following:

Intraoral studies
- Extraoral studies
- Cone beam scans
- Other computed tomography studies
- Angiograms
- Magnetic resonance imaging
- Arthrograms

When a patient presents with specific medical conditions that require laboratory testing or radiographic studies, one should use these modalities.

One specific challenge is how to provide anesthesia to women of childbearing age. Some individuals require pregnancy testing before any type of anesthetic delivery. Most practitioners will ask if there is a chance of the patient being pregnant. If there is not a likelihood of this, no specific laboratory testing is necessary.

Many patients are taking anticoagulants such as warfarin and their anticoagulation status can be accurately measured by using the International Normalized Ratio the day of surgery. In many cases minor treatment can be accomplished without discontinuing the warfarin. If more involved surgery is anticipated, medical consultation is in order. In high-risk cases a bridging therapy with low molecular weight heparin can be used.

There are new classes of anticoagulants including thrombin inhibitors that an increasing number of patients are taking that require specific types of laboratory tests that are not available in many locations. The drugs in this class do not have any way to be reversed should there be an overdose. One should consider a consultation with the patient's prescribing physician when there are questions about treating patients taking these drugs.

Patients undergoing sedation or anesthesia are asked to fast preoperatively. The American Society of Anesthesiologists has a publication entitled *Practice Guidelines for Preoperative Fasting and the Use of Pharmacologic Agents to Reduce the Risk of Pulmonary Aspiration: Application to Healthy Patients Undergoing Elective Procedures.*[1] For healthy patients undergoing sedation or anesthesia, a fasting time of 2 hours for clear liquids, water, juices without pulp, carbonated beverages, clear tea, and black coffee, is allowed. For nursing infants, at least 4 hours are necessary before anesthesia. For formula-fed infants, it is necessary to fast for at least 6 hours. Patients need to fast at least 6 hours before elective procedures after consuming an intake of a light meal, or nonhuman milk. A fasting time of 8 or more hours is necessary for patients eating meat or fatty foods.

Patients that have gastric motility disorders, gastroesophageal reflux disease, metabolic disorders such as diabetes mellitus or physical situations such as pregnancy or obesity should fast for increased lengths of time.

The routine use of gastrointestinal stimulants to decrease the risk of pulmonary aspiration in patients that have no obvious risk for aspiration is not necessary.

Airway evaluation of the patient before inducing sedation or anesthesia is essential. The Mallampati Classification is one of the most widely used scales used to assess the airway. There are increasing numbers of morbidly obese patients with body mass indices of 40 or more that are at significant risk for elective office surgery. There are patients with enlarged tonsils or adenoid tissue that are at increased risk for anesthesia. The patient with a short thyromental distance or who are severely retrognathic is at increased risk of airway problems. The patients that report or appear to have obstructive sleep apnea are at increased risk for airway obstruction during anesthesia. A child with a recent upper respiratory illness needs to be evaluated thoroughly before anesthesia.

One needs to evaluate the airway during a preoperative evaluation carefully and, if the risk to the patient seems to be great, be willing to postpone an elective surgery until the risks can be minimized or the surgery can be performed at another location where the difficult airway can be more adequately managed. Emergency treatment can also be performed using local anesthesia.

Baseline vital signs should be obtained and recorded at the initial consultation as well as the treatment appointment before sedation or anesthesia is induced. The minimal evaluations are blood pressure, pulse rate, respiratory rate, pulse oximeter reading, and temperature, if indicated. If any of these are significantly elevated or decreased from normal, one should continue to monitor the patient to see if the readings will become closer to a range that one could consider performing the anesthesia and procedure. One needs to consider whether the abnormal readings are a cause of some treatable condition (such as, pain or anxiety). One should not continue with sedation or anesthesia unless the abnormal readings can be explained or treated. Referral to the patient's attending physician or emergency department should be done at the earliest time available.

If a consultation appointment is made or the consultation is done by telephone and the treatment performed at the first visit, it is often appropriate to prescribe medications before surgery to eliminate a pharmacy stop after the surgery and anesthesia with the patient being left unattended in the car.

INTRAOPERATIVE ASSESSMENT AND MONITORING

On the day of the procedure one of the first things to assess is the NPO status. The office staff person seating the patient in the operatory or operating room can simply ask the patient when he/she last ate food or drink, or can ask the simple question, "what did you have for breakfast." The parents of a minor should be asked as well. Once the NPO status has been established, the patient can be connected to the monitoring devices.

Before the anesthesia team begins the procedure, a "time out" should be done. The patient should be positively identified. The exact procedure should be discussed with the patient or guardian. The medical history should be reviewed including medications being taken and allergies. The type of anesthesia to be delivered should be discussed. During the "time out" no other preparation should be done and the entire anesthesia and care team must be in attendance.

Once the "time out" is complete, the airway assessment should be performed as described earlier in the article. At the least a limited physical examination consisting of auscultation of the heart and lungs should be performed.

Intravenous access should be obtained by someone permitted by state law to do this. An appropriate size catheter should be introduced and stabilized and the fluid of choice should be attached and the patency of the catheter checked. The intravenous line must be secure because it may be a lifeline should an emergency occur. Straight steel needles and in most cases butterfly needles should not be used. In some patients it may be necessary to induce anesthesia using inhalation agents such as sevoflurane or intramuscular ketamine before starting the intravenous line. Before the induction of anesthesia many surgery teams will preoxygenate the patient using either a nasal canula or a nasal hood.

Preparation of the medications to be used in the anesthesia should be done by a member of the anesthesia team that is legally permitted to draw the drugs. Each state has individual regulations that describe who can withdraw the medications from the vial. In most jurisdictions the person withdrawing these medications is licensed by the state. Most states do not permit dental assistants to perform these tasks. The syringes should be labeled appropriately and stored according to the manufacturer's directions. The expiration

dates must be checked. Single-dose vials should be used on only one patient.

The anesthesia team should consist of a minimum of 3 individuals. The surgeon is the member that generally administers the anesthetic drugs. There must be one trained individual that monitors the patient's condition, vital signs, and respirations. If the patient is not breathing spontaneously or has some degree of obstruction, support of the airway can be accomplished by this individual. The third person on the team is the surgical assistant. There can be other members of the anesthesia team as well. On more challenging anesthesia cases or surgery cases another oral surgeon, nurse anesthetist, or dental or medical anesthesiologist will be in attendance. On more involved surgical procedures a circulating nurse or dental assistant will be present.

There are several monitoring devices that should be used on the patient to be anesthetized. Monitoring of the cardiovascular system should be done on most patients when appropriate. A baseline blood pressure, pulse rate, and respiratory rate should be obtained and recorded before the administration of any anesthetic agents. Blood pressure should be monitored and recorded at least every 5 minutes. The pulse rate and the SPO_2 should also be recorded on an anesthesia form or on a printout that can be stored in the patient chart.

The respiratory system should be evaluated and monitored with the pulse oximeter that measures the SPO_2 levels. There is a lag time in the actual SPO_2 level and the displayed numbers on the monitor. A historical method to monitor the rate and depth of respiration is by using a pretracheal stethoscope. There are traditional stethoscopes that are attached to the surgeon's ear and there are newer bluetooth-enabled electronic devices that will allow more than one individual to monitor the respirations. These devices can be left on the patient in the recovery area for monitoring of respiration. Monitoring of the color of the patient's blood is a primitive measure of the oxygenation but should still be used.

The use of a capnograph has been recommended for use in intubated patients for several years. It is also used for patients when a laryngeal mask airway (LMA) has been placed to administer inhalational agents. For several years practitioners have been using capnography on open airway anesthetics. A nasal cannula can be used that has been modified to accept a capnograph connection, which can be attached to obtain a relative carbon dioxide level and see a respiration wave. When a nasal hood is used, an attachment is available to connect it to the capnograph. The numbers displayed on the capnograph are used to detect changes in the rate and depth of respiration. When one sees an increase in the carbon dioxide level, airway manipulation may allow the rates to return to previous levels or more advanced airway management may be necessary.

Because the medical and dental anesthesia communities realized the importance of the rapid detection of respiratory depression or obstruction with the capnograph, in 2012 the American Association of Oral and Maxillofacial Surgeons (AAOMS) Office Anesthesia Evaluation Manual and the AAOMS Parameters of Care document were updated to recommend the capnograph be used on patients undergoing moderate sedation or deep sedation/general anesthesia in an open airway anesthetic. AAOMS members were informed of these recommendations, which will become effective in 2014.

The practice of using of supplemental oxygen in patients undergoing sedation or general anesthesia is still not universally accepted. Generally it is thought to be a good practice to preoxygenate patients before the induction of anesthesia. A nasal hood or nasal prongs should be placed unless a full mask is used before the induction of general anesthesia and LMA or endotracheal anesthesia is to be administered. Oxygen should be administered throughout the procedure as well as in the post operative recovery area. A backup oxygen supply must also be available in the post anesthesia care area should the primary supply fail.

One device that is sometimes used to monitor the patient's consciousness during anesthesia is the Bispectral Index monitor. This piece of equipment allows the provider administering the anesthesia to see a numerical level of brain wave activity to assess the level of consciousness during sedation or general anesthetic.

There should be a crash cart with emergency drugs and devices immediately available in the operatory suite. This cart should be inventoried weekly or daily to assure that the drugs are available and within the expiration date. Primary Advanced Cardiovascular Life Support (ACLS) drugs should be readily available and more advanced drugs can be stored. The ACLS protocols should be in this cart and readily available for immediate use. These templates can also be laminated and displayed on the walls of the operating suite. Before ACLS drug administration, basic cardiopulmonary resuscitation should be started and performed without delay or pause. Plans should be made as to how each individual on the anesthesia and office team will carry out their assigned tasks in an emergency. In addition to the resuscitation team, one person should be assigned to record the event and contact the emergency medical services team when the leader determines such a call is necessary.

If one is using malignant hyperthermia triggering agents, a supply of dantrolene (Dantrium) should be readily available. There is now a newer formulation of dantrolene for injection (Revonto) that is supplied in vials containing 20 mg dantrolene and 3000 mg mannitol in a formula that is easily reconstituted with 60 mL of sterile water in approximately 20 seconds. An emergency call should be made to Malignant Hyperthermia Association of the United States for additional instructions after the emergency medical services call has been made.

There should be a defibrillator readily available if a cardiac crisis occurs that can be treated with defibrillation. The automated external defibrillator can be used to treat cardiac defibrillation or pulseless ventricular tachycardia; however, a traditional cardiac monitor should be used when the patient is being sedated or undergoing general anesthesia because there are numerous other cardiac arrhythmias that can be diagnosed and treated. If an automated external defibrillator is not available, a cardiac monitor-defibrillator could be used. A printout from cardiac monitor could be attached to the patient chart. A rhythm strip can also be used to document a cardiac event.

Emergency airway devices should be readily available for use. The simple oral or nasal airways can easily be inserted when an obstruction is detected. The bag-valve-mask devise can also be used when necessary. This device, with a gauge that allows one to measure the millimeters of water pressure used, will allow one to keep from introducing an excessive amount of air into the stomach. Some of the newer second-generation LMA devices allow air to escape from the stomach or to have a nasogastric tube inserted to decompress the stomach during resuscitation. Endotracheal intubation equipment should be readily available. Periodically practicing intubating patients in the hospital or surgical center will help keep one's skills intact. Emergency surgical airway devices should be a part of the crash cart and be used if the airway cannot be established by any other approach. This device can be a large-bore intravenous catheter with jet ventilation placed through the cricothyroid membrane. A surgical cricothyrotomy can also be performed. If any advanced airway devise is used, it is necessary to assure the correct placement by checking for the presence of carbon dioxide in the exhaled air. This verification can be done with the capnograph, or by using a device that changes color when carbon dioxide is present in the expired ventilation.

Emergency drills should be staged in the office or clinic on a regular schedule and cover all types of situations from the simple to the complex. Each individual will have an assigned role to play in the simulated emergency so that when the actual situation arises the use of these drills will facilitate resuscitation of the patient.

Transportation of the patient from the primary surgical suite to the recovery area will be dependent on the type of sedation or anesthesia used and the conscious level of the patient. In most cases the patient will be transported to the recovery area on a gurney or operating table, moved in a wheelchair, or will be walked with assistance. Supplemental oxygen may or may not be necessary.

POSTOPERATIVE MONITORING AND EQUIPMENT

When deep sedation or general anesthesia is used and a surgical procedure is performed, generally a 2-stage recovery is used. This 2-stage recovery involves an intensive initial observation and treatment and then a less rigorous period after the patient regains consciousness.

At least one trained individual should be assigned to monitor the postoperative patient. Generally when the patient is transferred to the post anesthesia care area of the office or clinic, if general anesthesia has been used, the patient will have supplemental oxygen in place. This supplemental oxygen will be used until the patient has recovered and is able to keep the SPO$_2$ on room air greater than 90. A patent intravenous line must be maintained until the patient is awake.

The monitoring devices in the post anesthesia care unit may be the same as those used in the operating suite. If an endotracheal or LMA general anesthetic has been administered and the patient is still anesthetized, a cardiac monitor will be necessary. Blood pressure measurements should be taken at least every 5 minutes and recorded. The pulse rate, respiratory rate, and SPO$_2$ should be monitored and recorded. Supplemental oxygen must be available. A suction devise must be readily available as well.

During the first stage of recovery, the family members are generally left in the reception area and only the office staff is with the patient. When the patient is recovered to a state that they are conscious, can talk, and are not nauseous and relatively pain free, the responsible parties that accompanied the patient can be brought into the recovery area. This recovery area may be the primary post anesthesia care unit or a second area that is used for secondary recovery. Care must be taken to protect patient identity.

If moderate sedation or deep sedation is used and the primary recovery is done in the operating suite the patient can often walk with assistance to the secondary recovery area. There are also times that the patient may be fully recovered in and dismissed from the operating suite.

There must be defined criteria that can be used to determine if a patient is satisfactorily recovered before they are discharged. There are numerous scales that have been developed to assess the recovery status of a patient and to use to determine when he/she might be discharged. All the scales use a combination of stable vital signs, activity level, presence or absence of nausea and vomiting, pain level, lack of hemorrhage, oxygen saturation, level of consciousness, and rates of respiration to determine when the patient may be discharged.

The Modified Aldrete Scale is one scale that has been used in many oral and maxillofacial offices and clinics; however, there are others. The following lists some of the most commonly used scales:

- Aldrete Scale
- Modified Aldrete Scale
- Visual Analog Scale
- Procedure and Anesthesia Scoring System
- Post Anesthesia Discharge Scoring System
- Ramsey Sedation Schedule
- Pasero Opioid Agitation Scale
- Richmond Agitation Sedation Scale

Once discharge criteria have been satisfied, the patient may be released to a responsible adult that has been instructed with appropriate discharge procedures. A follow-up appointment should be made if necessary. Prescriptions should be given to the responsible adult accompanying the patient as well as contact information for after-hour problems. The properly written postoperative instructions must accompany the patient and responsible adult.

REFERENCE

1. American Society of Anesthesiologists (ASA). Practice guidelines for preoperative fasting and the use of pharmacologic agents to reduce the risk of pulmonary aspiration: application to healthy patients undergoing elective procedures. Anesthesiology 2011; 114:495.

Anesthesia Equipment for the Oral and Maxillofacial Surgery Practice

William L. Chung, DDS, MD

KEYWORDS

- Anesthesia • Equipment • Oral surgery • Maxillofacial surgery • Practice

KEY POINTS

- Consideration for emergency generator for lighting, suction, and monitors in event of a power outage.
- Portability of oxygen tank, lighting, and an aspiration unit essential during power outage.
- Multiple supraglottic airway devices available for office use and emergencies.
- Capnography capabilities mandatory for any planned deep sedation or general anesthetic.
- The surgical chair or operating table must allow for easy accessibility by surgeon and staff during an emergency.

INTRODUCTION

The physical design of an oral and maxillofacial surgeon's office is highly individualized and unique. Every office must incorporate certain essential equipment and features to safely deliver office anesthesia, regardless of the scope of anesthesia services provided. Furthermore, the office design and anesthesia armamentarium must take into account patient safety and comfort. This article discusses the necessary elements, ranging from preanesthesia assessment forms and intraoperative records to office design, anesthesia monitors, and equipment related to the safe and successful administration of office-based anesthesia by oral and maxillofacial surgeons and their staff.

MANIFOLD SYSTEM AND REMOTE GAS STORAGE

Specific building codes and local fire department regulations must be carefully adhered to before any plans are made to install remote gases. The gas manifold system is a piping network of valves, gauges, and regulators that allow a specific, desired gas to be released at the correct pressure. Most office manifold systems are located in an enclosure away from patient care areas (**Fig. 1**) to avoid potential injury from a possible fire, explosion, or sudden release of gas. During the soldering process of the copper pipes, nitrogen must be blown into the pipes to eliminate the oxidative by-products from within the pipes to avoid inadvertently delivering these harmful by-products to patients.

All gas tanks require easy accessibility by office staff to check the gauge and change it when the tank is empty. A minimum of 2 oxygen tanks needs to be connected to the system so that 1 tank can be activated if line pressure drops in the other. An audible or visible low-oxygen pressure warning device must be present if an automatic change-over system is used. The shutoff valves to each gas should be clearly labeled and easily accessible to any staff member in the event of an emergency (**Fig. 2**).

Department of Oral and Maxillofacial Surgery, University of Pittsburgh Medical Center, 3459 5th Avenue, Suite 202 South, Pittsburgh, PA 15213, USA
E-mail address: chungwl@upmc.edu

Oral Maxillofacial Surg Clin N Am 25 (2013) 373–383
http://dx.doi.org/10.1016/j.coms.2013.03.002
1042-3699/13/$ – see front matter © 2013 Elsevier Inc. All rights reserved.

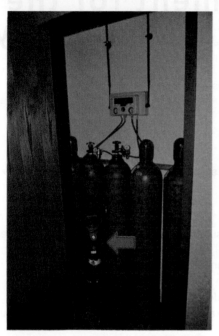

Fig. 1. Manifold system (Centurion II [Matrix Medical, Minneapolis, MN]). Nitrous oxide and multiple oxygen tanks as well as a portable oxygen tank (*arrow*), stored in a closet.

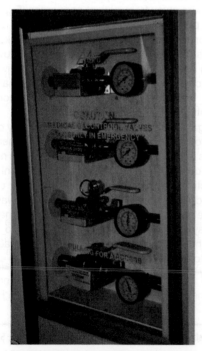

Fig. 2. Gas shutoff valves easily accessible and clearly labeled for each gas connected to the manifold system.

NITROUS OXIDE EXPOSURE CONTROL AND INHALATIONAL ANESTHETIC EXPOSURE CONTROL

The American Association of Oral and Maxillofacial Surgeons Committee on Anesthesia refers to the Centers for Disease Control and Prevention for recommendations on controls for exposure to nitrous oxide and other potential chemical hazards (http://www.cdc.gov/niosh/topics/nitrousoxide/).[1] A manual of the recommendations can be printed and kept with other office safety manuals for office staff to reference.

OFFICE FIRE SAFETY PROTOCOL

The exact location of an office's fire safety protocol (Rescue, Activate alarm, Confine the fire, Evacuate/Extinguish [RACE]) should be known by all staff and easily assessable for reference. If an office is not a free-standing facility, all other safety protocols should be clearly labeled and kept together.

COMMUNICATION EQUIPMENT

Telephone numbers of the local ambulance service and nearest hospital should be clearly displayed and their location known to all office staff. In larger office settings, an intercom system or call button facilitates communication between the surgical team and the office staff in the event of an emergency.

RECORD KEEPING/TIME-OUT FORMS

A preanesthesia assessment form is used to help identify any potential problems in a patient's medical history or physical examination prior to the administration of the anesthetic of choice (**Fig. 3**). The entire surgical team should be made aware of any potentially concerning history or examination findings before a patient even has an intravenous catheter placed.

Anesthesia records may vary in format but typically contain the same essential information (**Fig. 4**)—time and date, pertinent medical history, any patient medications and allergies, vital signs, type and amount of drugs administered, start and end times of anesthesia and surgery, surgeon and anesthetist names, and any complications. Vital signs are recorded every 5 minutes for deep sedation and general anesthetic cases. Cardiac rhythm, carbon dioxide levels, and temperatures are recorded during all general anesthetic cases until patients are extubated.

The consent form for surgery and anesthesia should be signed by the patient or responsible

UNIVERSITY OF PITTSBURGH SCHOOL OF DENTAL MEDICINE
DEPARTMENT OF ORAL AND MAXILLOFACIAL SURGERY
PRE-SEDATION ASSESSMENT

NOTES SHOULD BE SIGNED BY PHYSICIAN	
DATE/TIME	PRE-SEDATION ASSESSMENT—MUST BE COMPLETED ON THE DAY OF PROCEDURE

1. Is the patient's medical condition the same as it was on the date the history and physical was performed?
   ☐ Yes   ☐ No

2. Does patient meet NPO guidelines:
   ☐ Yes   ☐ No

Ingested Material	Minimum Fasting Period
Clear liquids	2 hours
Light meal (toast, clear liquids)	6 hours
Meal consisting of fried, fatty food or meat	6 hours

3. Airway assessment completed:
   ☐ Yes

   Airway management may be more difficult in the following conditions:
   - Dysmorphic features of the head and neck
   - Large tongue
   - Inability to visualize the uvula with mouth opening
   - Acute or chronic upper airway obstruction (i.e., sleep apnea)
   - Limited range of motion involving the neck or jaw
   - Prior history of difficult intubation

4. ASA physical status classification (check below):

Physical Status	Medical Description of Patient
☐ PS 1	No known systemic disease
☐ PS 2	Mild or well-controlled systemic disease
☐ PS 3	Multiple or moderate controlled systemic disease(s)
☐ PS 4	Severe life-threatening disease
☐ PS 5	Moribund patient
☐ E	Emergency

5. Plan for sedation:
   ☐ Moderate sedation

   Moderate sedation/analgesia (formerly conscious sedation)
   A drug-induced depression of consciousness during which patients respond purposefully to verbal commands, either alone or accompanied by light tactile stimulation. No interventions are required to maintain a patient airway, and spontaneous ventilation is adequate. Cardiovascular function is usually maintained.

   ☐ Minimal sedation

   Minimal sedation (anxiolysis)
   A drug-induced state during which the patients respond normally to verbal commands. Although cognitive function and coordination may be impaired, ventilatory and cardiovascular functions are unaffected.

6. Patient reassessed immediately prior to sedation and may proceed as planned.
   ☐ Yes   ☐ No

OMS Faculty/Resident Signature

UMC29338-0907

Fig. 3. Sample presedation assessment form. (*Courtesy of* University of Pittsburgh School of Dental Medicine, Pittsburgh, PA.)

party and be in plain view within the operating suite before a patient is placed under anesthesia. The Universal Protocol for Preventing Wrong Site, Wrong Procedure and Wrong Person Surgery must be performed before all surgeries. This information can be viewed at http://www.jointcommission.org/standards_information/up.aspx.

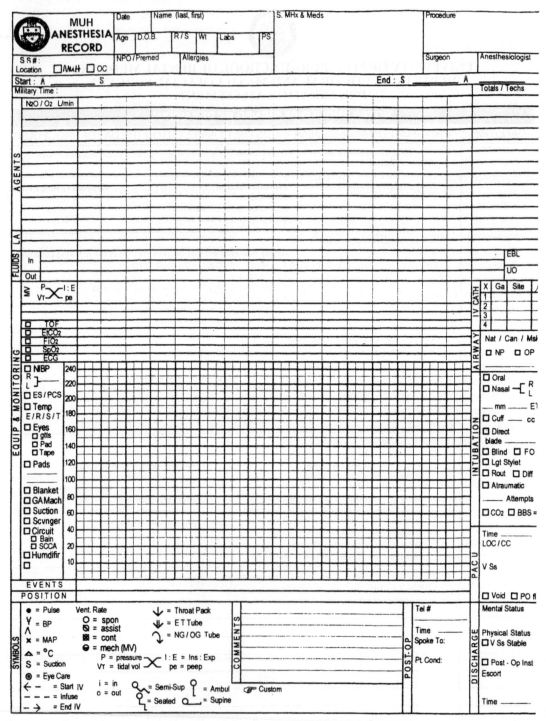

Fig. 4. Sample anesthesia record. (*Courtesy of* the Department of Oral and Maxillofacial Surgery, University of Pittsburgh Medical Center, Pittsburgh, PA.)

VENIPUNCTURE ARMAMENTARIUM AND INFUSION PUMPS

Peripheral venous access is commonly achieved with one of several different angiocatheters

(**Fig. 5**). One specific catheter system is the BD Insyte Autoguard (Becton Dickinson Infusion Therapy Systems, Sandy, Utah), which is a shielded intravenous catheter. This angiocatheter enables a surgeon to push a button on the catheter handle

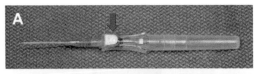

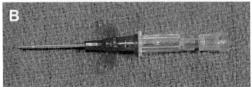

Fig. 5. (*A*) BD Insyte Autoguard Catheter (BD Infusion Therapy Systems, Sandy, Utah). When pushed, white button (*arrow*) safely retracts needle into handle. (*B*) B. Braun Introcan Safety IV Catheter Winged (B. Braun Melsungen AG, Melsungen, Germany).

after the needle is inserted into the vein, instantly retracting the needle into the handle and reducing the risk of a needlestick injury.

A winged infusion set, or butterfly needle, can be used during venipuncture for phlebotomy in patients with thin blood vessels that roll. The butterfly needle is not routinely used for the administration of intravenous fluids. If a butterfly needle is available and used because of difficult intravenous access, it may require the use of an arm board to prevent the upper extremity or hand from bending at the site of venipuncture.

A surgeon may choose to use an infusion pump to deliver intravenous medications rather than pushing intermittent boluses of the same drug (**Fig. 6**). Most infusion pumps provide similar safety and programmable features, such as accurate rapid occlusion detection and automated piggyback or concurrent delivery of a given drug. Some infusion pumps can also be programmed to accurately deliver intravenous fluids or blood products.

AIRWAY ARMAMENTARIUM

Emergency airway equipment must be both readily accessible and familiar to anyone providing anesthesia in the office. It is safe practice to keep airway equipment in both the operating suites and the recovery area. Airway equipment should include the following: a full face mask (preferably in multiple sizes with connectors); bag-valve-mask device with a pressure manometer, capable of providing positive pressure ventilation; oral and nasopharyngeal airways; a supraglottic airway; endotracheal tubes (various pediatric and adult sizes); laryngoscope in both pediatric and adult blades (with extra batteries and bulbs); and a cricothyrotomy kit.

Various supraglottic airway devices are available, and the specific device used in an office should preferentially be based on exposure and hands-on experience during a surgeon's anesthesia training. The laryngeal mask airway (LMA) is the most common supraglottic device and is available in several types. The LMA Classic is the original design and is the only reusable LMA. The LMA Supreme has a built-in bite block and an esophageal ventilation port (**Fig. 7**). The LMA Fastrach (**Fig. 8**) is an intubating LMA, which has a specific insertion handle and an epiglottic elevating bar designed to lift the epiglottis as the endotracheal tube passes. Another supraglottic airways is the King Airway (**Fig. 9**), which has the ability to provide positive pressure ventilation and spontaneous breathing. It has 2 cuffs that isolate the hypopharynx and laryngeal inlet, thus minimizing gastric insufflation. It does not pass below the vocal cords, so it is not a definitive airway. The King is more commonly used in the prehospital setting by emergency medical

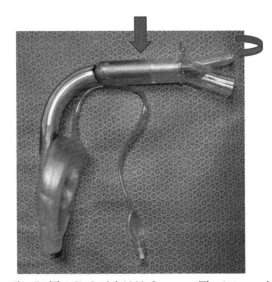

Fig. 7. (The Dr Brain) LMA Supreme (The Laryngeal Mask Company Limited, Victoria, Mahe, Seychelles) has a built-in bite block (*arrow*) and esophageal ventilation port (*curved arrow*).

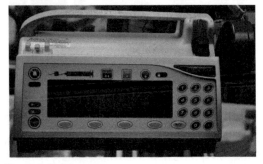

Fig. 6. Infusion pump.

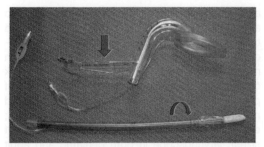

Fig. 8. LMA Fastrach ETT (The Laryngeal Mask Company Limited, Victoria, Mahe, Seychelles). Insertion handle (*arrow*) on LMA; accompanying endotracheal tube (*curved arrow*) in kit.

technicians and mobile intensive care practitioners and nurses.

A useful adjunct to airway armamentarium is an esophageal/precordial stethoscope. An array of precordial stethoscopes is available to anesthetists. These devices can be purchased with a custom molded earpiece for added comfort or even a wireless amplifier with Bluetooth technology to provide clear sound quality.

Another useful adjunct to airway armamentarium is transoral video laryngoscopy. Video laryngoscopy is a form of indirect laryngoscopy whereby a surgeon visualizes the larynx with a fiberoptic or digital laryngoscope. Two more common video laryngoscopes, the GlideScope (Verathon, Bothell, Washington) (**Fig. 10**) and McGrath (LMA North America, San Diego, California) (**Fig. 11**) both use a digital camera and rigid laryngoscopy to improve the view of the larynx.[2,3] The GlideScope is available in both single-use and reusable sets, whereas the McGrath is the first fully portable video laryngoscope and does not require focusing or image adjustment during use.

EMERGENCY DRUGS

The 8th edition of the American Association of Oral and Maxillofacial Surgeons *Office Anesthesia Evaluation Manual* provides a list of medications considered helpful in the event of an anesthetic

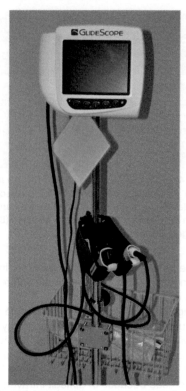

Fig. 10. GlideScope video laryngoscope (Verathon, Bothell, Washington).

emergency. This list is not considered all-inclusive or mandatory; it can be modified based on surgeon preference and experience level based on previous training (**Box 1**). An office should have a separate, clearly designated refrigerator for those medications that require storage in colder temperatures.

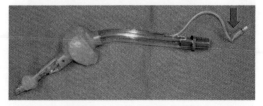

Fig. 9. King LT-D airway (King Systems, Noblesville, Indiana). Single valve (*arrow*) inflates both larger proximal cuff for oropharynx and smaller distal cuff, reducing possibility of gastric insufflation.

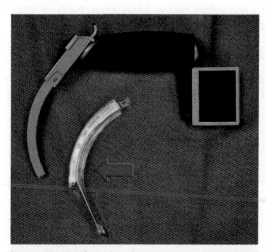

Fig. 11. McGrath video laryngoscope (LMA North America, San Diego, California) with single-use blade tip (*arrow*).

Box 1
Suggested drugs for treatment of anesthetic emergencies

- Intravenous fluids
  - Sterile water—inject or dilute drugs
  - Various intravenous fluids (normal saline, lactated Ringer, and so forth)
- Cardiovascular medications
  - Oxygen
  - Atropine (0.4 mg/mL)
  - Nitroglycerin (0.4 mg; 1/150 gR)
  - Dopamine (250 mg/5 mL)
  - Epinephrine (1 mg) (10 mL of 1:10,000)
  - Epinephrine (1:1000 or 1:10,000) (1 mg = 1:1000)
  - Dobutamine (1, 2, or 4 mg/mL)
  - Ephedrine (50 mg/mL)
  - Phenylephrine (Neo-Synephrine) (10 mg/mL)
  - Lidocaine (Xylocaine) (20 mg/mL)
  - Propranolol (Inderal) (1 mg/mL)
  - Procainamide (Procanbid) (100 mg/mL)
  - Verapamil (Calan) (5 mg/2 mL)
  - Amiodarone (Cordarone) (50 mg/mL)
  - Adenosine (3 mg/mL)
- Antihypertensive medications
  - Diazoxide (Hyperstat) (15 mg/mL)
  - Hydralazine (Apresoline) (20 mg/mL)
  - Esmolol (Brevibloc) (10 mg/mL)
  - Labetalol (Trandate) (5 mg/mL) (20-mL single-dose vial)
- Diuretics
  - Furosemide (Lasix) (10 mg/mL)
- Antiemetics
  - Prochlorperazine (Compazine) (5 mg/mL)
  - Ondansetron (Zofran) (2 mg/mL)
- Reversal agents
  - Naloxone (Narcan) (0.4 mg/mL)
  - Flumazenil (Romazicon) (0.1 mg/mL)
- Additional drugs
  - Dextrose 50%
  - Dexamethasone (Decadron) (4 mg/mL)
  - Hydrocortisone sodium succinate or methylprednisolone sodium succinate (Solu-Medrol) (125 mg)
  - Glycopyrolate (Robinul) (0.2 mg/mL)
  - Diazepam (Valium) (5 mg/mL)
  - Midazolam (Versed) (5 mg/mL)
  - Albuterol inhaler (Ventolin)
  - Succinylcholine (Anectine) (20 mg/mL)
  - Morphine sulfate (5 mg)
  - Dantrolene (Dantrium) (20-mg vials)
  - Lidocaine (10 mg/mL)
  - Nonenteric-coated aspirin (325 mg)
  - Famotidine (Pepcid)
  - Diphenhydramine (Benadryl) (50 mg/mL)

Data from American Association of Oral and Maxillofacial Surgeons. Office anesthesia evaluation manual. 8th edition. Rosemont (IL): American Association of Oral and Maxillofacial Surgeons; 2012.

OPERATING SUITE

The size of an operating room may be highly variable depending on surgeon preference and allotted floor space, but it must be able to readily accommodate an operating chair or table as well as an entire surgical team and anesthetist. Smaller operating spaces may make the resuscitation of a patient during an emergency unnecessarily challenging. The door width should be a minimum of 36 inches to allow for passage of any wheeled equipment and enable 2 adults to pass simultaneously through the doorway standing next to one another. Each suite requires electrical outlets in both the floor and wall for an operating table or chair as well as all anesthesia monitors.

MONITORS

Monitors do not eliminate a surgeon's need to directly observe patients during anesthesia. The ideal monitor enables a surgeon to analyze a patient's intended vital sign with ease and accuracy. Each office must be equipped with certain standard monitoring capabilities to provide a safe anesthetic. Standard office monitors include a noninvasive blood pressure monitor, a pulse oximeter, an ECG monitor, a capnography monitor, and either a basic monophasic defibrillator or automated external defibrillator. Most of the these standard monitors can be purchased with storage and printing features and should have a built-in rechargeable battery to run on an alternate power source in the event of a power outage. Patient monitors are also available in an array of combinations, so that each physiologic parameter does not require its own separate monitor. A common combination includes blood pressure, heart rate, pulse oximetry, and temperature and may be with (**Fig. 12**) or without (**Fig. 13**) ECG capabilities. Temperature monitoring is indicated or desirable depending on the type of anesthesia administered.

Capnography

A capnogram is a monitor of the inhaled and exhaled concentration or partial pressure of CO_2 and an indirect monitor of the CO_2 partial pressure in arterial blood.

Capnography provides valuable information regarding CO_2 production, pulmonary perfusion, alveolar ventilation, and elimination of CO_2 from the anesthesia circuit. Capnography also provides valuable clinical information, such as the frequency and regularity of ventilation during sedation cases. When capnography is monitored in an open circuit, such as during sedation, a nasal cannula with an attached gas sampling line can be used to monitor end-tidal CO_2 (**Fig. 14**).

The maintenance schedule for all monitors should be recorded in a log book and located in a common location known to all staff. Calibration of any monitor should be performed only by properly trained individuals and in accordance to the manufacturer's guidelines. During a loss of power in the office, the blood pressure monitor, pulse oximeter, ECG monitor, and defibrillator all need to be capable of being battery powered and portable.

SURGICAL CHAIR OR OPERATING TABLE

Many surgical chair and table designs are available to surgeons (**Fig. 15**). Surgeons must ensure that the surgical chair or operating table of preference has certain essential features. The design of

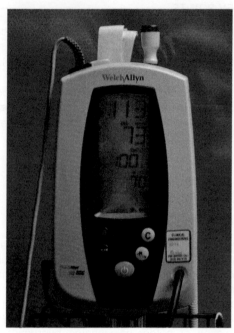

Fig. 13. Welch Allyn monitor (Welch Allyn, Skaneateles Falls, New York). Provides noninvasive blood pressure, pulse oximetry, heart rate, and temperature.

the chair or table must allow surgeon and anesthetist ease of accessibility to patients to allow for positional changes and maintaining a patient's airway. The chair and table should have a wide height range for the surgeon and staff, and both must be capable of resisting the pressure of performing cardiopulmonary resuscitation as well as placing patients in Trendelenburg position (**Fig. 16**). The headrest of a chair needs to have a secure, tight lock to avoid an unexpected release during the procedure, which could cause a

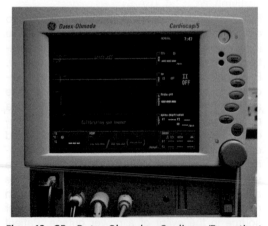

Fig. 12. GE Datex-Ohmeda Cardiocap/5 patient monitor (GE Healthcare, Waukesha, Wisconsin). This compact monitor allows full vital sign monitoring, including noninvasive blood pressure, pulse oximetry, heart rate, temperature, and 5-lead ECG.

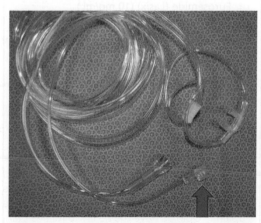

Fig. 14. Hudson RCI Softech Bi-Flo EtCO$_2$ Cannula (Teleflex Medical, Research Triangle Park, North Carolina). *Arrow* depicts attachment to CO_2 monitor.

A   **B**

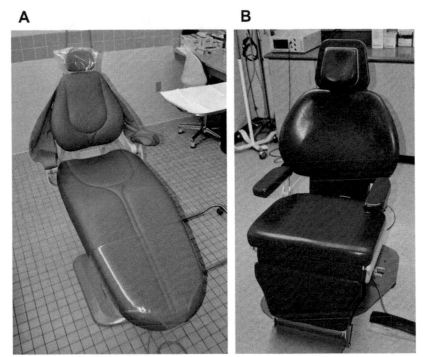

Fig. 15. (*A*) J/V-Generation Chair (DentalEZ Group, Bay Minette, Alabama). (*B*) Ritter 391 surgical chair (Midmark, Versailles, Ohio).

potential cervical injury (**Fig. 17**). Surgeons may also want to consider purchasing a surgical chair that is not only wider for heavier patients but also one that is also handicapped accessible. Such chairs have a low starting height to allow for wheelchair accessibility and adjustable and/or removable arms to allow for easy access/egress by patients. Some chairs are designed as a prototypical examination chair, which is upright and has a base for a patient's feet (see **Fig. 15**). These chairs can be adjusted to recline patients and also place patients in Trendelenburg during rescusitative

measures. Lastly the chair or table should be made of a material that is easy to clean and maintain.

OXYGEN AND SUPPLEMENTAL GAS DELIVERY SYSTEM

Most oxygen and anesthetic gas machines are fairly similar in design and function. The most essential feature of any oxygen delivery system is that it can deliver metered oxygen under positive pressure to a patient. All gas delivery machines have standard fail-safe mechanisms that prevent the delivery of any gas if the concurrent amount of oxygen administered is below a level that would ultimately deliver a hypoxic amount of gases. Furthermore, the gas outlets must be pin-indexed to prevent accidental administration of an incorrect gas. These machines require periodic calibration by appropriately trained individuals, and any maintenance records should be properly documented and stored in a log book located in an area known to all office staff.

LIGHTING SYSTEM

Operating light systems are typically wall or ceiling mounted but are also available on a mobile stand. The specific lighting system must allow a surgeon

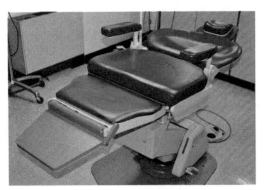

Fig. 16. Surgical chair in supine position to allow for cardiopulmonary resuscitation maneuvers.

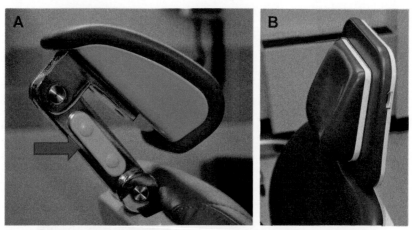

Fig. 17. (*A*) Headrest lock (*arrow*) on surgical chair. (*B*) Headrest that is not capable of tilting, avoiding risk of unintentional cervical injury if lock unexpectedly releases.

to accurately view the color of a patient's skin and mucosa. Other desirable features for a given lighting system are its abilities to provide cool and color-corrected light; enable deep cavity illumination; allow focus control, pattern size adjustment, and shadow reduction; and enable easy positioning of the light heads. Surgeons may also choose to use a headlight for additional lighting. Auxiliary lighting is mandatory in the event of a power failure in the operating suite or entire office. Most outpatient offices do not have an emergency generator that activates immediately to provide lighting, such as in ambulatory surgical centers. Thus, any backup lighting should be battery powered, portable, and able to provide enough lighting to enable surgeons to complete the procedure or safely stop at a point where a surgery can be completed when power eventually returns.

SUCTION EQUIPMENT

An office suction system may operate through either a central suction installation or a portable unit. Most offices incorporate a central installation with the pump located remote from the operating room to reduce noise. During a power outage or pump failure, a portable aspiration unit must be readily accessible. These portable units can be battery powered. Portable suction should also be available in the recovery area during such emergencies. Ofice staff should adhere to a routine schedule and keep detailed records for maintenance of the suction system.

TRANSPORT EQUIPMENT

Patients typically are transferred from an operating suite to a recovery area by a portable chair.

Desirable features of a transfer/recovery chair are capability of recliner positions and Trendelenburg position, transport handle on back, attached intravenous hanger, and construction with a material that is easy to clean and maintain. If a surgeon does not choose to fully recover a patient in the operating suite, then a surgical staff member must be present in the recovery area to monitor the patient's airway and vital signs. The ideal recovery scenario involves patients who walk with assistance to the recovery area.

RECOVERY ROOM

The design of the recovery area must allow the staff to observe patients after an anesthetic in an unobstructed manner. The staff also requires clear access to the patient for resuscitation purposes in the event of an anesthetic emergency. Essential equipment and features that need to be available in any recovery area are oxygen under pressure, suction, sufficient lighting, a pulse oximeter, a cardiac monitor, and a defibrillator. All monitors require an electrical outlet,and battery-powered lighting as well as portable suction, and oxygen should be accessible during a power outage. Most offices design the recovery area to be located remote or at the opposite end of the corridor from the operating suites. Patients should also exit the office through a door that is situated nearest the recovery area and opposite that of the entrance to the operating suites.

SUMMARY

The surgical equipment and anesthesia-related monitors in an oral and maxillofacial surgeon's office are highly individualized. The specific floor plan is also variable and may be partly influenced by the availability of floor space. Regardless, certain features are required for the safe practice of office-based anesthesia. The blood pressure monitor, pulse oximeter, ECG, and defibrillator must each have a built-in rechargeable battery to maintain functionality in the event of a power outage. Portable oxygen, suction, and lighting are essential safe measures as well. Surgeons may opt to purchase an emergency generator to provide power during an emergency. Otherwise, battery powered equipment must be available.

REFERENCES

1. Office Anesthesia Evaluation Manual. 8th edition. American Association of Oral and Maxillofacial Surgeons; 2012.
2. Rai MR, Dering A, Verghese C. The Glidescope system: a clinical assessment of performance. Anaesthesia 2005;60(1):60–4.
3. Serocki G, Bein B, Scholz J, et al. Management of the predicted difficult airway; a comparison of conventional blade laryngoscopy with video-assisted blade laryngoscopy and the Glidescope. Eur J Anaesthesiol 2010;27(1):24–30.

Adult Airway Evaluation in Oral Surgery

James C. Phero, DMD[a],*, Morton B. Rosenberg, DMD[b],
Joseph A. Giovannitti Jr, DMD[c]

KEYWORDS

• Airway • Thyromental distance • Laryngoscopy • Cormack and Lehane • Intubation • Ventilation
• Oxygenation • Obstructive sleep apnea

KEY POINTS

- Patients with a history of difficult ventilation and/or intubation should be treated as having a difficult airway, even though the physical appearance and physical examination may be unremarkable.
- Preparedness for potential difficult mask ventilation airway rescue is one of the most important aspects in assuring patient safety in the deep sedation/general anesthesia techniques performed routinely in oral and maxillofacial surgical outpatient settings.
- Unexpected failed ventilation and intubation may result from oropharyngeal, laryngeal, or tracheal abnormalities and disease processes that may not be identified by classic examination.
- The identification of patients with possible or potential difficultly in ventilation and intubation may be aided with the preoperative assessment of the airway, including the Mallampati test; evidence of receding mandible; limited mouth opening as a result of tissue or temporomandibular joint restriction; enlarged teeth; high-arched palate; narrow, small mouth; and/or restricted cervical spine movement.
- All current tests to predict difficulty with airway management are associated with a high incidence of false-positive and false-negative results and have low predictive value. To minimize airway-related complications, it is optimal to accept this high incidence of false-positive predictions using the classic evaluation tests and treat any patient identified as having a potential difficult intubation with caution and care.

SCOPE OF THE PROBLEM AND INCIDENCE

A challenging airway may present as difficulty with ventilation, difficulty with tracheal intubation, or both. The American Society of Anesthesiologists' (ASA) *Practice Guidelines for Management of the Difficult Airway* has defined difficult ventilation as a circumstance whereby "it is not possible for the unassisted anesthesiologist to prevent or reverse signs of inadequate ventilation during positive pressure ventilation."[1]

The precise frequency of difficult mask ventilation is unknown, but an Australian study indicated that 15% of difficult intubations were also associated with difficult mask ventilation.[2] In an evaluation of 22 600 attempts at mask ventilation at the University of Michigan, 1.4% (313 cases) were difficult to ventilate and 0.16% (37 cases) were impossible to ventilate. A total of 0.37% (84 cases) of the cases that were difficult and impossible to mask ventilate were also observed to be a difficult

[a] Anesthesiology Department, College of Medicine, University of Cincinnati Academic Medical Center, 231 Albert Sabin Way, Cincinnati, OH 45267-0531, USA; [b] Division of Anesthesia and Pain Control, Tufts University Schools of Dental Medicine and Medicine, 1 Kneeland Street, Boston, MA 02111, USA; [c] Department of Dental Anesthesiology, Center for Patients with Special Needs, University of Pittsburgh School of Dental Medicine, 3501 Terrace Street, Pittsburgh, PA 15261, USA
* Corresponding author.
E-mail address: james.phero@uc.edu

Oral Maxillofacial Surg Clin N Am 25 (2013) 385–399
http://dx.doi.org/10.1016/j.coms.2013.04.005
1042-3699/13/$ – see front matter © 2013 Elsevier Inc. All rights reserved.

intubation. Of the 37 cases that were impossible to ventilate, only 1 patient required surgical airway access.[3]

"Difficult rigid laryngoscopy is defined as a situation in which it is not possible to visualize any portion of the vocal cords with conventional laryngoscopy."[1] A difficult intubation is defined as a circumstance in which "the proper insertion of an endotracheal tube using conventional laryngoscopy requires more than three attempts, or greater than 10 minutes."[1]

The incidence of difficult intubation by rigid laryngoscopy varies from 0.5% to 13.6% in published studies.[4–10] These discrepancies in the reported incidence of difficult intubation are expected because most reports are retrospective studies and apply different definitions of what constitutes a difficult intubation.[11] Thirty percent to 50% of all anesthetic deaths have been attributed to the inability to manage a difficult airway.[12]

GRADING THE DIFFICULTY OF MASK VENTILATION

The ability to predict the difficulty of mask ventilation as an airway rescue technique is especially important in the contemporary oral and maxillofacial surgical office using open airway techniques for deep sedation/general anesthesia. In the adult population, difficult mask ventilation was seen in 5% of the patients studied.[13] Unfortunately, research in this area has not been as vigorous as with intubation. However, there are scoring systems in use.[3,14] Common risk factors include a body mass index (BMI) of more than 30 kg/m, male sex, presence of a beard, high Mallampati classification, snoring, decreased thyromental distance, and neck radiation. Factors that may prevent adequate mask ventilation include a good mask fit, adequate positioning of a supraglottic

airway, proper positioning of the head and neck, and opening of the mouth. Inability to ventilate the lungs or intubate the trachea may, of course, also result from poor technique and/or lack of technical expertise.[15]

GRADING THE DIFFICULTY OF TRACHEAL INTUBATION

Cormack, Lehane, and others have developed classifications determined by the view obtained at laryngoscopy.[16] The Cormack and Lehane classification uses 4 grades as follows: grade I, a full view of glottis; grade II, only the posterior commissure is visible; grade III, only the tip of the epiglottis is visible; grade IV, no glottic structures are visible (**Fig. 1**). The use of the original Cormack and Lehane scoring system led Yentis and Lee[17] to develop a modified Cormack and Lehane scoring system in which grade II (only part of the glottis visible) was divided into IIa (part of the cords are visible) and IIb (only the arytenoids or the very posterior origin of the cords are visible) (**Fig. 2**). In this system, grade IIb denotes a laryngoscopic view that is relatively common and often associated with difficulty passing a tracheal tube. This system is now commonly used for recording the ease or difficulty in laryngoscopic view in hospital anesthetic records and in studies of tracheal intubation.

EVALUATION OF THE POTENTIALLY DIFFICULT AIRWAY

All patients receiving sedation and general anesthesia should receive an airway assessment as part of their focused physical examination before surgery. To identify patients with potentially difficult-to-manage airways, a careful history regarding patient breathing, sleep position, and voice quality is taken. During physical examination, patients should be viewed from a frontal

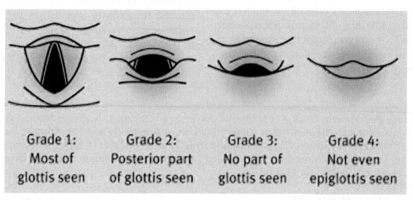

Grade 1:
Most of
glottis seen

Grade 2:
Posterior part
of glottis seen

Grade 3:
No part of
glottis seen

Grade 4:
Not even
epiglottis seen

Fig. 1. The Cormack and Lehane grading system. (*From* Grover A, Canavan C. Tracheal intubation. Anaesth Intensive Care Med 2007;8(9):347–51.)

Original Cormack and Lehane system	I	II		III	IV
	Full view of the glottis	Partial view of the glottis or arytenoids		Only epiglottis visible	Neither glottis nor epiglottis visible
View at laryngoscopy	E — Li				
Modified system	I	IIa	IIb	III	IV
	As for original Cormack and Lehane above	Partial view of the glottis	Arytenoids or posterior part of the vocal cords only just visible	As for original Cormack and Lehane above	As for original Cormack and Lehane above

Fig. 2. Original versus modified Cormack and Lehane scoring system. Description of the 2 scoring systems used for recording laryngoscopy view. E, epiglottis; LI, laryngeal outlet. (*From* Phero JC, Ovassapian A, Hurford WE. Evaluation of the patient with a difficult airway. In: Longnecker DE, Brown DL, Newman MF, et al, editors. Anesthesiology. New York: McGraw Hill; 2008. p.116–31.)

and profile view to assess mandibular size. Thyromental distance is measured; neck rotation, flexion, and extension mobility are evaluated and graded. The neck is palpated for the identification of the cricothyroid membrane. Additionally, one should check for temporomandibular joint (TMJ) problems, mouth opening, loose or protruding teeth, degree of overbite, size of the tongue, visibility of faucial structures, and patency of the nares.

Several predictive tests have been described that detect potentially difficult intubation (**Box 1**). These clinical examinations are straightforward. Although useful in airway evaluation, all of these tests are associated with relatively high rates of false-positive and false-negative predictions (**Box 2**).

Anatomic Considerations

Certain anatomic features are recognized as contributing to the difficulty of intubation.[18]

Atlantooccipital mobility

Adequate cervical mobility and mouth opening are essential for the alignment of the oral, pharyngeal, and laryngeal axes required for visualization of the glottis during laryngoscopy.[18,19] Decreased neck mobility also limits maneuvers that can be used to keep the airway open, thereby predisposing to difficult mask ventilation.

The evaluation of atlantooccipital extension is performed by having patients sit straight and extend the head while maintaining the cervical spine in a neutral position.[19] The greater the atlantooccipital distance in the neutral position, the greater the possible degree of head extension and the more likely the ease of intubation. A

reduction of atlantooccipital extension by one-third or more will contribute to the difficulty of intubation.[19] If the posterior tubercle of the atlas is in contact with the occiput in the neutral position, attempts to extend the head result in anterior bowing of the cervical spine and forward displacement of the larynx.[20] Limitations in head extension may occur secondary to anatomic variations of the

---

Box 1
Categories of difficult airway

Known or expected difficult airway

    History of difficult or failed intubation

    History of difficult or failed mask ventilation

    Conditions associated with difficult airway

        Acquired

        Congenital

Potentially difficult airway

    Limited neck extension

    Limited mouth opening

    Receding mandible

    Mallampati class III or IV

    Short thyromental distance

Unexpected difficult airway

    Unknown supraepiglottic mass

        Hyperplasia of lingual tonsils

        Supraepiglottic cyst or tumor

    Missed evidence of difficult airway

        Poor preoperative evaluation

        Ignoring presence of evidence

Box 2
Tests applied to predict difficult intubation

External anatomic features

Head and neck movement (atlantooccipital joint)

Jaw movement (TMJ)

Mouth opening

Subluxation of mandible

Receding mandible

Protruding maxillary incisors

Obesity

Thyromental distance

Sternomental distance

Visualization of the oropharyngeal structures

Anterior tilt of larynx

Radiographic assessment

atlantooccipital gap in otherwise healthy people or secondary to pathologic conditions, such as rheumatoid arthritis.

Mouth opening, dentition, mandibular space

Other anatomic factors may interfere with the line of vision from the mouth opening to the vocal cords. The TMJ hinge movement of the mandible controls mouth opening. The horizontal gliding TMJ movement allows for subluxation of the mandible, which permits additional anterior displacement of the tongue during laryngoscopy. A mouth opening (distance between mandibular and maxillary central incisors) limited to 3.5 cm or less tends to make intubation more difficult. TMJ dysfunction, congenital fusion of the joints, trauma, tissue contracture around the mouth, and trismus may limit the mouth opening. Trismus secondary to pain associated with infection usually relaxes under general anesthesia, but this cannot be assured if the infection has been long standing or involves the pterygoid space.

Protruding maxillary anterior teeth may interfere with the laryngoscope placement and passage of the endotracheal tube during intubation. During laryngoscopy, the tongue is displaced into the mandibular space, opening the line of vision from the mouth to the larynx. A small mandibular vault may not adequately accommodate tongue displacement, thus interfering with the visualization of the larynx.

Thyromental distance

Patil and colleagues[21] reported that rigid laryngoscopy may be impossible in adults if the thyromental distance is less than 6.0 cm (3 finger breadths). The thyromental distance is measured between the bony point of the mentum of the mandible and the thyroid notch with the head fully extended.

Visibility of Oropharyngeal Structures

Mallampati and others[22] described examination signs and related them to intubation difficulty. They correlated the degree of visibility of the oropharyngeal structures with the difficulty of rigid laryngoscopy.[22] A sitting patient is asked to open his or her mouth as wide as possible and maximally protrude the tongue. The visibility of the faucial pillars, soft palate, and uvula was noted. The airway was classified into 3 categories: class I, soft palate, fauces, uvula, and pillars are visualized; class II, soft palate, fauces, and pillars are visualized, but the uvula is masked by the base of the tongue; and class III, only the soft palate can be visualized. In class III, visualization of the glottis with rigid laryngoscopy is expected to be difficult.[22] Samsoon and Young[6] extended the oropharyngeal exposures to include a fourth class. This 4-category system is in common use and classified as follows: class I, soft palate, fauces, uvula, and pillars are visualized; class II, soft palate, fauces, uvula are seen; class III, only the soft palate and base of the uvula are observed; class IV, the soft palate is not visible (**Fig. 3**). A further modification of the Mallampati visualization scoring included a class zero view.[23,24] Class zero is defined as the ability to see any part of the epiglottis on mouth opening and tongue protrusion. Ezri and colleagues[25] evaluated 764 patients and reported that 1.18% of patients had a class zero airway. A class zero airway was noted to be an excellent predictor of uncomplicated laryngoscopy.

The Mallampati score has become a standard part of a comprehensive airway evaluation, although its predictive value for difficult intubation has proven to be low. Additionally, the American Society of Anesthesiologists Task Force On the Management of the Difficult Airway also recommended including the assessment of dentition, thyromental distance, and neck extension.[1]

In summary, the Mallampati test has been broadly applied, even though its predictive value for difficult intubation is low. The practitioner should rely on a combination of tests and the results of a focused physical examination and history.[26]

A stepwise approach to decision making incorporating evaluation of the airway is crucial in the ASA's airway approach algorithm.[27] This algorithm is based on 5 clinical questions: Is airway

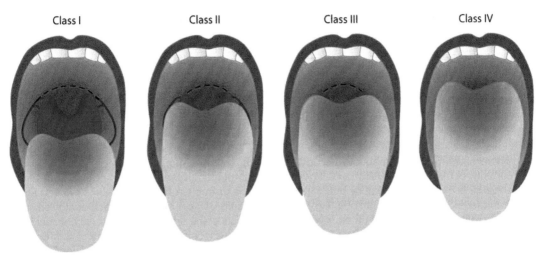

Fig. 3. Classification of pharyngeal structures as proposed by Mallampati and Samsoon. Note: Class III, soft palate visible; class IV, soft palate not visible. (*From* Phero JC, Ovassapian A, Hurford WE. Evaluation of the patient with a difficult airway. In: Longnecker DE, Brown DL, Newman MF, et al, editors. Anesthesiology. New York: McGraw Hill; 2008. p. 116–31.)

control necessary? Is there potential for difficult laryngoscopy? Can supralaryngeal ventilation be used? Is there an aspiration risk? Will the patient tolerate an apneic period? Answers to these basic questions can help guide the practitioner in the potential use of the ASA's difficult airway algorithm.

EVALUATION OF THE COMPLEX AIRWAY

Patients with a history of difficult ventilation or intubation and patients with anatomic or abnormal conditions associated with a complex airway fall into the category of known difficult airway.[28] The causes of the expected difficult airway may be grouped into congenital or acquired conditions and be further classified by the location of involvement or disease. These patients are generally not considered acceptable risks for office-based sedation/anesthetic procedures.

Increased frequency of ventilation, chest retractions, increased use of accessory muscles, stridor, voice weakness, or hoarseness, alone or in combination, may indicate a potential airway problem (**Table 1**). Stridor is a particularly important sign and may provide evidence of the site and severity of airway obstruction related to severe oropharyngeal, glottic, and/or upper tracheal occlusion. Stridor during inspiration generally indicates an obstruction at or above the larynx. Expiratory stridor is most often associated with intrathoracic or subglottic obstructions. Obstruction associated with the larynx or glottic region may produce biphasic stridor, although either inspiratory or expiratory sounds may predominate. In adults, stridor at rest indicates a serious degree of obstruction with a cross-sectional airway opening of less than 4 mm or an irregularly narrowed airway several centimeters in length.

Obesity

Airway assessment of obese patients should be performed with patients in both the sitting and supine positions. Respiratory function and airway

Table 1
History findings that suggest difficult airway management

Finding	Implication
Dry cough	Possible tracheobronchial compression
Easy bleeding	Epistaxis risk
Gastroesophageal reflux	Aspiration risk
Long-standing diabetes mellitus	Limited cervical mobility
Loud snoring	Prone to soft tissue obstruction
Major trauma	Unstable neck, limiting safe mobility
Radiation to neck	Fibrosis, immobility
Recent temporal craniotomy	Limited mandibular motility
Smoking	Salivation, cough, laryngospasm
Undigested food returning to mouth	Aspiration risk from pharyngeal pouch

patency can be significantly altered by this change in position.[29] A large neck circumference is associated with obstructive sleep apnea (OSA) in obese patients. In evaluating 123 patients with thick necks for OSA, Katz and colleagues[30] found that the sleep apnea–hypopnea index correlated with external neck circumference, BMI, and the internal circumference of the distal pharynx. Men more commonly have sleep-disordered breathing than women and the sleep-disordered breathing tends to be more severe.[31] In a prospective study of 100 morbidly obese patients (BMI >40 kg/m^2), the preoperative measurements of height, weight, neck circumference, width of mouth opening, sternomental distance, thyromental distance, and Mallampati score were recorded.[32] The view during direct laryngoscopy was graded, and the number of attempts at tracheal intubation was recorded. Neither absolute obesity nor BMI was associated with intubation difficulties. Large neck circumference and high Mallampati score were the only predictors of potential intubation problems.

In the supine position, changes in chest compliance and vital capacity may interfere with adequate spontaneous ventilation. The incidence of hiatal hernia, gastric pH of 2.5 or lower, and reduced functional residual capacity found in obese patients places these patients at an increased risk for the consequences of aspiration of gastric contents.[33,34]

There is consensus that airway management is more difficult in morbidly obese patients. Body weight may not be as critical as the location of excess weight. Massive weight in the lower abdomen and hip area may be less important than when the weight is in the upper body area. A short, thick, immobile neck caused by cervical spine fat pads will interfere with rigid laryngoscopy. Furthermore, the redundancy of soft tissue structures inside the oropharyngeal and supralaryngeal area may make mask ventilation and intubation difficult. When high positive pressure is required to ventilate patients, the chance of inflating the stomach is increased. Rapid oxygen desaturation during apnea, secondary to reduced functional residual capacity, limits available intubation time. In the case of the cannot intubate–cannot ventilate situation, access to the neck for transtracheal jet ventilation or establishing a surgical airway (eg, emergency tracheostomy or cricothyroidotomy) will also be more complex.

Rheumatoid Arthritis

The airway management of these patients should be based on an understanding of the pathologic changes affecting the airway. In patients with advanced rheumatoid arthritis and spondylosis, airway management may be extremely difficult. Rheumatoid arthritis may involve any joint of the body, including the cervical spine, TMJ, and cricoarytenoid joint. A change in voice, the presence of dysphagia, dysarthria, stridor, or a sense of fullness in the oropharynx may indicate laryngeal involvement.

Physical examination of patients with rheumatoid arthritis should include flexion, extension, and rotation of the head with palpation of the larynx and trachea for evidence of deviation and/or limitation. Upper extremity radiculopathy suggests cervical spine arthritis. Progressive cervical spondylosis associated with rheumatoid arthritis leads to severe flexion deformity of the cervical spine, which complicates airway management.[35] Although chin lift and jaw thrust are commonly used to improve mask ventilation and oxygenation, these maneuvers may increase the possibility of spinal cord compression and damage.[36]

Congenital Disease

Anomalies of the cardiovascular, nervous, musculocutaneous, endocrine, or excretory systems may produce abnormalities of the head, neck, or upper airway. Rosenberg and Rosenberg[28] have tabulated the syndromes most often accompanied by aberrations of the upper airway. These syndromes include Crouzon, Goldenhar, Pierre Robin, and Treacher Collins syndromes, which are known for their grossly abnormal head and neck anatomy. Patients with congenital malformations associated with micrognathia, retrognathia, and macroglossia have a smaller oropharyngeal cross section and are prone to soft tissue upper airway obstruction.[37,38] Patients with severe congenital anomalies are often not candidates for office sedation/anesthesia procedures.

Airway Infection

Inflammation and edema can distort anatomy, fix soft tissues, and compress the airway, interfering with ventilation and intubation.[39,40] Airway compromise by infection poses a major airway management problem in patients younger than 10 years. Of 90 deaths resulting from upper airway obstruction in children, 36 were related to airway infections.[41,42] Anesthetics and surgical care involving acute, potentially airway-threatening infections, such as peritonsillar abscess, retropharyngeal abscess, submandibular abscess, Ludwig angina, croup, and epiglottitis, are reserved for skilled anesthesia/surgical teams in a hospital setting.

Trauma

Trauma to the head and neck may produce major acute or chronic anatomic changes. These changes may affect airway accessibility, making tracheal intubation or mask ventilation difficult. Blunt or penetrating trauma to the larynx, trachea, hyoid structure, and facial bones can result in a complex, difficult-to-manage airway.[43,44] Subcutaneous emphysema, hoarseness, stridor, and tracheal deviation are warning signs of airway injury. Such patients should be observed closely because progression of the condition may lead to airway obstruction.

The signs and symptoms of laryngeal trauma may be quite subtle. Patients with laryngeal trauma are often hoarse or short of breath, although this clinical presentation may not correlate with the severity of injury. Dysphagia is not a common symptom of laryngotracheal injury. Nevertheless, esophageal injury should be strongly considered in patients with laryngotracheal trauma. On physical examination, the presence of hemoptysis may indicate laryngeal or tracheal injury. External palpation of the neck should include evaluation of the hyoid bone and thyroid and cricoid cartilages. The skin should be examined for abrasions and subcutaneous air. Open wounds should not be probed, but entrance and exit wounds should be noted to better understand the trajectory of the injury, particularly with bullet wounds. Cricotracheal separation should be suspected when the mechanism of injury is via a clothesline or hanging injury. In these patients, stridor and subcutaneous emphysema should prompt immediate evaluation, and orotracheal intubation is contraindicated because it may cause more harm than good. In these cases, an endotracheal tube can migrate through a perforation into the cervical soft tissues or mediastinum, creating a tenuous and possibly dangerous airway for patients.[45] Thus, awake tracheostomy below the site of injury remains the mainstay of airway management in these cases.

Trauma patients should also be examined for cervical spine injuries because movement of the neck during intubation may lead to irreversible paralysis. Maintaining cervical collar placement or applying axial traction may minimize spinal cord injury during intubation.[46] Acute airway management for trauma patients is beyond the scope of this article but requires meticulous physical examination and advanced airway management techniques.

Tumors

Head and neck tumors, both benign and malignant, may make intubation difficult. Tumors, surgical scars, or radiation fibrosis of head and neck tissues can limit mouth opening and proper positioning of the head and neck for rigid laryngoscopy (**Table 2**).[4,47] Tumors of the oral cavity and oropharynx may create trismus caused by invasion of the muscles of mastication.

Foreign Body

Foreign bodies in the upper aerodigestive tract are an important cause of morbidity and mortality for patients at both age extremes. Both the elderly and children younger than 3 years are at risk for foreign-body ingestion. Impacted food in the upper aerodigestive tract tends to be a problem in the elderly. These patients may have dentures that prevent the detection of a small bone fragments or proper mastication of food. In addition, elderly patients are more likely to suffer from esophageal dysmotility, Zenker diverticulum, malignancy or stricture, all of which predispose to esophageal foreign bodies. Symptoms of an impacted bone include stabbing pain on swallowing. Typically the bone protrudes from the lingual or palatine tonsil. Generally, when a foreign body is lodged in the upper esophagus, patients can point to the level of obstruction. Dysphagia, regurgitation of food, bloody secretions, and an inability to tolerate secretions may be noted. Removal of an impacted foreign body may be performed under general anesthesia depending on the patient's age, material that is impacted, and location. In these situations, it is imperative to control the airway to prevent aspiration. Even if the foreign body is noted on laryngoscopy, unless it is obstructing the airway, tracheal intubation should be achieved before removal.

Children, particularly those younger than 3 years, can also present with an upper airway foreign body in addition to the more common esophageal foreign body. Airway foreign bodies may involve the larynx, trachea, or bronchi. Most inhaled foreign bodies enter the right mainstem bronchus, which is larger and has a straighter takeoff from the carina than the left. The symptoms associated with aspiration can include gagging, coughing, spasmodic choking, stridor, wheezing, tachypnea, tachycardia, and decreased breath sounds on auscultation.[48] Removal of an inhaled foreign body may involve a general anesthetic, depending on the patient's age as well as the location and material of the foreign body. Careful control of the airway in these situations is imperative. The anesthetist should work closely with the otolaryngologist to perform laryngoscopy and bronchoscopy for removal of the foreign body.

Table 2
Physical findings that suggest difficult airway management

Finding	Implication
Obesity	Easily obstructed airway, aspiration risk, diminished chest wall compliance, difficult laryngoscopy because of macroglossia and immobile head
Pregnancy	All the problems associated with obesity, especially aspiration risk; large breasts impair laryngoscope insertion; swollen mucosa bleed easily
Ascites	Aspiration risk, diminished chest wall compliance
Whiskers, flat nasal bridge, large face	Difficult mask seal
Mouth opens less than 40 mm	Glottic exposure blocked by maxillary teeth
Cervico-occipital extension limited to an angle at the hyoid less that 160°	Difficult to align mouth and pharynx for glottic exposure
Short, thick, muscular neck	Prone to soft tissue obstruction, difficult to extend neck for intubation or mask ventilation
Thyromental distance less than 60 mm, receding chin	Difficult to mobilize tongue for glottic exposure, glottis too anterior to visualize
Maxillary gap from missing incisors with other teeth present to the right	Laryngoscope fits into gap while adjacent teeth, lip, or gums block view of glottis and passage of tracheal tube
Edentulous with atrophic mandible	Small face and furrowed cheeks impair mask fit, tongue and soft palate block exhalation
Prominent or protruding maxillary incisors	Teeth block view of glottis
Advanced caries, loose teeth, caps, bridges	Dentition can be damaged or aspirated, rough edges can tear tube cuff
Stridor, retractions	Risk or insurmountable airway obstruction
Hoarseness	Chance of vocal cord dysfunction or airway masses
Underwater voice	Vallecular or epiglottic cysts
Nasogastric tube in situ	Difficult to seal mask
Poorly visualized soft palate and fauces in upright patients with mouth fully open (Mallampati sign)	Difficult to expose glottis with rigid laryngoscopy
Large goiter or immobile tumor displacing trachea	Difficult to expose glottis, airway obstruction, or tracheal collapse
Tracheostomy scar	Possible tracheal stenosis

IMPORTANCE OF PREOPERATIVE AIRWAY EVALUATION

The ASA's Closed Claims Project evaluated adverse anesthetic outcomes obtained from the closed claim files of 35 US liability insurance companies. This database dates from 1985 and accrues about 300 cases per year. One of the first reviews of this data evaluated respiratory events, the most common cause of adverse outcomes. This study found respiratory events to be the single largest class of injury, accounting for 34% of all claims. Eighty-five percent of these adverse outcomes resulted in death or brain damage. Critical review found that most outcomes could have been prevented. It is not surprising that 30% of the mortalities in these claims were attributable to an anesthetic malpractice and were the result of an inability to manage a difficult airway. More recent examination of the data looked at outcomes from perioperative airway claims from 1985 to 1999. In this series, 57% of claims resulted in brain damage or loss of life with the difficult airway being encountered on induction. In an effort to improve the management of the difficult airway, the ASA released their original airway algorithm in 1993, which has been updated to include newer advanced airway adjuncts.[49]

EMERGENCY MANAGEMENT TASK TRAINING AND TEAM CRISIS SIMULATIONS

National and international professional society emergency simulation education workshops are evolving to meet the patient safety need for practitioners and their office teams to provide prompt and effective management of patient airway, ventilation, and oxygenation. The American Association of Oral and Maxillofacial Surgeons continues to offer hands-on small-group emergency management workshops at their annual meeting for practitioners with American Heart Association (AHA) Basic Life Support for Health care Providers (BLS HP), AHA Advanced Cardiac Life Support (ACLS), and general anesthesia permits. The American Dental Society of Anesthesia (ADSA) continues to offer hands-on small-group emergency management workshops at their annual and regional meetings for 3 groups of practitioners and their office staff: (1) BLS HP training, (2) BLS HP/ACLS training, and (3) BLS HP/ACLS training and the general anesthesia permit. In 2011, the ADSA also began supporting these emergency simulation education workshops at the component level to provide improved access to practitioners closer to their practice settings. The ADSA Anesthesia Research Foundation has developed the format for coordinated and calibrated emergency education workshops that focus on standardized recommendations for training, emergency management protocols, equipment, drugs, and supplies to optimize team care for the 10-minute period from the recognition of a patient's emergency until emergency medical services arrives to assist in patient care. This patient safety initiative is trademarked *Ten Minutes Saves A Life!* and began in 2011. Appendix 1 is an example of the checklists used in the ADSA workshops. These checklists are for the practitioner with BLS HP/ACLS training plus the general anesthesia permit and the office staff. Ideally, these hands-on team crisis resource management emergency workshops will be offered throughout the United States and abroad in simulation education centers to make this training readily accessible.

SUMMARY

Patients with a history of difficult intubation or with conditions associated with difficult airway management should be approached with organized primary and secondary plans for airway management. The detection of these problems may result in patients being referred to centers with appropriate clinicians and equipment. The authors' rule of thumb is that if it cannot be predicted that patients can be easily ventilated by mask ventilation and rescued, then consideration should be given to the use of advanced techniques or further evaluation.

REFERENCES

1. American Society of Anesthesiologists Task Force on Management of the Difficult Airway. Practice guidelines for management of the difficult airway: an updated report by the American Society of Anesthesiologists Task Force on Management of the Difficult Airway. Anesthesiology 2003;98(5): 1269–77.
2. Williamson JA, Webb RK, Szekely S, et al. The Australian Incident Monitoring Study. Difficult intubation: an analysis of 2000 incident reports. Anaesth Intensive Care 1993;21(5):602–7.
3. Kheterpal S, Han R, Tremper KK, et al. Incidence and predictors of difficult and impossible mask ventilation. Anesthesiology 2006;105(5):885–91.
4. Latto IP. Management of difficult intubation. In: Latto IP, Rosen M, editors. Difficulties in tracheal intubation. London: Balliere Tindall; 1985. p. 141.
5. Lyons G. Failed intubation. Six years' experience in a teaching maternity unit. Anaesthesia 1985;40(8): 759–62.
6. Samsoon GL, Young JR. Difficult tracheal intubation: a retrospective study. Anaesthesia 1987; 42(5):487–90.
7. Savva D. Prediction of difficult tracheal intubation. Br J Anaesth 1994;73(2):149–53.
8. Wilson ME, Spiegelhalter D, Robertson JA, et al. Predicting difficult intubation. Br J Anaesth 1988;61(2): 211–6.
9. Crosby ET, Elliott RD. Anaesthesia for caesarean section in a parturient with quintuplet gestation, pulmonary oedema and thrombocytopaenia. Can J Anaesth 1988;35(4):417–21.
10. Rocke DA, Murray WB, Rout CC, et al. Relative risk analysis of factors associated with difficult intubation in obstetric anesthesia. Anesthesiology 1992;77(1): 67–73.
11. Rosenstock C, Hansen EG, Kristensen MS, et al. Qualitative analysis of unanticipated difficult airway management. Acta Anaesthesiol Scand 2006; 50(3):290–7.
12. Caplan RA, Posner KL, Ward RJ, et al. Adverse respiratory events in anesthesia: a closed claims analysis. Anesthesiology 1990;72(5):828–33.
13. Langeron O, Masso E, Huraux C, et al. Prediction of difficult mask ventilation. Anesthesiology 2000; 92(5):1229–36.
14. Kheterpal S, Martin L, Shanks AM, et al. Prediction and outcomes of impossible mask ventilation: a review of 50,000 anesthetics. Anesthesiology 2009; 110(4):891–7.

15. Henderson JJ, Popat MT, Latto IP, et al. Difficult Airway Society guidelines for management of the unanticipated difficult intubation. Anaesthesia 2004;59(7):675–94.

16. Cormack RS, Lehane J. Difficult tracheal intubation in obstetrics. Anaesthesia 1984;39(11):1105–11.

17. Yentis SM, Lee DJ. Evaluation of an improved scoring system for the grading of direct laryngoscopy. Anaesthesia 1998;53(11):1041–4.

18. Bannister FB, Macbeth RG. Direct laryngoscopy and tracheal intubation. Lancet 1944;244(6325): 651–4.

19. Bellhouse CP, Dore C. Criteria for estimating likelihood of difficulty of endotracheal intubation with the Macintosh laryngoscope. Anaesth Intensive Care 1988;16(3):329–37.

20. Nichol HC, Zuck D. Difficult laryngoscopy–the "anterior" larynx and the atlanto-occipital gap. Br J Anaesth 1983;55(2):141–4.

21. Patil VU, Stehling LC, Zauder HL. Predicting the difficulty of intubation utilizing an intubation gauge. Anesthesiol Rev 1983;X(8):32–3.

22. Mallampati SR, Gatt SP, Gugino LD, et al. A clinical sign to predict difficult tracheal intubation: a prospective study. Can Anaesth Soc J 1985;32(4):429–34.

23. Ezri T, Cohen I, Geva D, et al. Pharyngoscopic views. Anesth Analg 1998;87(3):748.

24. Maleck WH, Koetter KK, Less SD. Pharyngoscopic views. Anesth Analg 1999;89(1):256–7.

25. Ezri T, Warters RD, Szmuk P, et al. The incidence of class "zero" airway and the impact of Mallampati score, age, sex, and body mass index on prediction of laryngoscopy grade. Anesth Analg 2001;93(4): 1073–5.

26. Wilson ME. Predicting difficult intubation. Br J Anaesth 1993;71(3):333–4.

27. Rosenblatt WH. The airway approach algorithm: a decision tree for organizing preoperative airway information. J Clin Anesth 2004;16(4):312–6.

28. Rosenberg H, Rosenberg H. Syndromes associated with upper airway abnormalities. In: Orkin FK, Cooperman LH, editors. Complications in anesthesiology. Philadelphia: Lippincott, J.B.; 1983.

29. Paul DR, Hoyt JL, Boutros AR. Cardiovascular and respiratory changes in response to change of posture in the very obese. Anesthesiology 1976; 45(1):73–8.

30. Katz I, Stradling J, Slutsky AS, et al. Do patients with obstructive sleep apnea have thick necks? Am Rev Respir Dis 1990;141(5 Pt 1):1228–31.

31. Bixler EO, Vgontzas AN, Lin HM, et al. Prevalence of sleep-disordered breathing in women: effects of gender. Am J Respir Crit Care Med 2001; 163(3 Pt 1):608–13.

32. Brodsky JB, Lemmens HJ, Brock-Utne JG, et al. Morbid obesity and tracheal intubation. Anesth Analg 2002;94(3):732–6.

33. Bond A. Obesity and difficult intubation. Anaesth Intensive Care 1993;21(6):828–30.

34. Buckley FP, Robinson NB, Simonowitz DA, et al. Anaesthesia in the morbidly obese. A comparison of anaesthetic and analgesic regimens for upper abdominal surgery. Anaesthesia 1983;38(9):840–51.

35. Ovassapian A, Land P, Schafer MF, et al. Anesthetic management for surgical corrections of severe flexion deformity of the cervical spine. Anesthesiology 1983;58(4):370–2.

36. Hastings RH, Kelley SD. Neurologic deterioration associated with airway management in a cervical spine-injured patient. Anesthesiology 1993;78(3): 580–3.

37. Brock-Utne JG, Downing JW, Seedat F. Laryngeal oedema associated with pre-eclamptic toxaemia. Anaesthesia 1977;32(6):556–8.

38. Finer NN, Muzyka D. Flexible endoscopic intubation of the neonate. Pediatr Pulmonol 1992;12(1):48–51.

39. Heindel DJ. Deep neck abscesses in adults: management of a difficult airway. Anesth Analg 1987; 66(8):774–6.

40. Prakash UB, Abel MD, Hubmayr RD. Mediastinal mass and tracheal obstruction during general anesthesia. Mayo Clin Proc 1988;63(10):1004–11.

41. Baxter FJ, Dunn GL. Acute epiglottitis in adults. Can J Anaesth 1988;35(4):428–35.

42. Schwartz HC, Bauer RA, Davis NJ, et al. Ludwig's angina: use of fiberoptic laryngoscopy to avoid tracheostomy. J Oral Surg 1974;32(8):608–11.

43. Flood LM, Astley B. Anaesthetic management of acute laryngeal trauma. Br J Anaesth 1982;54(12): 1339–43.

44. Seed RF. Traumatic injury to the larynx and trachea. Anaesthesia 1971;26(1):55–65.

45. Lee WT, Eliashar R, Eliachar I. Acute external laryngotracheal trauma: diagnosis and management. Ear Nose Throat J 2006;85(3):179–84.

46. Hastings RH, Marks JD. Airway management for trauma patients with potential cervical spine injuries. Anesth Analg 1991;73(4):471–82.

47. Keenan MA, Stiles CM, Kaufman RL. Acquired laryngeal deviation associated with cervical spine disease in erosive polyarticular arthritis. Use of the fiberoptic bronchoscope in rheumatoid disease. Anesthesiology 1983;58(5):441–9.

48. Gregori D, Salerni L, Scarinzi C, et al. Foreign bodies in the upper airways causing complications and requiring hospitalization in children aged 0-14 years: results from the ESFBI study. Eur Arch Otorhinolaryngol 2008;265(8):971–8.

49. American Society of Anesthesiologists Task Force on Management of the Difficult Airway. Practice guidelines for management of the difficult airway. A report by the American Society of Anesthesiologists Task Force on Management of the Difficult Airway. Anesthesiology 1993;78(3):597–602.

APPENDIX 1

<table>
<tr><td colspan="2" align="center">

Adult Respiratory Management - The Unresponsive Patient
Ten Minutes Saves A Life!®

</td></tr>
<tr><td colspan="2">Monitoring (blood pressure, heart rate, pulse oximetry, respiratory rate) ongoing throughout evaluation and management. All initial actions are performed simultaneously after verification of unresponsiveness by stimulating the patient including head tilt and jaw lift. Reversal agents (naloxone and flumazenil) may be administered at any time.</td></tr>
</table>

No Respiratory Depression and Unresponsive

Respiratory rate >10 and Oxygen saturation > 95%	Step 1	Verify unresponsiveness. Call for emergency equipment. Monitor patient.
	Step 2	Open the airway with head tilt, chin lift, and jaw thrust. Ammonia vaporole respiratory stimulant (optional). Supplemental oxygen with Non-rebreathing face mask 15 L/minute or Nasal cannula/Nasal hood 4 L/minute.
	Step 3	Reversal agent(s) if indicated.
	Step 4	Respiratory deterioration - begin **Ventilation Management** * - see below.

Respiratory Depression and Unresponsive

Respiratory rate <10 and/or Oxygen saturation <95%	Step 1	Verify unresponsiveness. Call for emergency equipment. Monitor patient.
	Step 2	Open the airway with head tilt, chin lift, and jaw thrust. Ammonia vaporole respiratory stimulant **Ventilation Management*** - see below.
	Step 3	Reversal agent(s) if indicated.

Apnea with Carotid Pulse

Respiratory rate 0	Step 1	Verify unresponsiveness. Call for emergency equipment. Monitor patient.
	Step 2	Open the airway with head tilt, chin lift, and jaw thrust. Verify not breathing. Check Pulse oximeter (BP >80 systolic) and/or Carotid pulse present (BP >60 systolic) which indicate chest compressions not needed.
	Step 3	**Ventilation Management*** - see below.
	Step 4	Reversal agent(s) if indicated.

Apnea without Carotid Pulse - see Adult Cardiac Management

Ventilation Management - Apnea / Hypoventilation / Obstruction

Step 1	Open the airway with head tilt, chin lift, and jaw thrust.
Step 2	Consider oral or nasal airway if apneic.
Step 3	Bag Mask ventilation - preferably two person. One breath every 6 seconds, breath volume 400-600 mL, pressure <20 cm H_2O, oxygen flow 15 L/minute.
Step 4	Confirm chest rise with each breath.
Step 5	Consider advanced supraglottic airway with gastric venting capacity if unable to ventilate with bag mask easily.
Step 6	Confirm supraglottic airway placement with chest rise.
Step 7	If no chest rise seen after advanced airway placement, continue with evaluation for larynospasm, foreign body, bronchospasm, or chest wall rigidity.

Ten Minutes Saves A Life! is a registered trademark of the ADSA Anesthesia Research Foundation   © 2013 EmergSim LLC / 10Min Resp Mgmt 130320

Oxygenation - Airway - Ventilation Algorithm
Office Team with AHA BLS HP Training
Ten Minutes Saves A Life! ®

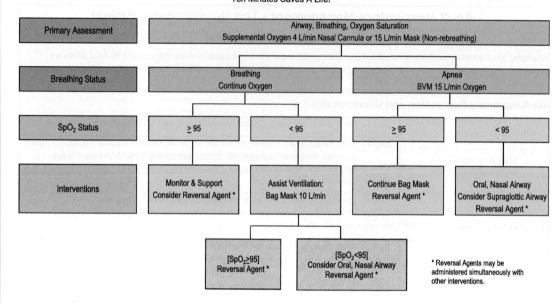

Primary Assessment	Airway, Breathing, Oxygen Saturation Supplemental Oxygen 4 L/min Nasal Cannula or 15 L/min Mask (Non-rebreathing)			
Breathing Status	Breathing Continue Oxygen		Apnea BVM 15 L/min Oxygen	
SpO₂ Status	≥ 95	< 95	≥ 95	< 95
Interventions	Monitor & Support Consider Reversal Agent *	Assist Ventilation: Bag Mask 10 L/min	Continue Bag Mask Reversal Agent *	Oral, Nasal Airway Consider Supraglottic Airway Reversal Agent *

[SpO₂≥95]
Reversal Agent *

[SpO₂<95]
Consider Oral, Nasal Airway
Reversal Agent *

* Reversal Agents may be administered simultaneously with other interventions.

Ten Minutes Saves A Life! is a registered trademark of the ADSA Anesthesia Research Foundation

© 2013 EmergSim LLC / 10Min Airway Vent Team 130320

Drug Management for Adult Emergencies (Not including CPR)
Provider with AHA BLS HP and ACLS + General Anesthesia Permit
Ten Minutes Saves A Life! ®

Drug	Action	Supplied	Administration
Respiratory Depression / Over Sedation / Respiratory Soft Tissue Obstruction			
Naloxone	Opioid antagonist	0.4 mg/mL	IV or IM: 0.4 mg (1 mL) q 2-3 minutes
Flumazenil	Benzodiazepine antagonist	0.1 mg/mL	IV: 0.2 mg (2 mL) q 1 minute
Bradycardia			
Drug	**Action**	**Supplied**	**Administration**
Atropine	Anticholinergic	1 mg/mL	IV or IM: 0.5 mg (5 mL) q 3-5 minutes
	Anticholinergic	0.1 mg/mL 10 mL prefilled syringe	IV: 0.5 mg (5 mL) q 3-5 minutes
Hypotension			
Drug	**Action**	**Supplied**	**Administration**
Ephedrine	Alpha and beta agonist	50 mg/mL	IV: 10-25 mg (0.2-0.5 mL) q 3-5 minutes
Hypoglycemia			
Drug	**Action**	**Supplied**	**Administration**
Glucose oral	Carbohydrate	15 or 24 gram tube	Contents slowly swallowed. Only for conscious patient.
Glucagon (optional)	Induces liver glycogen breakdown and glucose release	1 mg with 1 mL diluent	IV, IM or SC 1 mg (1mL)
Bronchospasm			
Drug	**Action**	**Supplied**	**Administration**
Albuterol	Selective beta-2 agonist	90 mcg/dose metered inhaler	2 inhalations. Epinephrine IM if ineffective.
Epinephrine Severe bronchospasm	Alpha and beta agonist	1:1000 in 1 mg/mL	IM: 0.3 mg (0.3 mL). May need to repeat. Cardiovascular compromised patient consider reduced dose.
		1:1000 auto-injector adult 0.3 mg	Auto-inject IM: 0.3 mg. May need to repeat.
Allergic Reaction Mild			
Drug	**Action**	**Supplied**	**Administration**
Diphenhydramine	Histamine H1 antagonist	50 mg/mL	IM: 25 mg (0.5 mL). May need to repeat.
Anaphylaxis / Laryngeal Edema			
Drug	**Action**	**Supplied**	**Administration**
Epinephrine	Alpha and beta agonist	1:1000 in 1 mg/mL vial	IM: 0.3 mg (0.3 mL). May need to repeat.
		1:1000 auto-injector adult 0.3 mg	Auto-inject IM: 0.3 mg. May need to repeat.
Laryngospasm			
Drug	**Action**	**Supplied**	**Administration**
Succinylcholine	Paralysis	20 mg/mL	IV or IM: 20 mg (1 mL)

Ten Minutes Saves A Life! is a registered trademark of the ADSA Anesthesia Research Foundation

© 2013 EmergSim LLC / 10Min Emerg ACLS GA 130320

Adult Cardiac Emergency Management
Office Team with AHA BLS HP and ACLS Training
Ten Minutes Saves A Life! ®

Responsive with Chest Pain: ACS Diagnosis	
Acute Coronary Syndrome (ACS) symptoms Chest, arm, or face discomfort / pressure Diaphoresis Syncope Hemodynamic instability	**Step 1** Assistance and Emergency Medical Service (EMS) called. Call for emergency equipment. Monitor patient.
	Step 2 Nitroglycerin 0.4 mg tablet sublingual or metered spray dose Aspirin 325 mg tablet chew and swallow. Supplemental oxygen: Face mask non-rebreathing 15 L/min or Nasal cannula/Nasal hood 4 L/min
	Step 3 Repeat nitroglycerin 0.4 mg in 5 minutes if pain persists and blood pressure >90 systolic

Unresponsive with Apnea and Carotid Pulse Absent	
Apnea No pulse oximeter reading Carotid pulse absent	**Step 1** Assistance and EMS called. Call for emergency equipment.
	Step 2 Begin chest compression at 100/minute for 30 compressions. Turn on AED and follow directions.
	Step 3 Insert oral airway and deliver 2 bag-mask ventilations at the end of each 30 chest compression cycle. Advanced Airway placement as soon as possible - See Adult Respiratory Management.
	Step 4 Continue with 30 chest compressions and 2 bag-mask ventilations five (5) times or until AED says stop to analyze rhythm.
	Step 5 AED will indicate either shock recommended (V-fib or pulseless V-tach) or no shock recommended (PEA/Asystole) - see below.

Optimizing CPR	AED Indicates Shock	AED Indicates No Shock
AED 2 minute timer is activated once unit is turned on. Practitioner should check carotid pulse at end of each 2 minute interval of chest compressions while AED is analyzing ECG rhythm. With bag-mask ventilation the 2 minute interval of chest compressions to ventilations at a ratio of 30-2 for 5 cycles provides 150 chest compressions and 10 ventilations. Additionally, the coronary and cerebral perfusion pressures drop with each pause and require ~ 3 compressions to peak again. With placement of an LMA/advanced airway, compressions and ventilations are continuous resulting in 200 compressions and 20 ventilations for the 2 minute interval. Additionally, the coronary and cerebral perfusion pressures are maintained throughout the 2 minute interval. Chest compressions are optimized at a depth of at least 2 inches / 50 mm and a rate of 100/minute. Good chest recoil is necessary to fill the heart. Change the individual performing chest compressions at the end of each 2 minute interval.	**Step 1** AED charges and practitioner clears and defibrillates #1. **Step 2** Resume CPR for 2 minutes per AED timer. **Step 3** Two minute interval complete. AED analyzes ECG rhythm and carotid pulse absent. AED indicates shock. **Step 4** AED charges and practitioner clears and defibrillates #2. **Step 5** Resume CPR and administer epinephrine 1 mg in prefilled syringe 1:10,000 10 ml IV followed by flush. **Step 6** Two minute interval complete. AED analyzes ECG rhythm and caroitid pulse absent. **Step 7** AED charges and practitioner clears and defibrillates #3. **Step 8** Resume CPR and administer amiodarone 300 mg/IV followed by flush. **Step 9** Two minute interval complete. AED analyzes ECG rhythm and carotid pulse absent. AED indicates shock. **Step 10** AED charges and practitioner clears and defibrillates #4. **Step 11** Resume CPR and administer epinephrine 1 mg in prefilled syringe 1:10,000 10 mL IV followed by flush. **Step 12** CPR continues at 2 minute intervals until EMS arrives.	**Step 1** Resume CPR and administer epinephrine 1 mg in prefilled syringe 1:10,000 10 mL IV followed by flush. **Step 2** Two minute interval complete. AED analyzes ECG rhythm and carotid pulse absent. AED still indicates no shock. **Step 3** Resume CPR. **Step 4** Two minute interval complete. AED analyzes ECG rhythm and carotid pulse absent. AED still indicates no shock. **Step 5** Resume CPR and administer epinephrine 1 mg in prefilled syringe 1:10,000 10 mL IV followed by flush. **Step 6** CPR continues at 2 minute intervals until EMS arrives.

Ten Minutes Saves A Life! is a registered trademark of the ADSA Anesthesia Research Foundation   © 2013 EmergSim LLC / 10Min Cardiac ACLS 130320

Emergency Drugs – Adult Medical Emergency Management
Practitioner with AHA BLS HP and ACLS Training
Ten Minutes Saves A Life! ®

Drugs		
Albuterol inhalation aerosol (90 mcg/actuation)	Ephedrine 50 mg/mL 1 mL vial	Naloxone 0.4 mg/mL 1 mL vial
Amiodarone 50 mg/mL 3 mL vial – three	Epinephrine 1:1,000 1 mg/mL 1 mL vial – two (Optional) Epinephrine auto-injectors (0.3 mg/actuation) - two	Nitroglycerin 0.4 mg tablets. (Optional) Nitroglycerine 0.4 mg/dose pump spray bottle
Aspirin 325 mg tablets (not enteric coated) unit dose package	Epinephrine 1:10,000 0.1 mg/mL 10 mL prefilled syringe – two	Succinylcholine 20 mg/mL 10 mL vial - Refrigerate. (Practitioner with general anesthesia permit)
Atropine 1 mg/mL 1 mL vial (Optional) Atropine 0.1 mg/mL 10 mL prefilled syringe	Flumazenil 0.1 mg/mL 10 mL vial (or 5 mL vials – two)	**Optional**
Diphenhydramine 50 mg/mL 1 mL vial	Glucose oral 15 gram tube – two (or 24 gram tube – one)	Aromatic ammonia inhalant vaporole(s) – two
		Glucagon Kit 1 mg vial + 1 mL sterile water (vial or syringe)
		Vasopressin 20 units/mL 1 mL vial – two

Syringes and Needles for Administration	
1 mL syringe with 21 gauge 1 inch needle – five \n\n5 mL syringe with 21 gauge 1.5 inch needle – four	20 mL syringe + 21 gauge 1 inch needle (Optional Vasopression use)

Oxygenation, Ventilation, Airway Equipment
Adult Emergency Management
Office Team with AHA BLS HP and ACLS Training
Ten Minutes Saves A Life! [®]

Oxygen E tank (alloy) with regulator (integral or detachable with key), pressure gauge, and flow meter (1–15L/minute)

Suction handle with Yankauer tip, suction tubing, and vacuum high volume system adapter

Nasal cannula adult

Face mask non-rebreather adult

Resuscitation bag adult 1900 mL with pressure manometer, face mask, oxygen reservoir bag, and oxygen tubing

Nasopharyngeal airways (polyvinyl chloride): 24 Fr / 6.0 mm I.D.,
    26 Fr / 6.5 mm I.D., 28 Fr / 7.0 mm I.D., and 30 Fr / 7.5 mm I.D.

Oropharyngeal airways (Guedel): 80 mm, 90 mm, and 100 mm

Laryngeal Supraglottic Airways – gastric venting
        Size 3 (30-60 kg)
        Size 4 (50-90 kg)
        Size 5 (90 kg+)

Stethoscope

Magill forceps

Practitioner with advanced airway intubation training:
        Laryngoscope handle
        Laryngoscope blades(s)
        Endotracheal tubes: 6.0, 6.5, 7.0, 7.5
        Endotracheal tube stylet
        Eschmann introducer/bougie
        10 mL syringe
        End-tidal carbon dioxide detector

Management of Allergy and Anaphylaxis During Oral Surgery

Morton B. Rosenberg, DMD[a],*, James C. Phero, DMD[b],
Joseph A. Giovannitti Jr, DMD[c]

KEYWORDS

- Allergy • Anaphylaxis • Anaphylactoid • Epinephrine

KEY POINTS

- Minor and major allergic reactions occur during oral and maxillofacial treatment.
- Immediate diagnosis and pharmacologic intervention are imperative.
- Signs and symptoms may be variable.
- The early administration of epinephrine is critical.

Allergic reactions can and do occur during routine oral and maxillofacial surgery and dental treatment.[1] These reactions can vary from mild to life threatening, and the clinical manifestations of a reaction to an antigen may vary from mild (with minor skin manifestations occurring over time) to those requiring immediate diagnosis and aggressive treatment to prevent ultimate respiratory and cardiovascular collapse, leading to death.

MILD ALLERGY

Mild allergic reactions that are slow in onset and consist primarily of itching, hives, and/or rash and are not associated with respiratory or cardiovascular issues are usually initiated by the body's histamine release response. As with any medical emergency, consciousness should be ascertained and vital signs monitored. Treatment is symptomatic and involves the administration of a histamine blocker, such as diphenhydramine by the intramuscular (IM), intravenous (IV), or oral route. Because drugs given via the oral route are slow in onset, the parenteral route is preferred for immediate relief. It is imperative to appreciate that even after initial treatment, histamine may continue to circulate for 3 or more days and an oral prescription of diphenhydramine should be prescribed to manage this time period. A verbal and written warning of the sedating effects of histamine blocking drugs must be given to the patient.

SEVERE ALLERGY (ANAPHYLAXIS/ANAPHYLACTOID REACTIONS)

Anaphylaxis is an acute life-threatening systemic reaction with varied mechanisms, clinical presentations, and involvement of multiple organ systems. It has recently been defined "as a serious allergic reaction that is rapid in onset and may cause death."[2] Anaphylaxis occurs when antigen-specific IgE molecules, which are bound to mast cells and basophils, are cross-linked by the specific antigen and on antigenic re-exposure causes these cells to degranulate. It takes an extremely small

[a] Division of Anesthesia and Pain Control, Tufts University School of Dental Medicine, Tufts University School of Medicine, 1 Kneeland Street Boston, MA 02111, USA; [b] Department of Anesthesiology, University of Cincinnati College of Medicine, Academic Health Center, 231 Albert Sabin Way, Cincinnati, OH 45267-0531, USA; [c] Department of Dental Anesthesiology, University of Pittsburgh School of Dental Medicine, 3501 Terrace Street Pittsburgh, PA 15261, USA
* Corresponding author.
E-mail address: morton.rosenberg@tufts.edu

Oral Maxillofacial Surg Clin N Am 25 (2013) 401–406
http://dx.doi.org/10.1016/j.coms.2013.04.001

amount of antigen to trigger the releases of a combination of biochemical mediators, such as histamine, neutral proteases, prostaglandins, leukotrienes, and other chemokines and cytokines.[3] These mediators are responsible for the signs and symptoms of anaphylaxis. Anaphylactoid reactions are not IgE related, but they release similar mediators and can cause identical symptoms and pathology. Symptoms usually occur with 20 minutes to an anaphylactic or anaphylactoid reaction, but the time course may be variable.

Although many drugs and substances (**Table 1**) can trigger acute hypersensitivity reactions, the most commonly involved substances and drugs during perioperative anaphylaxis are neuromuscular blocking agents, antibiotics, and latex.[4] Data concerning the incidence and severity of anaphylaxis are limited; the estimated incidence during anesthesia ranges from 1 in 10,000 to 1 in 20,000 anesthesia cases.[5] Anaphylaxis reactions triggered by antibiotics are of special concern to oral and maxillofacial surgeons and primarily involve penicillins and cephalosporins, which contain a β-lactam ring. Reactions from the rapid IV administration of vancomycin are rare and should be differentiated from red man syndrome that is a nonallergic phenomenon.[6] Publication of the Federal Drug Administration medical alert on this documented the increasing number of allergic reactions to medical products composed of latex during the perioperative period.[1]

Certain subsets of patients have a higher risk of latex allergy and can exhibit any of the 3 types of reactions to natural rubber products. The first type is a nonallergic irritant dermatitis; the second is a type IV T cell-mediated delayed hypersensitivity reaction, is due to the chemicals added to the latex during manufacturing, and is usually a delayed localized dermatitis; and the most serious one—type I—is an immediate hypersensitivity reaction mediated by IgE antibodies specifically toward low molecular weight antigens in latex and can range

from mild to severe. Populations at risk include (1) patients with histories of myelodysplasia, bladder extropy, and multiple surgeries; (2) health care workers; (3) atopic individuals (those with asthma, rhinitis, eczema, or food allergies, especially tropical ones); and (4) workers in the rubber industry.[7] There is a growing trend in creating latex-free oral surgical environments to reduce the incidence of latex issues relating to both the surgical team and patients.[8]

The clinical signs of an anaphylaxis/anaphylactoid reaction usually occur within minutes after the agent is injected IV. The clinical signs can be varied and either cascade from one system to another or appear simultaneously in many organs. The primary target organs are the skin, mucous membranes, gastrointestinal tract, and cardiorespiratory systems. Clinical cutaneous-mucous signs may include erythema, pruritus, and edema, with or without angioedema. Moderate multivisceral signs include hypotension, tachycardia, dyspnea, and gastrointestinal disturbances. The most serious manifestations involve swelling of the airway, severe bronchospasm, cardiac dysrhythmias, and cardiovascular collapse (**Table 2**).

The appearances of signs can also be classified and graded on a clinical severity scale:

Grade I, involving cutaneous-mucous features
Grade II, having cutaneous-mucous features with accompanying cardiovascular and/or respiratory signs
Grade III, cardiovascular collapse with multivisceral signs
Grade IV, cardiac arrest[9]

The rapid, initial diagnosis of an anaphylactic/anaphylactoid reaction is critical and early intervention is the key to successful management. The immediate removal or discontinuing of the triggering agent, early administration of epinephrine, maintenance of the airway and ventilation with 100% oxygen, and calling for help are fundamental. Epinephrine is the primary and first drug of

Table 1
Triggering agents of anaphylactic and anaphylactoid reactions

Common	Food (eg, peanuts, fish, shellfish, milk, eggs, bisulfites) Insect stings Medications: antibiotics, nonsteroidal anti-inflammatory drugs, aspirin, opioids, general anesthetic agents, radiocontrast dye, protamine, neuromuscular blocking agents Latex Exercise
Uncommon	Local anesthetics
Rare	Nitrous oxide, benzodiazepines, antihistamines

Table 2
Clinical characteristics of anaphylaxis/anaphylactoid reactions

System	Signs	Symptoms
Pulmonary	Increased respiratory rate Laryngeal edema Bronchospasm Pulmonary edema	Wheezing, stridor, coughing, dyspnea, chest tightness
Cardiovascular	Hypotension, tachycardia, cardiac Dysrhythmias, cardiac arrest	Chest tightness and pain
Mucocutaneous	Urticaria, flushing, diaphoresis, Periorbital and gingival edema	Itching, burning
Neurologic	Altered mentation Unconsciousness	Dizziness, loss of orientation, fatigue
Gastrointestinal	Vomiting, diarrhea	Nausea, cramping
Renal	Decrease in urine output	
Hematologic	Disseminated intravascular coagulation	Bleeding from mucosal surfaces

choice in the treatment of anaphylaxis due to its α_1 effects of supporting the blood pressure while its strong β_2 effects provide bronchial smooth muscle relaxation. In addition, epinephrine also effectively blocks the deleterious effects of circulating mediators.[10] If epinephrine is administered via an autoinjector or needle and syringe IM, absorption is more rapid and plasma levels are higher when in the thigh (vastus lateralis) than when injected IM into the arm (deltoid). IM injection into the thigh (vastus lateralis) is also superior to IM or subcutaneous injection into the arm (deltoid).[11,12]

No established dosage or regimen for IV epinephrine in anaphylaxis is recognized. Because of the risk for potentially lethal arrhythmias, epinephrine should be administered IV only during cardiac arrest or to profoundly hypotensive patients who have failed to respond to IV volume replacement and several injected doses of IM epinephrine. Poor outcomes during anaphylaxis are often associated with late, absent, inadequate, or excessive doses of epinephrine. When anaphylaxis is suspected, however, early intervention is the key to a successful outcome. The American Academy of Allergy, Asthma and Immunology practice parameter on the diagnosis and management of anaphylaxis is an excellent reference and should be reviewed.[2] If the reaction is severe, the patient has lost, or soon will lose, consciousness and laryngeal edema may occur. The patency of the airway should be immediately verified and basic airway rescue techniques used, beginning with basic head tilt and chin lift and escalating, if unsuccessful, to positive pressure ventilation via a bag-valve-mask device, advanced airway adjuncts (eg, supraglottic airways, endotracheal

intubation, and, in rare exceptional cases, a surgical airway (**Box 1**).[13]

Although the injection of epinephrine usually reverses systemic vasodilation and inhibits the release of mediators from mast and basophil cells, there are episodes where the circulatory system function continues to deteriorate. The use of vasopressin, in cases where patients seem refractory to epinephrine and where fluid therapy is unable to counteract profound hypotension, has been put forward as a possible intervention.[4,14]

PATIENT EVALUATION FOR LOCAL ANESTHETIC REACTIONS

Although adverse reactions to local anesthetics are frequently reported, true documented immune-mediated reactions to local anesthetics are rare.[15] Often the allergic response is not even reproduced with subsequent testing/challenge.[16,17] There are also many confounding factors in these reactions, such as the presence of epinephrine, latex, and other possible triggers often found in environments where local anesthetics are used.[18] As a result, the mechanism behind local anesthetic reactions is poorly understood, and there is often confusion about the safety of using local anesthetics in patients who previously experienced a reaction. Patients with a suspected history of local anesthetic allergy must be thoroughly questioned to determine the nature of the response. The vast majority of patients labeled as allergic to local anesthetics have experienced adverse reactions related to a direct pharmacologic effect of the local anesthetic and/or vasoconstrictor, suffered an acute anxiety reaction, or experienced syncope. In a

---

Box 1
Pharmacologic management of anaphylaxis/anaphylactoid reactions

Primary Treatment

IV fluids (25–50 mL/kg of crystalloid solution)

Epinephrine Intramuscular

Autoinjection of 1:1000 solution

> Weight 10–25 kg: 0.15 mg epinephrine IM (deltoid or vastus lateralis) autoinjector or needle

> Weight >25 kg: 0.3 mg epinephrine IM (deltoid or vastus lateralis) autoinjector or needle

> Repeated doses of epinephrine may be needed every 5–15 minutes

Epinephrine Intravenous

(for profound bronchospasm or hypotension)

Use epinephrine 1:10,000 in prefilled syringe for IV use

Begin at dose of 50–200 μg IV (0.5–2 mL), increase as needed

Secondary Treatment

Bronchodilator (β$_2$-agonist)

> Albuterol (90 μg per inhalation puff)

H$_1$-blocker (antihistamine)

> Diphenhydramine (Benadryl) (IV 0.5 mg/kg), requires dilution to avoid vein damage

Optional H$_2$-blocker

> Famotidine (Pepcid) (20 mg IV)

(Optional) steroids

> Hydrocortisone (1–2.5 mg/kg)

> Methylprednisolone (1 mg/kg)

Data from Refs.[2,4,21]

---

review of 5018 patients receiving local anesthetics, 25 experienced an adverse reaction. Two were determined to have possible allergic reactions, which were later ruled out by intradermal and challenge testing.[19,20]

Most commonly, patients screened for local anesthetic allergy are tested solely with intradermal local anesthetic injections. Unfortunately, this testing may produce false results, and patients do not have the knowledge that receiving a local anesthetic is safe.

A multimodal testing approach has been used for local anesthesia evaluation/screening at the University of Cincinnati Medical Center to permit patient screening to rule out agent sensitivity,

anxiety leading to syncope, amide tachyphylaxis, catecholamine sensitivity, and possible poor technique for injection; patients with known allergy to local anesthetics have been screened over a 20-year period.

This program involved testing patients in a controlled setting at the medical center due to potential adverse reaction requiring immediate emergency medical care. Patient monitoring for local anesthetic screening included pulse, ECG, blood pressure, pulse oximeter, and respirations. An IV line was started before local anesthetic screening. No alcohol or antiseptic was applied to the skin before start of the IV.

There were 3 parts to the evaluation protocol: intradermal screening, IV lidocaine challenge, and right and left posterior superior alveolar (PSA) nerve blocks.

Intradermal Screening Protocol

For the intradermal screening, 27-gauge needles with fixed volume of 0.05 mL of agent were used. Scratch test and progressive challenge were not used. Skin sites were evaluated 5 minutes after injection using the HollisterStier grading system (Allergy Skin Test Guide/HollisterStier - Sliding Guide Miles [www.hsallergy.com]). Grading included evaluation of erythema and weal by size in centimeters and regular versus irregular wheal shape. This screening provided background information on potential patient agent sensitivities and likelihood of a vasovagal syncope response to injection being the reason for the prior "allergic reaction".

Agents used for intradermal testing included

1. Normal saline (control)
2. 1% Lidocaine
3. 2% Mepivacaine
4. 0.5% Bupivacaine
5. 1% Lidocaine with 1:100:000 epinephrine
6. 4% Articaine with 1:100,000 epinephrine
7. 5% Diphenhydramine (Benadryl)
8. 1% Lidocaine with methylparaben
9. 3% 2-Chloroprocaine (Nesacaine)
10. 1% Tetracaine/procaine
    - With no skin reaction to intradermal lidocaine, IV lidocaine 30-mg challenge was given 15 minutes after the last intradermal skin weal. This screening permitted patients to observe that the most commonly used local anesthetic in health care was safe for them.
    - Actual injection/block using local anesthetic agents was performed 15 minutes after the IV lidocaine challenge. Right and left PSA nerves were blocked using 3 mL of different local anesthetics, each at 15-minute

intervals. The choice of local anesthetics for the PSA blocks was based on patient response to the intradermal testing and IV challenge: 2% lidocaine with 1:100,000 epinephrine and 0.5% bupivacaine with 1:200,000 epinephrine were used most often for the PSA blocks

Initial Results

1. One patient demonstrated a 4+ irregular weal and 4+ erythema to lidocaine. This patient did not receive the lidocaine IV challenge.
2. All patients screened, including the patient who that reacted to intradermal lidocaine, were found able to receive at least one amide local anesthetic per the PSA block screening.
3. Diphenhydramine (Benadryl) has not been recommended as a local anesthetic because the injection is painful and gives a poor response of limited duration.

Long-Term Results

In 2012, this group of 55 patients (tested from 1981 to 2003) was contacted to verify that ongoing use of the screened and recommended local anesthetic was acceptable: 13 patients were successfully contacted; 41 patients were not able to be reached for follow-up; 3 of the 13 patients (23%) answered "no" when asked whether they had been exposed to local anesthetics since their screening at the medical center; 10 of the 13 patients (77%) stated they had subsequent exposure to local anesthetics; 8 of these patients denied having a subsequent reaction to local anesthetics; 2 of the 10 patients with subsequent local anesthetic exposure stated they had a reaction to the local anesthetic; and 1 patient stated the reaction consisted of pain in her chest and throat, but she could not recall if this was the same reaction that she had experienced with her previous exposure—she stated the medication was Novocaine, which is unlikely given that Novocaine is not commonly available and used. The second patient with a subsequent reaction experienced an "increased heart rate." This was the same reaction that the patient had experienced with her initial exposure. This patient recalled that the reaction was to either lidocaine or bupivacaine.

Even after patients have been screened and found to safely tolerate a particular local anesthetic or anesthetic, significant anxiety about re-exposure may persist. To effectively maximize the subsequent exposure to a local anesthetic for an oral surgical procedure, sedation may be beneficial in treatment planning.

SUMMARY

Anaphylaxis and anaphylactoid reactions can be life threatening even to healthy patients during oral and maxillofacial procedures done with or without sedation and/or anesthesia. With such a rapid onset and the potential for a rapid dangerous cascade to respiratory compromise and cardiac arrest, especially when medications are administered IV, immediate diagnosis and treatment is imperative. Although these conditions can arise suddenly and without warning, a meticulous history focusing on drug reactions and allergies and latex exposure assists in identifying atopic individuals. Anaphylaxis/anaphylactoid reactions are uncommon and their courses may be unpredictable, but luckily most episodes respond to treatment to epinephrine and fundamentals of basic life support.

REFERENCES

1. Malamed SF. Managing medical emergencies. J Am Dent Assoc 1993;124(8):40–53.
2. Joint Task Force on Practice Parameters, American Academy of Allergy, Asthma and Immunology, American College of Allergy, Asthma and Immunology, Joint Council of Allergy, Asthma and Immunology. The diagnosis and management of anaphylaxis: an updated practice parameter. J Allergy Clin Immunol 2005;115(3 Suppl 2):S483–523.
3. Rusznak C, Peebles RS Jr. Anaphylaxis and anaphylactoid reactions. A guide to prevention, recognition, and emergent treatment. Postgrad Med 2002; 111(5):101–4, 107–8, 111–4.
4. Dewachter P, Mouton-Faivre C, Emala CW. Anaphylaxis and anesthesia: controversies and new insights. Anesthesiology 2009;111(5):1141–50.
5. Mertes PM, Laxenaire MC, Alla F. Groupe d'Etudes des Reactions Anaphylactoides Peranesthesiques. Anaphylactic and anaphylactoid reactions occurring during anesthesia in France in 1999–2000. Anesthesiology 2003;99(3):536–45.
6. Ebo DG, Fisher MM, Hagendorens MM, et al. Anaphylaxis during anaesthesia: diagnostic approach. Allergy 2007;62(5):471–87.
7. Vassallo SA. Perioperative care of latex-allergic patients. In: Lake ED, editor. Advances in anesthesia. St Louis (MO): Mosby-Year Book; 1998. p. 107–31.
8. Desai SV. Natural rubber latex allergy and dental practice. N Z Dent J 2007;103(4):101–7.
9. Ring J, Messmer K. Incidence and severity of anaphylactoid reactions to colloid volume substitutes. Lancet 1977;1(8009):466–9.
10. Hepner DL, Castells MC. Anaphylaxis during the perioperative period. Anesth Analg 2003;97(5): 1381–95.

11. Simons FE, Roberts JR, Gu X, et al. Epinephrine absorption in children with a history of anaphylaxis. J Allergy Clin Immunol 1998;101(1 Pt 1):33–7.

12. Simons FE, Gu X, Simons KJ. Epinephrine absorption in adults: intramuscular versus subcutaneous injection. J Allergy Clin Immunol 2001;108(5):871–3.

13. Reed KL. Basic management of medical emergencies: recognizing a patient's distress. J Am Dent Assoc 2010;141(Suppl 1):20S–4S.

14. Schummer W, Schummer C, Wippermann J, et al. Anaphylactic shock: is vasopressin the drug of choice? Anesthesiology 2004;101(4):1025–7.

15. Gall H, Kaufmann R, Kalveram CM. Adverse reactions to local anesthetics: analysis of 197 cases. J Allergy Clin Immunol 1996;97(4):933–7.

16. Berkun Y, Ben-Zvi A, Levy Y, et al. Evaluation of adverse reactions to local anesthetics: experience with 236 patients. Ann Allergy Asthma Immunol 2003;91(4):342–5.

17. Incaudo G, Schatz M, Patterson R, et al. Administration of local anesthetics to patients with a history of prior adverse reaction. J Allergy Clin Immunol 1978;61(5):339–45.

18. Phillips JF, Yates AB, Deshazo RD. Approach to patients with suspected hypersensitivity to local anesthetics. Am J Med Sci 2007;334(3):190–6.

19. Baluga JC. Allergy to local anesthetics in dentistry. Myth or reality? Rev Alerg Mex 2003;50(5):176–81.

20. Mertes PM. Recognition and management of anaphylactic and anaphylactoid reactions during anesthesia. Anesthesiology News 2005.

21. Boyce JA, Assa'ad A, Burks AW, et al. Guidelines for the Diagnosis and Management of Food Allergy in the United States: summary of the NIAID-Sponsored Expert Panel Report. J Allergy Clin Immunol 2010;126(6):1105–18.

Common Medical Illnesses that Affect Anesthesia and Their Anesthetic Management

Ravi Agarwal, DDS*, Michael H. Porter, DDS,
George Obeid, DDS

KEYWORDS

- Office anesthesia • Preoperative evaluation • Common medical illnesses • Anesthetic management

KEY POINTS

- Oral and maxillofacial surgeons must have an understanding of the background, treatment modalities, and medications of various medical illnesses and their impact on the anesthetic management of their patients.
- By and large, in most medical illnesses minimal anesthetic modifications are needed if the disease is found to be well controlled.
- There are few evidence-based guidelines on anesthetic considerations of medical illnesses for office-based open-airway anesthetics.

Any patient undergoing an office-based anesthetic will require a thorough preoperative evaluation to identify medical illnesses that can affect the anesthetic management. The literature is abundant with information about general anesthetic management of patients with medical illnesses. However, some of such considerations may not be applicable to the open-airway office-based anesthesia. This article addresses common medical illnesses seen in oral surgery offices, with specific focus on the preoperative and perioperative anesthetic considerations of open-airway office-based anesthesia.

HYPERTENSION
Background

Hypertension is a common disease affecting more than 30% of adults in America. The diagnosis of hypertension is having a blood pressure higher than 140/90 mm Hg measured on a minimum of 2 occasions over a 1- to 2-week span.[1] Classifications of hypertension are listed in **Table 1**.

Hypertension is a risk factor for ischemic heart disease, congestive heart failure, cerebral vascular accident, arterial aneurysm, and end-stage renal disease. Essential hypertension is a diagnosis obtained when a true identifiable cause cannot be found, and accounts for more than 95% of diagnoses. Most often there are familial factors and/or biochemical factors leading to the hypertension. Biochemically, hypertension is a result of a disruption in the complex interplay of endogenous vasoconstrictors and the hormones within the renin-angiotensin system. Other major medical contributors in causing and perpetuating hypertension are involved in 5% of cases; this is known as secondary hypertension. The most common cause of secondary hypertension is renovascular disease.

Disclosures: None.
Department of Oral & Maxillofacial Surgery, Medstar Washington Hospital Center, 110 Irving Street Northwest, GA-144, Washington, DC 20010, USA
* Corresponding author.
E-mail address: ravi.agarwal@medstar.net

Oral Maxillofacial Surg Clin N Am 25 (2013) 407–438
http://dx.doi.org/10.1016/j.coms.2013.03.001

Table 1
Classification of systemic blood pressure in adults

Category	Systolic Blood Pressure (mm Hg)	Diastolic Blood Pressure (mm Hg)
Normal	<120	<80
Prehypertension	120–139	80–89
Stage 1	140–159	90–99
Stage 2	≥160	≥100

Data from Matei V, Sami Haddadin A. Systemic and pulmonary arterial hypertension. In: Hines RL, Marschall KE, editors. Stoelting's anesthesia and co-existing disease. 6th edition. Philadelphia: Elsevier Saunders; 2012. p. 104–19.

Treatment of hypertension usually begins with lifestyle modifications that include weight loss, moderation of alcohol, physical activity, moderation of dietary salt intake, and smoking cessation.[2] In addition, pharmacologic therapy should be initiated and managed by the primary care physician. Initial therapy for uncomplicated hypertension is a thiazide diuretic such as hydrochlorothiazide.[1] Other classes of medications such as angiotensin-converting enzyme (ACE) inhibitors, Angiotensin receptor blockers (ARBs), β-blockers, or calcium-channel blockers may be added if necessary. Commonly used antihypertensive agents are listed in **Table 2**. If patients have other comorbidities, specific classes of drugs may be selected for their pleiotropic benefits.[2]

Table 2
Commonly used antihypertensive drugs

Class	Subclass	Generic Name	Trade Name
Diuretics	Thiazides	Hydrochlorothiazide	HydroDiuril
		Metolazone	Lozol
	Loop	Bumetanide	Bumex
		Furosemide	Lasix
	Potassium sparing	Amiloride	Midamor
		Spironolactone	Aldactone
		Triamterene	Dyrenium
Adrenergic antagonists	β-Blockers	Atenolol	Tenormin
		Metoprolol	Lopressor
		Propranolol	Inderal
	α1-Blockers	Doxazosin	Cardura
		Prazosin	Minipress
		Terazosin	Hytrin
	α- and β-Blockers	Carvedilol	Coreg
		Labetalol	Normodyne
	Central acting	Clonidine	Catapres
Vasodilators		Hydralazine	Apresoline
ACE inhibitors		Benzepril	Lotensin
		Captopril	Capoten
		Enalapril	Vasotec
		Lisinopril	Prinvil
		Ramipril	Altace
Angiotensin receptor blockers		Candesartan	Atacand
		Irbesartan	Avapro
		Losartan	Cozaar
		Olmesartan	Benicar
		Telmisartan	Micardis
		Valsartan	Diovan
Calcium-channel blockers	Dihyropyridine	Amlodipine	Norvasc
		Nicardipine	Cardene
		Nifedipine	Procardia
		Felodipine	Plendil
	Nondihydropyridine	Diltiazem	Cardizem
		Verapamil	Tiazac

Data from Matei V, Sami Haddadin A. Systemic and pulmonary arterial hypertension. In: Hines RL, Marschall KE, editors. Stoelting's anesthesia and co-existing disease. 6th edition. Philadelphia: Elsevier Saunders; 2012. p. 104–19.

Anesthetic Management

Preoperative

- Determine adequacy of blood pressure control by asking if the patient checks the blood pressure at home and have knowledge of its average range.
  - Preanesthesia blood pressure can often be elevated, and is noted with increased age.[3]
- Review pharmacology of the drugs used in control.
  - Often the more severe cases require multiple classes of drugs.
- Perform thorough history and physical examination evaluating the heart, kidney, or eyes for end-organ damage (left ventricular hypertrophy, proteinuria, reduced renal function, and retinopathy).
- Assume that the patient may have some form of ischemic heart disease or renal dysfunction.
- Continue all prescribed home medications; office-based procedures are of low surgical risk.
  - Although ACE inhibitors/ARBs have been associated with intraoperative hypotension with general anesthesia, they are continued for outpatient sedation. Hypotension associated with ACE inhibitors/ARBs is more common with patients experiencing high intraoperative blood loss, hypovolemia, or fluid shifts.[1] In the oral surgery office, these risks are negligible and the hazards of increase in blood pressure would be more concerning when stopping these medications.
- There are no universal guidelines on when to postpone elective procedures, but anecdotally a diastolic pressure higher than 110 mm Hg would be a reason to delay the procedure. A diastolic pressure lower than 110 mm Hg has been shown not to have any increased incidence of postoperative complications.[1]

Perioperative

- Most classes of anesthetic drugs used in the oral surgery office such as benzodiazepines, opioids, propofol, and barbiturates are safe.
- Ketamine is a general anesthetic agent used as an adjunct during office anesthesia. However, its indirect effects of increasing heart rate and blood pressure should deter its use in patients with hypertension and other cardiovascular diseases.
- Pain control with local anesthesia and/or sedation is important in preventing stimuli-induced hypertension.

- Management of persistent hypertension is not addressed in this article. However, drugs to consider in the office would be medications such as hydralazine or labetalol.
- Hypotension may be seen with the use of propofol/barbiturates, opioids, and benzodiazepines. However, the hypotension is usually transient and can be addressed, if necessary, with the administration of intravenous fluid. Sympathomimetic medications such as phenylephrine or ephedrine may be used if intravenous fluids fail to address the problem.
- Local anesthesia is safe, and dosages are known to most practitioners. In patients with poorly controlled hypertension (Stage II or upward), consider eliminating the use of epinephrine if possible. If vasoconstriction is needed, consider a maximum dose of 0.04 mg epinephrine.

CORONARY ARTERY DISEASE
Background

Coronary artery disease (CAD), also known as ischemic heart disease, often manifests itself through angina, acute myocardial infarction (MI), and sudden cardiac death. Risk factors for CAD include male gender, increasing age, dyslipidemia, hypertension, smoking, diabetes, obesity, sedentary lifestyle, and family history.[4]

Angina is retrosternal chest discomfort, pain, pressure, or heaviness caused by imbalance from coronary blood flow and consumption of myocardial oxygen. Pain may radiate to the neck, left shoulder, left arm, jaw, and sometimes the back. When classified as stable angina this pain lasts several minutes and is often triggered by physical exertion, emotional tension, and cold weather. It is best relieved with rest and/or nitroglycerin. Chronic stable angina is pain that occurs with a repeatable level of exertion or stimulation for more than 2 months. Unstable angina is classified as pain at rest, new onset, or increasing in severity or frequency.

Treatment consists of lifestyle changes, pharmacologic therapy, and coronary revascularization. Often patients will be on a statin drug to reduce low-density lipoprotein to less than 100 mg/dL, and this has been shown to aid in secondary prevention.[4] Hypertension is controlled with β-blockers, calcium-channel blockers, or ACE inhibitors. Patients with stable disease should be on low-dose aspirin therapy (commonly 81 mg). If a patient has undergone revascularization with an intracoronary stent then often aspirin and an adenosine diphosphate blocker such as clopidogrel (Plavix) or ticlopidine (Ticlid) are prescribed.

Patients with bare-metal stents will require uninterrupted antiplatelet therapy for a minimum of 6 weeks, whereas patients with drug-eluting stents will require uninterrupted antiplatelet therapy for a minimum of 1 year. Thus if the patient has received these interventions within these time frames the antiplatelets should not be stopped, owing to the risk of stent thrombosis. If possible, surgery should be deferred until after the dual antiplatelet therapy is complete.[5]

Anesthetic Management

Preoperative

- A thorough history and physical examination can determine the severity, progression, and any functional limitations caused by CAD.
- Assess if any cardiac clinical risk factors (**Box 1**) are present, in which case cardiac consultation may be needed for risk stratification.
  - Determine the patient's functional status using activities of daily living and metabolic equivalents (METs). A patient capable of performing activities of greater than 4 METs is considered to have a good functional capacity (**Table 3**).
- If there is a positive history for an MI, elective procedures should be delayed at least 6 weeks following the incident and after clearance from the cardiologist.[6] This recommendation of 6 weeks of waiting has changed from the previously recommended delay of 6 months after MI.
- Recommendations for timing of elective noncardiac surgery after coronary intervention are listed in **Table 4**. Any deviations should be carried out in consultation with the cardiologist.
- Using the guidelines published by the American College of Cardiology/American Heart Association, most oral surgery office-based procedures are low risk. If a patient has had coronary revascularization within the past 5 years or has had an appropriate coronary evaluation (ie, physical/chemical stress test or appropriate nuclear imaging) in the past 2 years, with no subsequent deterioration of cardiac status, further cardiac evaluation is not warranted.[6]
  - If the patient has any clinical risk factors, consultation with the cardiologist is recommended.
- Continue all home medications including antiplatelets.
  - The decision to hold any antiplatelet should be based on the risk of surgical bleeding and discussion with the cardiologist.

Box 1
Clinical predictors of increased perioperative cardiovascular risk

Major

    Unstable coronary syndromes

    Acute or recent MI with evidence of important ischemic risk based on clinical symptoms or noninvasive study

    Unstable or severe angina

    Decompensated heart failure

    Significant dysrhythmias

    High-grade atrioventricular block

    Symptomatic ventricular dysrhythmias in the presence of underlying heart disease

    Supraventricular dysrhythmias with uncontrolled ventricular rate

    Severe valvular disease

Intermediate

    Mild angina pectoris

    Previous MI based on history or Q waves on electrocardiogram (ECG)

    Compensated or previous heart failure

    Diabetes mellitus (particularly insulin dependent)

    Renal insufficiency

Minor

    Advanced age (>70 years)

    Abnormal ECG (left ventricular hypertrophy, left bundle branch block, ST-T abnormalities)

    Rhythm other than sinus

    Low functional capacity

    History of stroke

    Uncontrolled systemic hypertension

Data from Fleisher LA, Beckman JA, Brown LA, et al. ACC/AHA 2007 guidelines on perioperative cardiovascular evaluation and care for noncardiac surgery: a report of the American College of Cardiology/American Heart Association Task Force on Practice Guidelines (Writing Committee to Revise the 2002 Guidelines on Perioperative Cardiovascular Evaluation for Noncardiac Surgery). Circulation 2007;116(17):e418–99.

- For most oral surgical procedures it is suggested to continue antiplatelets, as the risk of significant bleeding on dual antiplatelets is not well established.[7]
- In cases of bleeding risk and with cardiology consultation, it is possible to stop the clopidogrel 5 days before the procedure

Table 3
Metabolic equivalents (METs) based on activities of daily living

>4 METs	<4 METs
Climb flight of stairs	Walking indoors
Walking speed >4 mph	around the house
Run short distances	Walking speed
Yard work (raking,	2–3 mph
mowing)	Light household
Household work	work (dusting,
(lifting/moving	dishes)
furniture)	Personal care (dress,
Recreational sports	eat, bath, toilet)
(golf, tennis,	Walk 1–2 blocks on
swimming)	level ground

Data from Fleisher LA, Beckman JA, Brown LA, et al. ACC/AHA 2007 Guidelines on perioperative cardiovascular evaluation and care for noncardiac surgery: a report of the American College of Cardiology/American Heart Association Task Force on Practice Guidelines (Writing Committee to Revise the 2002 Guidelines on Perioperative Cardiovascular Evaluation for Noncardiac Surgery). Circulation 2007;116(17):e418–99.

while maintaining aspirin.[5] The oral medications should be resumed as soon as possible after the procedure.

Perioperative

- Prevent any myocardial ischemia by limiting tachycardia, sympathetic nervous system responses, hypotension, arterial hypoxemia, and systolic hypertension.
- Monitor for myocardial injury by electrocardiogram (ECG) monitoring of ST-segment elevations or depression, the most commonly monitored leads being II and V5.

Table 4
Recommended timing of elective noncardiac surgery after coronary interventions

Procedure	Time Interval to Wait
Angioplasty without stenting	2–4 wk
Bare-metal stent	At least 6 wk, consider 12 wk
Drug-eluting stent	At least 1 y
Coronary artery bypass grafting	At least 6 wk, consider 12 wk

Data from Akhtar S. Ischemic heart disease. In: Hines RL, Marschall KE, editors. Stoelting's anesthesia and co-existing disease. 6th edition. Philadelphia: Elsevier Saunders; 2012. p. 1–3.

- Considerations for anesthetic choice are similar to those for patients with hypertension.
  - Avoid ketamine, as tachycardia and hypertension may occur as a result of sympathetic stimulation
  - Moderate sedation for anxiolysis can be beneficial by reducing stress and oxygen demands
  - Fentanyl or propofol to prevent hypotension should be used with caution
  - Anticholinergics such as glycopyrrolate should be avoided because of tachycardia and increased chronotrophy

VALVULAR HEART DISEASE
Background

At present, the prevalence of valvular heart disease in the United States is approximately 2.5% and increases with age. Valvular disease is a significant risk factor for perioperative complications during anesthesia. The common valve disorders may cause a pressure-overload problem (mitral/aortic stenosis) or a volume-overload problem (mitral/aortic regurgitation).

Heart murmurs are a common physical finding, and represent turbulent blood flow. During systole, murmurs arise from stenosis of the aortic/pulmonary valves or incompetent closure of mitral/tricuspid valves. Diastolic murmurs usually arise from incompetent aortic/pulmonary valves or stenosed mitral/tricuspid valves. Commonly these murmurs decrease myocardial work, so the patient may develop symptoms such as dyspnea, orthopnea, fatigue, anxiety, diaphoresis, or resting tachycardia. In addition to valvular heart disease, congestive heart failure or cardiac dysrhythmias (especially atrial fibrillation in mitral diseases) are commonly found.

ECG findings include enlarged P waves suggesting left atrial enlargement, and findings of left ventricular hypertrophy that can include increase voltage in precordial waves or deviation of the left axis.

Mitral stenosis is most commonly caused by rheumatic heart disease. Often symptoms arise 20 to 30 years after experiencing rheumatic fever, owing to its slow progression. The stenosis occurs from leaflet thickening, calcifications, and decreased orifice size. The high atrial pressure causes increased pulmonary pressure, the symptoms of which are dyspnea on exertion, orthopnea, and paroxysmal nocturnal dyspnea. Mild mitral stenosis can be treated with diuretics.

Mitral valve prolapse (MVP) is the most common valvular heart disease, affecting 1% to 2.5% of the United States population, and found more often in young women.[8] It can be associated with Marfan syndrome, rheumatic carditis, myocarditis, thyrotoxicosis, and systemic lupus erythematosus. Usually MVP is a benign condition, but it can give rise to serious events such as thromboembolic stroke, infective endocarditis, dysrhythmias, and so forth. Clinically a midsystolic click and late systolic murmur are noted. The diagnosis is based on echocardiographic findings.

In addition, there can be mitral regurgitation associated with mitral valve diseases, commonly from papillary muscle dysfunction or ruptured chordae tendineae. The left atrial volume overload from the incompetent valve can lead to slow progression of pulmonary overload. On physical examination, a holosystolic murmur can be heard radiating to the axilla. Asymptomatic patients often do not need treatment; symptomatic patients require surgery for mitral valve replacement.

Aortic stenosis is an increasingly common valvular lesion in the United States. Increasing age results in degeneration and calcification of the aortic leaflets. Patients with congenital bicuspid aortic valves can develop aortic stenosis earlier in life. The stenosis leads to ventricular hypertrophy and increases the risk for MI. Symptoms include angina, syncope, and dyspnea on exertion. About 75% of symptomatic patients will succumb to death within 3 years if their valve is not replaced.[8] A systolic murmur radiating to the neck can be auscultated, mimicking a carotid bruit. Asymptomatic patients are treated with medical management, whereas symptomatic patients should have valve surgery.

Prosthetic valves may be mechanical or bioprosthetic. Mechanical valves are very durable, lasting at least 20 to 30 years, whereas bioprosthetic valves last about 10 to 15 years. Mechanical valves are highly thrombogenic and require long-term anticoagulation. Because bioprosthetic valves have a low thrombogenic potential, long-term anticoagulation is not necessary; however, future replacement valves are required. Mechanical valves are preferred in patients who are young, have a life expectancy of more than 10 to 15 years, or require long-term anticoagulation therapy for another reason such as atrial fibrillation. Bioprosthetic valves are preferred in elderly patients and in those who cannot tolerate anticoagulation. The risk of a thromboembolic event with a mechanical heart valve is 5% to 8%, compared with chronic atrial fibrillation which has an embolic stroke rate of 7% to 15%.[8]

Medical management of valve disease usually requires heart-rate control with β-blockers, calcium-channel blockers, or digoxin. Blood pressure should be controlled with ACE inhibitors or vasodilators. Congestive heart failure can be controlled with diuretics or inotropes.

Anesthetic Management

Preoperative

- A thorough evaluation includes assessment of the severity of the disease, degree of impaired myocardial contractility, and presence of any major organ disease. Also, define a patient's exercise tolerance using the METs scale (see **Table 3**), as with ischemic heart disease.
- Obtain a cardiology consult if there is any evidence of symptomatic heart disease.[6] In general, asymptomatic systolic clicks or murmurs may not require preoperative cardiology consultation.[8]
- Consider ECG if there is concern for any arrhythmias associated with valvular disease. Be wary of atrial fibrillation in mitral diseases or left atrial abnormalities.
- In general, aortic stenosis carries a high risk for perioperative complications. For patients with anything more than mild, asymptomatic diseases, consider hospital-based surgery.[8]
- If a patient has a prosthetic heart valve or another high-risk condition for endocarditis (**Box 2**), provide the appropriate antibiotic prophylaxis (**Table 5**).[9]
- In general, continue all home medications to maintain a controlled rate and normotension.
- Check for diuretic-induced hypokalemia (if applicable).

Perioperative

In aortic and mitral stenosis the filling time of the chamber is compromised, so these patients generally require a slow heart rate to allow adequate filling.[8]

- Avoid anticholinergics and ketamine.
- Most other intravenous medications are safe.
- Treat tachycardias with short-acting β-blockers.

In aortic and mitral regurgitations a slow heart rate or hypertension accentuates the regurgitation, so bradycardia and hypertension must be avoided.[8]

- Avoid potent narcotic-induced bradycardia.
- Maintain intravascular volume with intravenous fluids.
- Provide good local anesthetic to reduce sympathetic stimulation.
- Avoid ketamine in patients with MVP.

Box 2
Cardiac conditions associated with the highest risk of adverse outcome from endocarditis for which prophylaxis with dental procedures is reasonable

- Prosthetic cardiac valve or prosthetic material used for cardiac valve repair
- Previous infective endocarditis
- Congenital heart disease (CHD)[a]
- Unrepaired cyanotic CHD, including palliative shunts and conduits
- Completely repaired congenital heart defect with prosthetic material or device, whether placed by surgery or by catheter intervention, during the first 6 months after the procedure[b]
- Repaired CHD with residual defects at the site or adjacent to the site of a prosthetic patch or prosthetic device (which inhibit endothelialization)
- Cardiac transplantation recipients who develop cardiac valvulopathy

[a] Except for the conditions listed above, antibiotic prophylaxis is no longer recommended for any other form of CHD.
[b] Prophylaxis is reasonable because endothelialization of prosthetic material occurs within 6 months after the procedure.
Adapted from Wilson W, Taubert KA, Gewtiz M, et al. Prevention of infective endocarditis: guidelines from the American Heart Association: a guideline from the American Heart Association Rheumatic Fever, Endocarditis, and Kawasaki Disease Committee, Council on Cardiovascular Disease in the Young, and the Council on Clinical Cardiology, Council on Cardiovascular Surgery and Anesthesia, and the Quality of Care and Outcomes Research Interdisciplinary Working Group. Circulation 2007;116:1736–54.

CONGESTIVE HEART FAILURE
Background

Congestive heart failure (CHF) is a complex disease process whereby the heart is unable to fill with or eject blood to meet bodily demands. Etiology most often involves impaired contractions secondary to ischemic heart disease, valve abnormalities, systemic hypertension, and disease of the pericardium or cor pulmonale.

The most common aspect of CHF is systolic heart failure caused by decreased ventricle wall motion, often secondary to ischemic complications. Left heart failure shows signs of pulmonary edema (orthopnea, dyspnea, paroxysmal nocturnal dyspnea), whereas right heart failure results in venous hypertension and peripheral edema.[10] A commonly used classification of heart failure is that of the New York Heart Association (NYHA), and is based on functional status:

> Class I: Ordinary physical activity does not cause symptoms
> Class II: Symptoms occur with ordinary exertion
> Class III: Symptoms occur with less than ordinary exertion
> Class IV: Symptoms occur at rest

Symptoms are dyspnea on exertion (an early symptom), orthopnea (typically dry nonproductive cough when supine), paroxysmal nocturnal dyspnea, fatigue, weakness, nausea, and abdominal pain (from liver congestion). On examination, the physician may note tachypnea, "moist" rales (mostly in lung bases), resting tachycardia, third heart sound, cool and pale extremities, right upper quadrant pain, and/or bilateral lower extremity pitting edema.

Typical treatment depends on symptoms and staging of heart failure. The primary treatment is lifestyle modifications consisting of low sodium diet, weight control, smoking cessation, and glycemic control. Patients with heart failure will be under treatment with various classes of cardiac medications. Classes may include ACE inhibitors/ARBs, aldosterone antagonists, β-blockers, diuretics, vasodilators, and statins.

Anesthesia Management

Preoperative

- It is important to assess precipitating factors for heart failure, and confirm control and management. Heart failure can be one of the most important risk factors for perioperative cardiac morbidity.[10] Common signs and symptoms of poor control can include:
  - Shortness of breath with minimal exertion (use METs criteria)
  - Peripheral edema: look for swollen ankles and feet
  - Orthopnea: ask about the use of 2 or more pillows
  - Fluctuations in body weight
- Obtain cardiology clearance and classification of disease.
- If on diuretics, check potassium and electrolytes for disturbances. Remember the need for frequent urination when administering intraoperative fluids.
- For the office-based patient, continue all medication unless there is concern for diuretic hypokalemia or volume depletion.[10]

Table 5
Antibiotic regimens for a dental procedure, single dose 30 to 60 minutes before procedure

		Adults	Children
Oral	Amoxicillin	2 g	50 mg/kg
Oral (allergic to PCN)	Cephalexin[a]	2 g	50 mg/kg
	Clindamycin	600 mg	20 mg/kg
	Azithromycin	500 mg	15 mg/kg
Unable to take orally	Ampicillin	2 g IM or IV	50 mg/kg IM or IV
Unable to take orally (allergic to PCN)	Cefazolin[a]	1 g IM or IV	50 mg/kg IM or IV
	Ceftriaxone[a]	1 g IM or IV	50 mg/kg IM or IV
	Clindamycin	600 mg IM or IV	20 mg/kg IM or IV

Abbreviations: IM, intramuscular; IV, intravenous; PCN, penicillin.
[a] Cephalosporins should not be used with history of anaphylaxis, angioedema, or urticaria with penicillins or ampicillin.
Adapted from Wilson W, Taubert KA, Gewtiz M, et al. Prevention of infective endocarditis: guidelines from the American Heart Association: a guideline from the American Heart Association Rheumatic Fever, Endocarditis, and Kawasaki Disease Committee, Council on Cardiovascular Disease in the Young, and the Council on Clinical Cardiology, Council on Cardiovascular Surgery and Anesthesia, and the Quality of Care and Outcomes Research Interdisciplinary Working Group. Circulation 2007;116:1736–54.

- Consider only moderate sedation for patients with stable heart failure who can tolerate ordinary activities (NYHA Class I).

Perioperative

- Moderate-sedation drugs are safe and well tolerated.
- Minimize fluctuations in blood pressure and heart rate with gradual titration of sedation and careful selection of anesthetics.[11] Compensated heart failure can easily decompensate.
- Carefully administer intravenous fluids.
- As for other cardiac conditions, avoid medications that have significant hemodynamic effects (eg, ketamine, glycopyrrolate, atropine).

ATRIAL FIBRILLATION
Background

Atrial fibrillation occurs when multiple areas within the atria depolarize, causing a quivering of the atrium. The atrioventricular (AV) node sporadically reacts, leading to an irregular heart rate usually in the 180s.

Signs and symptoms of atrial fibrillation include palpitations, fatigue, weakness, CHF, and hypotension. The most important consequence is an increased risk for thromboembolic events, which are often prevented by anticoagulation therapy. Long-term anticoagulation is commonly managed with warfarin (Coumadin), a vitamin K antagonist that has many drug interactions and a narrow therapeutic window requiring frequent monitoring. Recently a new oral anticoagulant, dabigatran (Pradaxa), was approved in 2010. Dabigatran is a direct thrombin inhibitor with half-life of 12 to 17 hours; however, there is no available reversal agent apart from plasma replacement products.[12]

New-onset atrial fibrillation is treated by either electrical cardioversion (if within 24–48 hours) or pharmacologic cardioversion (if within 7 days). In either case, rate control is necessary and is accomplished with β-blockers, calcium-channel blockers, or digoxin. Clinically the palpable pulse will be "irregularly irregular."

Anesthesia Management
Preoperative

- Continue all antiarrhythmic medications.
- Check electrolytes, specifically magnesium and potassium, if the patient is on digoxin.
- Coordinate care with the primary care team for anticoagulation management or transitions if needed for surgical procedures.

Perioperative

- Maintain rate control; use β-blockers or calcium-channel blockers if necessary.
- Avoid use of medications that can induce tachycardias (ketamine, glycopyrrolate, atropine).

PACEMAKERS AND IMPLANTABLE CARDIOVERTER-DEFIBRILLATORS
Background

Pacemakers
Permanently implanted pacemakers are most commonly used for patients with sick sinus syndrome, and are the only long-term treatment

for symptomatic bradycardia.[12] Improvements in pacemakers now allow for dual-chamber sensing, pacing, and variable response. Pacing modes are designated by a 5-letter generic code of which the first 3 letters give the most important information.

> First letter denotes the chamber being paced (A atrium, V ventricle, D dual chamber)
> Second letter denotes chamber being sensed (A atrium, V ventricle, D dual chamber)
> Third letter denotes the response to sensed signals (I inhibition, T triggering, D both)

For example, DDI pacing paces both chambers, senses both chambers, and only inhibits if it senses a response. The mode can give insight for the reason for pacing, such as AV dyssynchrony, atrial tachyarrhythmias, or sinoatrial node disease.

Implanted cardioverter-defibrillators

The implanted cardioverter-defibrillator (ICD) can be used independently from a pacemaker, and provides a shock within 15 seconds of sensing a dysrhythmia. Timely defibrillation is the most important factor in survival from cardiac arrest. ICDs are typically given to patients at significant risk for sudden cardiac death, patients with advanced heart failure (ejection fraction <30%), or patients at high risk for ventricular tachycardia/fibrillation.

Anesthetic Management

Preoperative

- Focused history and physical examination in coordination with the patient's cardiologist is necessary.
  - Determine the reason for pacemakers/ICD.
    - Ask about bradyarrhythmias, AV nodal ablation, or lack of escape rhythm
  - Assess current function, and check ECG to determine pacing spikes.
- Battery depletion may be seen through decreases in heart rate, often 10% lower than the initial planned rate (commonly 70–72 beats/min).[12]
- The ECG may not show pacemaker function if intrinsic heart rate is adequate.
- If there is no plan for electromagnetic interference (EMI) such as cautery use, then no modifications are required. If EMI is planned then determining pacemaker or ICD function is important; in coordination with cardiology determine a plan to reprogram the pacemaker, suspend rate-adaptive functions, or suspend antiarrhythmia function.[13]

Perioperative

- Monitor ECG for proper functioning of the pacemaker.
- Ensure backup equipment is available in case of unexpected failure.
- There is no evidence that anesthetic drugs alter the stimulation threshold for pacemakers.
- A magnet can be placed externally over the pacemaker to convert it to asynchronous mode. Although this is unnecessary for most office-based procedures, if required its use needs to be coordinated with the patient's cardiologist.[14]
- Avoid monopolar electrocautery if possible by using a bipolar or harmonic scalpel to reduce any potential damage to the pulse generator.
  - Of note, new shielding reduces problems associated with electrocautery. However, this cannot be guaranteed, so consultation with the patient's cardiologist and the manufacturer is recommended.[14]

ACUTE RESPIRATORY INFECTION
Background

Uncomplicated upper respiratory infection (URI), also known as the common cold or infectious nasopharyngitis, is a viral infection that comprises 95% of URIs. Symptoms include sneezing, runny nose, fever, purulent discharge, cough, and general malaise. Noninfectious nasopharyngitis, with a somewhat similar presentation without the fever, often has an allergic or vasomotor origin; diagnosis is based on the clinical history and the variety of symptoms.

Anesthetic Management

Preoperative

- In pediatric patients there is an increased risk of respiratory complications associated with the copious amount of secretions during a URI,[15] which lead to airway irritability and increase the risk of laryngospasm and bronchospasm.
- It is recommended to delay the procedure in patients with obvious symptoms such as rhinitis, cough, rhonchi, and/or fever, for ideally 6 weeks,[15] but the procedure can be completed once most symptoms have resolved.
- For URI patients who are improving and on the latter end of symptoms, consider proceeding with the procedure. The rationale for this is that it takes 6 weeks for airway

hyperreactivity to resolve, by which point another URI can take effect.[15]

- For patients who have preexisting airway comorbidity such as asthma or chronic obstructive pulmonary disease (COPD), the procedure should be postponed until they are asymptomatic.

Perioperative

- Adequately hydrate with intravenous fluids.
- Manage secretions judiciously, taking care to monitor secretions from the nasopharynx.
- The use of bronchodilators to reduce bronchospasm prophylactically has not been established.[15]
- The use of Afrin (oxymetazoline hydrochloride) or decongestants preoperatively to reduce nasal secretions has not been well studied.

ASTHMA
Background

Asthma affects 4% to 5% of the United States population and is characterized by chronic airway inflammation, temporary expiratory airflow obstruction, and bronchial mucosal reactivity.[15] Acute exacerbations of asthma are short lived, usually lasting minutes to hours. Signs and symptoms include wheeze, cough (productive or nonproductive), dyspnea, and chest tightness. The greatest risk factor for asthma is atopy. Asthmatic disease can be seen in patients with allergic diseases such as rhinitis, urticaria, and eczema. Symptoms of asthma, which can occur during the day or even at night, may be provoked by exercise, viral infections, inhalant allergens (animal dander, dust, pollen), irritants (smoke, chemicals), changes in weather, strong emotions, stress, and/or menstrual cycles.

The diagnosis of asthma is typically based on quantifying the obstruction using spirometry, commonly using the forced expiratory volume in 1 second.[16] Other classifications may be based on symptoms (**Table 6**).

Treatment of asthma is based on preventing and controlling bronchial inflammation. **Table 7** lists common medications used in the treatment of obstructive airway diseases.

There are 2 component strategies in the treatment:

- Control airway inflammation and irritability using inhaled/systemic steroids, antileukotrienes, and theophylline.
- Provide rescue relief during acute phases, often using inhaled β-adrenergic agonists.

Anesthetic Management

Preoperative

- Preoperative evaluation is needed to determine the severity of the disease and effectiveness of medication. **Box 3** lists questions to ask patients to determine the severity of their disease.
    - Poorly controlled disease can be indicated by a recent visit to the emergency room or hospitalization within the past month, increasing use of short-acting inhalers, and/or recent flare-ups requiring oral corticosteroids.

Table 6
Classification of asthma for patients older than 12 years

	Intermittent	Mild Persistent	Moderate Persistent	Severe Persistent
Symptoms	≤2 d/wk	>2 d/wk but not daily	Daily	Throughout the day
Night-time awakenings	≤2×/mo	3–4×/mo	>1×/wk but not nightly	Often 7×/wk
Rescue inhaler use for symptoms	≤2 d/wk	>2 d/wk but not daily	Daily	Several times per day
Interference with daily activities	None	Minor limitation	Some limitation	Extremely limited
Lung function	FEV$_1$ >80% predicted FEV$_1$/FVC normal	FEV$_1$ >80% predicted FEV$_1$/FVC normal	FEV$_1$ >60% predicted FEV$_1$/FVC reduced 5%	FEV$_1$ <60% predicted FEV$_1$/FVC reduced >5%

Abbreviations: FEV$_1$, forced expiratory volume in 1 second; FVC, forced vital capacity.

Adapted from National Institutes of Health (2007). National Asthma Education and Prevention Program Expert Panel Report 3: Guidelines for the Diagnosis and Management of Asthma (NIH Publication No. 08–5846). Available at: http://www.nhlbi.nih.gov/guidelines/asthma/index.htm. Accessed December 1, 2012.

Table 7
Common drugs used in treatment of obstructive airway disease

Drug Class Generic (Trade Name)	Action	Adverse Effects
Corticosteroids Beclomethasone (Qvar) Mometasone (Asmanex) Flunisolide (Aerobid) Fluticasone (Flovent) Budesonide (Pulmicort) Ciclesonide (Alvesco) Triamcinolone (Azmacort)	Decrease airway inflammation, reduce airway hyperresponsiveness	Dysphonia, myopathy of laryngeal muscles, oropharyngeal candidiasis
Cromolyn	Inhibits mediator release from mast cells, stabilizes membranes	
Leukotriene Modifiers Zafirlukast (Accolate) Motelukast (Singulair) Zileuton (Zyflo)	Reduce synthesis of leukotrienes by inhibiting 5-lipoxygenase enzyme	Minimal
β-Adrenergic Agonists Short acting: Albuterol (Proventil) Metaproterenol (Alupent) Levalbuterol (Xopenex) Pirbuterol (Maxair) Long acting: Salmeterol (Serevent) Formoterol (Foradil)	Bronchodilator Stimulate β2-receptors of tracheobronchial tree	Tachycardia, tremors, dysrhythmias, hypokalemia
Anticholinergics Ipratropium (Atrovent) Tiotropium (Spiriva)	Bronchodilator Decrease vagal tone by blocking muscarinic receptors in airway smooth muscle	Dry mouth, cough, blurred vision
Theophylline	Increases levels of cyclic adenosine monophosphate by inhibiting phosphodiesterase, releases endogenous catecholamines	Disrupted sleep cycle, nervousness, nausea, vomiting, anorexia, headache, dysrhythmias

Data from Al-Ruzzeh S, Kurup V. Respiratory diseases. In: Hines RL, Marschall KE, editors. Stoelting's anesthesia and co-existing disease. 6th edition. Philadelphia: Elsevier Saunders; 2012. p. 181–217.

- Auscultate lungs for wheezing/crepitation and look for use of accessory muscles.
- Pulmonary function tests can be reviewed; however, in the office-based setting these are unlikely to change management.
- All medications should be continued throughout the preoperative and perioperative period.[16]

Perioperative

- Before induction, use a short-acting inhaler if the patient has any evidence of wheezing.[15] Do not start anesthesia until wheezing has resolved.
- Common office-based medications are safe to use in asthmatics; propofol has bronchodilating effects, ketamine produces smooth-muscle relaxation.[16]

- Drugs that induce histamine release such as morphine, meperidine, and succinylcholine should be avoided except in emergent situations.[17]
- Consider the use of a precordial stethoscope to monitor airway resistance.

SMOKING
Background

Tobacco smokers can have a significant impact on both anesthetic and surgical management. The risk of pulmonary complications can be 5 to 7 times higher in smokers than in nonsmokers. The effects of smoking on the heart and lung are listed in **Box 4**.

The carbon monoxide in smoke preferentially binds hemoglobin, decreasing oxygen delivery

Box 3
Characteristics of asthma to be evaluated preoperatively

- Age at onset
- Triggering events
- Hospitalization for asthma
- Frequency of emergency department visits
- Need for intubation and mechanical ventilation
- Allergies
- Cough
- Sputum characteristics
- Current medications
- Anesthetic history

Data from Al-Ruzzeh S, Kurup V. Respiratory diseases. In: Hines RL, Marschall KE, editors. Stoelting's anesthesia and co-existing disease. 6th edition. Philadelphia: Elsevier Saunders; 2012. p. 181–217.

and shifting the oxygen dissociation curve to the left. These effects are short term, usually 4 to 6 hours, and normal hemoglobin function can return in 48 hours.

Nicotine, another component, has known sympathomimetic effects and also can induce hepatic enzyme function, which can elevate metabolism.[15] The half-life of nicotine is 20 to 50 minutes.

Box 4
Effects of smoking on different organ systems

Cardiac

   Smoking is a risk factor for cardiovascular disease

   Carbon monoxide decreases oxygen delivery and increases myocardial work

   Smoking releases catecholamines and causes coronary vasoconstriction

   Smoking decreases exercise capacity

Respiratory

   Smoking is a major risk factor for chronic pulmonary disease

   Smoking decreases mucociliary activity

   Smoking results in hyperreactive airways

   Smoking decreases pulmonary immune function

Data from Al-Ruzzeh S, Kurup V. Respiratory diseases. In: Hines RL, Marschall KE, editors. Stoelting's anesthesia and co-existing disease. 6th edition. Philadelphia: Elsevier Saunders; 2012. p. 181–217.

The long-term effects of decreased mucociliary function, hyperreactivity of the airway, and reduced immune function caused by smoking can take up to 6 weeks to resolve after smoking cessation.[15] Thus short-term cessation before an anesthetic may not be as beneficial as was once thought.

Smoking cessation may be advised through counseling, nicotine replacement therapies, or use of the antidepressant bupropion.

Anesthetic Management

Preoperative

- If surgery is more than 4 weeks away, smoking cessation should be advised.[15]
- Immediate cessation before surgery:
    - Can be detrimental owing to increased sputum production, nicotine withdrawal, irritability, restlessness, sleep disturbances, and anxiety[15]
    - Can improve carboxyhemoglobin levels and improve oxygenation[15]
- Auscultate lungs and question the patient regarding the degree of dyspnea (if any) with various levels of activity.

Perioperative

- Management of the patient who smokes is similar to that for the asthmatic patient.

CHRONIC OBSTRUCTIVE PULMONARY DISEASE
Background

COPD is a disease process largely related to smoking, hallmarked either by chronic productive cough or progressive exercise limitations. Symptoms include cough, dyspnea, and orthopnea. COPD often can be categorized as chronic bronchitis, emphysema, or a combination of both (**Table 8**).

Patients with chronic bronchitis, sometimes called "blue bloaters," often are noted for chronic productive cough and frequent respiratory infections, and can be barrel chested. It is also important to bear in mind that chronic hypoxemia and hypercapnia causes respiratory acidosis, pulmonary hypertension, cor pulmonale (right heart failure), and secondary erythrocytosis.

Patients with emphysema, sometimes called "pink puffers," are typically thin, often have distant breath sounds, and show hyperlucency on chest radiographs. In emphysema, the alveolar walls and pulmonary capillaries are destroyed. This process reduces oxygen diffusion capacity but does not lead to pulmonary vasoconstriction and its secondary effects.

Table 8
Features of chronic obstructive pulmonary disease

Feature	Chronic Bronchitis	Emphysema
Mechanism	Mucus and inflammation of airway lumen	Loss of elastic recoil
Dyspnea	Moderate	Severe
FEV_1	Decreased	Decreased
Pa_{O_2}	Marked decrease (blue bloater)	Modest decrease (pink puffer)
Pa_{CO_2}	Increased	Normal to decreased
Diffusing capacity	Normal	Decreased
Hematocrit	Increased	Normal
Cor pulmonale	Marked	Mild
Prognosis	Poor	Good

Data from Al-Ruzzeh S, Kurup V. Respiratory diseases. In: Hines RL, Marschall KE, editors. Stoelting's anesthesia and co-existing disease. 6th edition. Philadelphia: Elsevier Saunders; 2012. p. 181–217.

Smoking cessation is the ultimate goal, as this can alter the progression of COPD. Home oxygen is often used, especially in cases of chronic hypoxemia with arterial oxygen pressure (Pa_{O_2}) less than 55 mm Hg. Oxygen via nasal cannula at 2 L/min can restore Pa_{O_2} to between 60 and 80 mm Hg.

Symptomatic relief is accomplished using bronchodilator therapy; however, unlike asthma, anticholinergics may be more effective than β2-agonists. Inhaled steroids are also used in COPD to reduce airway inflammation. Another common finding is frequent respiratory infections, which are managed with intermittent antibiotic therapy.

Anesthetic Management

Preoperative

- Determine the severity of exercise tolerance, chronic cough, wheezing, and incidence of respiratory tract infections.
- Risk factors for pulmonary complications include age older than 60 years, American Society of Anesthesiologists (ASA) Class II or higher, smoking, pulmonary disease, surgery longer than 3 hours, and general anesthesia.[15]
- Continue all home medications. **Table 7** lists common drugs used in obstructive pulmonary diseases.
- Patients may be referred to their pulmonologist for optimization if home medications are ineffective or there is clinical evidence of poor lung function.

Perioperative

- Inhalation anesthesia with nitrous oxide should be avoided because of the risk of gas being trapped within the bullae, which can potentially rupture.[15]
- Supplemental oxygen can be used, and should be titrated to maintain adequate oxygen saturation.
- Note that in advanced disease, patients adapt to hypercarbia and then rely on arterial oxygen levels to trigger their respiratory drive (hypoxemic drive). Excess administration of oxygen could lead to bradypnea, especially if under the influence of anesthetic medications.[17]
- Opioids should be used cautiously, as central nervous system depression can reduce any hypercapnic respiratory drive and cause prolonged ventilatory depression.
- In severe disease, consider minimal conscious sedation and good local anesthesia.
- Avoid early-morning appointments, as patients can have significantly increased coughing as they clear excess mucus accumulated overnight.[17]

OBESITY AND OBSTRUCTIVE SLEEP APNEA
Background

Obesity is an epidemic with significant comorbidities including cardiovascular, pulmonary, and metabolic diseases. As the age and weight of the United States population increases, the incidence of obstructive sleep apnea (OSA) also increases. Obesity currently is best measured with body mass index, calculated as weight in kilograms divided by height in meters squared.

OSA is characterized by 5 or more episodes of apnea, each lasting 10 seconds or more, or a decrease in oxygen saturation of 4% or more from baseline. The polysomnogram is the gold standard for the diagnosis of OSA. The severity of obstructions is measured by the average number of apnea-hypopnea episodes per hour, the apnea-hypopnea index. Alternatively, a screening tool such as the STOP-BANG questionnaire (**Table 9**) is helpful in identifying patients at risk and stratifying risk management.

Comorbidities associated with obesity and OSA that require investigation include hypertension, pulmonary hypertension, heart failure, dysrhythmias, MI, stroke, diabetes, nutritional deficiencies, and fatty liver infiltration.

Patients with obesity and OSA are at risk for both difficult mask ventilation and difficult airway intubations. Because of increased abdominal fat the functional residual capacity will be reduced, thus leading to quicker desaturation as a result of decreased reserves. The risk of pulmonary aspiration is increased, owing to incidence of hiatal hernias or acid reflux disease from increased intragastric pressures associated with obesity.

Many OSA patients are treated with nighttime dental appliances or continuous positive airway pressure (CPAP), and some receive upper airway surgery to relieve obstructions. Obesity management includes weight loss, medical therapy, and surgery.

Anesthetic Management

Preoperative

- If OSA is suspected or the STOP-BANG questionnaire suggests high risk, avoid

Table 9 STOP-BANG questionnaire	
Snoring: Do you snore loudly (louder than talking or loud enough to be heard through closed doors?)	Yes or No
Tired: Do you often feel tired, fatigued, or sleepy during the daytime?	Yes or No
Observed: Has anyone observed you stop breathing during your sleep?	Yes or No
Blood pressure: Do you have or are you being treated for high blood pressure?	Yes or No
Body mass index: >35 kg/m^2?	Yes or No
Age: Older than 50 y?	Yes or No
Neck circumference: >40 cm?	Yes or No
Gender: Male?	Yes or No

Three or more Yes answers indicate high risk for obstructive sleep apnea (OSA). Less than 3 indicate low risk for OSA.

From Chung F, Yegneswaran B, Liao P, et al. STOP questionnaire: a tool to screen patients for obstructive sleep apnea. Anesthesiology 2008;108:812–21; with permission.

sedation and have the patient undergo a formal assessment.[18] Alternatively, proceed with local anesthesia only if feasible.

- Assess the cardiorespiratory system by conducting a thorough cardiac and respiratory review of systems including symptoms of chest pain, shortness of breath, sleeping position, exertional dyspnea, fatigue, and so forth.
- Assess the risk of pulmonary aspiration by questioning for symptoms of gastroesophageal reflux disease (GERD) (coughing, inability to lie flat without coughing, heartburn).
- Perform a thorough airway examination looking for a short neck, large tongue, small mouth, large tonsils, and/or excessive palatal soft tissues.[15]
- If a cephalometric radiograph is available, measure the distance from hyoid to mandibular plane. A distance greater than 20 mm has been correlated with OSA.[19]
- For OSA patients who are successfully treated using CPAP and whose coexisting illnesses are effectively managed, outpatient sedation can be considered.[18]
  - Keep in mind that patients must be able to use their CPAP machine during the postoperative period

Perioperative

- Keep the patient in a sitting position to minimize the effects of gravity on airway collapse.
- A dedicated head holder is crucial in helping to maintain a patent airway.
- If possible, use conscious sedation only with anesthetics such as midazolam or dexmedetomidine to limit respiratory depression.[20]
- Avoid opioids, owing to the risk of pharyngeal collapse and respiratory depression.
  - Also must be considered during the postoperative period, as respiratory events can occur even 1 week after anesthesia[18]
  - It is important to maintain a closely monitored follow-up period and to manage analgesia with nonopioids when possible postoperatively[18]
- Adjust medications to ideal body weight (110 lb [50 kg]+ 5 lb [2.3 kg] for every inch [2.54 cm] above 5 feet [152.4 cm]); see **Table 10**.
- Have the patient bring the CPAP machine to the office; use postoperatively if necessary.

DIABETES
Background

Diabetes mellitus (DM) is a result of either an inadequate production of insulin (type 1) or inadequate

Table 10
Recommended weight basis for dosing of common outpatient anesthetic drugs

Total Body Weight	Lean Body Weight
Propofol: loading dose	Propofol: maintenance dose
Midazolam	Fentanyl
Succinylcholine	Remifentanil

Data from Al-Ruzzeh S, Kurup V. Respiratory diseases. In: Hines RL, Marschall KE, editors. Stoelting's anesthesia and co-existing disease. 6th edition. Philadelphia: Elsevier Saunders; 2012. p. 181–217.

use of the insulin produced (type 2). Type 1 DM is caused by autoimmune destruction of β cells within the pancreas, resulting in essentially a complete absence of circulating insulin. Patients with type 1 DM require exogenous insulin for survival.

Type 2 DM results from defect(s) in the insulin receptors or pathways, making insulin ineffective and secondarily decreasing its production. Type 2 DM accounts for almost 90% of diabetics.

The diagnosis of diabetes requires 1 of the following criteria[21]:

- Hemoglobin A$_{1c}$ (HbA1c) greater than 6.5%
- Fasting glucose greater than 126 mg/dL
- Two-hour plasma glucose greater than 200 mg/dL after 75 g oral glucose tolerance test
- Symptoms of hyperglycemia with random glucose greater than 200 mg/dL

Symptoms of hyperglycemia can include polyphagia, polydipsia, polyuria, fatigue, and unexplained weight loss.

Acute hyperglycemia causes dehydration, impaired wound healing, and an increased rate of infection and hyperviscosity with thrombogenesis. The possibility of infection (especially skin and soft tissue) and the delay in wound healing result from a reduction in neutrophil number, impaired chemotaxis/phagocytosis, a reduction in capillary volume, a decrease in tensile wound strength, a decrease in fibroblast and collagen synthesis, and an increase in edema.[21]

Chronic hyperglycemia in diabetics has long-term consequences.[21]

- Microvascular complications include nephropathy, peripheral neuropathy, retinopathy, and autonomic nephropathy.
- Macrovascular complications are associated with dyslipidemia leading to cardiovascular, cerebrovascular, and peripheral vascular diseases.

- Untreated hyperglycemia can lead to diabetic ketoacidosis (mostly type 1 patients) or hyperglycemic hyperosmolar syndrome (mostly type 2 patients).

Treatment of diabetics is often multifold. Type 2 diabetics often need weight loss, exercise therapy, and antidiabetic agents. Further comorbidities of the disease, or those associated with it, may necessitate other medications such as antihypertensives and statins. Common antidiabetic drugs and insulin preparations are listed in **Tables 11** and **12**.

It is important to remember that the stress response of anesthesia and surgery creates a hyperglycemic challenge through activation of the sympathetic nervous system. This process can turn a well-controlled diabetic into one with hyperglycemia or turn a poorly controlled diabetic into one with severe metabolic effects, including ketoacidosis.

Anesthetic Management

Preoperative

- The following areas should have a complete physical examination and review of systems, as they have implicit effects on the anesthetic management[21]:
  - Cardiac
    - Be wary of silent ischemia in chronic diabetics and keep a high suspicion for myocardial disease
    - Patients should be on β-blockers if CAD is present
    - Patients with concomitant renal disease should be on ACE inhibitors
    - Autonomic neuropathy predisposes patients to dysrhythmias and associated hypotension
  - Renal
    - Maintain adequate hydration
    - Avoid nephrotoxins
    - Maintain renal blood flow with adequate perfusion from fluid and blood pressure
  - Neurologic
    - Gastroparesis is common, thus patients can have an increased risk of aspiration
    - In chronic diabetes, autonomic dysfunction may lead to hypoglycemic unawareness
  - Musculoskeletal
    - Patients may have limited joint mobility of the neck secondary to glycosylation of proteins within the joints
      - This can result in increased difficulty with intubation

Table 11
Common noninsulin antidiabetic medication

Drug Class Generic (Trade) Name	Mechanism of Action	Half-Life (h)	Side Effects
Biguanides Metformin (Glucophage)	Decreases hepatic gluconeogenesis, increases insulin sensitivity	6–18	Diarrhea, nausea, vomiting, lactic acidosis (avoid in renal, liver, and congestive heart failure patients)
Sulfonylureas Chlorpropamide (Diabenese) Tolbutamide (Orinase) Glimperide (Amaryl) Glipizide (Glucotrol) Glyburide (DiaBeta, Micronase)	Stimulate insulin secretion, decrease insulin resistance	2–10	Hypoglycemia, gastrointestinal disturbance
Meglitinides Repaglinide (Prandin) Nateglinide (Starlix)	Stimulate pancreatic insulin secretion	1	Hypoglycemia (less than sulfonylureas)
Thiazolidinediones Rosiglitazone (Avandia) Pioglitazone (Actos)	Regulate carbohydrate and lipid metabolism, reduce insulin resistance, and hepatic glucose production	3–8	Fluid retention, increased cardiac risk, hepatotoxicity.
α-Glucosidase Inhibitors Acarbose (Precose) Miglitol (Glyset)	Reduce intestinal absorption of ingested glucose	2–4	Gastrointestinal irritation, flatus
Dipeptidyl Peptidase-4 Inhibitors Sitagliptin (Januvia) Saxagliptin (Onglyza)	Reduce breakdown of gastrointestinal hormones (incretins), enhance insulin secretion, decrease glucagon	8–14	Infection
Noninsulin Injectables Exenatide (Byetta) Pramlintide (Symlin)	Suppress glucagon secretion and hepatic glucose production, suppress appetite, delay gastric emptying	6–10 2–4	Nausea, vomiting, weight loss

Data from Joshi GP, Chung F, Vann MA, et al. Society for Ambulatory Anesthesia consensus statement on perioperative blood glucose management in diabetic patients undergoing ambulatory surgery. Anesth Analg 2010;111(6):1378–87; with permission.

- ■ Ask the patient to put palms of hands together (Prayer sign) and assess if the palms of the hands are touching. If the palms are unable to touch because of stiff joints, be wary of limited neck mobility
- Question the patient on history of hypoglycemia at night, in the morning, or with missed meals, as this will give insight regarding any necessary modification of medication regimens.
- In general, modification of a patient's medication regimen for diabetes is based on whether a normal diet can be resumed that day. If a procedure is short and the patient can resume normal oral intake, minimal modifications are necessary.[22]

- ○ The medications of concern that require modifications are those that can directly cause hypoglycemia (sulfonylureas, meglitinides, insulin preparations)
- ○ These medications may need to be held until after the patient resumes normal intake

Noninsulin medications
- All medications can be taken the day before surgery and on the morning of surgery; however:
- Consider holding sulfonylureas, meglitinides, and noninsulin injectables on the morning of surgery, owing to potential risk of hypoglycemia.[22]

Table 12
Common insulin medications

Drug Class Generic (Trade) Name	Onset	Duration (h)
Rapid acting	5–15 min	4–6
Lispro (Humalog)		
Aspart (Novolog)		
Glulisine (Apidra)		
Short acting	30–60 min	6–8
Regular (Novolin R, Humulin R)		
Intermediate acting		
NPH (Novolin N, Humulin N-NF)	2–4 h	4–10
Zinc insulin (Lente)	2–4 h	4–10
Extended zinc insulin (Ultralente)	6–10 h	10–16
Long acting (peakless)	2–4 h	20–24
Glargine (Lantus)		
Detemir (Levemir)		
Mixed insulins		
NPH/regular	30–90 min	10–16
Novolin 70/30		
Humulin 70/30		
Humulin 50/50		
Aspart protamine/Aspart	5–15 min	10–16
Novolog mix 70/30		
Lispro protamine/Lispro	5–15 min	10–12
Humalog 75/25		
Humalog 50/50		

Data from Joshi GP, Chung F, Vann MA, et al. Society for Ambulatory Anesthesia consensus statement on perioperative blood glucose management in diabetic patients undergoing ambulatory surgery. Anesth Analg 2010;111(6):1378–87; with permission.

- Metformin has a concern for lactic acidosis; however, there seems to be a lack of evidence regarding this problem unless the patient has renal dysfunction or use of intravenous contrast.[23] If there is a concern for renal dysfunction, hold metformin 24 to 48 hours before surgery.

Insulin medications
- Insulin doses on the day before surgery do not require change unless the patient suggests a history of hypoglycemia at night, in the morning, or without meals (**Table 13**).[22]
- On the morning of surgery all rapid-acting and short-acting insulin should be held. Intermediate-acting insulin should be reduced to 50% to 75% and long-acting insulin, if taken in the morning, can be reduced to 75%.[22]
- Check blood sugar on initial office visit and on the day of surgery.

- If the patient is hyperglycemic, try to determine if it is from poor long-term control or poor medication management preoperatively
- There is no consensus or evidence to suggest that preoperative blood glucose is necessary for elective procedures[22]
  - If a patient is hyperglycemic, practitioners can consider treating the patient with a rapid-acting insulin to lower blood sugar to less than 180 mg/dL before proceeding[22]
- Ask about recent HbA1c.
  - Evidence suggests that HbA1c less than 7% has reduced incidence of infections and hospital stays[22]

Preoperative hyperglycemia management
- Typically, 1 unit of insulin will lower blood glucose levels by approximately 25 to 30 mg/dL.[22]

Table 13
Instructions for injectable antidiabetic medications

Insulin Regimen	Day Before Surgery	Day of Surgery
Insulin pump	No change	Use sick day or sleep basal rates
Long-acting peakless	No change	75%–100% of morning dose
Intermediate acting	No change in daytime dose 75% of dose if taken in evening	50%–75% of morning dose
Fixed combinations	No change	50%–75% of intermediate acting (may have to substitute NPH)
Short and rapid acting	No change	Hold the dose
Noninsulin injectables	No change	Hold the dose

Data from Joshi GP, Chung F, Vann MA, et al. Society for Ambulatory Anesthesia consensus statement on perioperative blood glucose management in diabetic patients undergoing ambulatory surgery. Anesth Analg 2010;111(6):1378–87; with permission.

- There are many methods to approximate an appropriate correction factor for insulin. One recommendation is the "rule of 1500" for surgical patients.
  - Take 1500 and divide it by the total number of units of insulin taken daily by the patient. The resulting correction factor is the expected decrease in blood glucose with each unit of insulin
- With an appropriate correction factor, administer the amount of short-acting or rapid-acting insulin required to obtain a serum glucose level of less than 200 mg/dL.
- If the patient has never taken insulin before (insulin-naïve type II DM), a sliding-scale dose regime with rapid-acting insulin can be used without any detrimental effects.
- It is recommended to use rapid-acting insulin for correctional doses as opposed to regular insulin because the peak blood level occurs earlier, thus reducing the observation time; this helps prevent "stacking" of correctional insulin doses.

Perioperative

- If patients are at risk for hypoglycemia, consider using a 5% dextrose solution to prevent a "catabolic" state (hypoglycemia, ketosis, and protein breakdown).
  - Normal saline is a good alternative given the nature of short procedures and minimal blood loss in outpatient offices
  - Avoid lactated Ringer solution in poorly controlled diabetics, owing to concern of hepatic conversion of lactate to glucose
- It is important to provide adequate intravenous hydration, especially if the patient is hyperglycemic and/or NPO (nothing by mouth).

- Check serum glucose hourly until discharge (coincide serum glucose checks with the peak effects of any correctional insulin administered).
- To provide adequate nausea prophylaxis dexamethasone may be considered, although the practitioner should be prepared to manage elevated blood sugar over the next 4 hours.
  - If not needed to prevent postoperative inflammation, suitable nausea prophylaxis may be achieved with 4 mg dexamethasone, and will result in less elevation of blood sugar in comparison with 8 mg.[22]

CHRONIC LIVER DISEASE
Background

Chronic liver diseases are further classified based on etiology such as viral hepatitis, autoimmune hepatitis, drug-induced hepatitis, and alcoholic hepatitis. Symptoms of chronic liver diseases may be minimal but can be complicated with malaise, jaundice, ascites, or cirrhosis. Common physical findings can include fetor hepaticus, spider angiomas, engorged abdominal veins (caput medusa), hemorrhoids, enlargement of the liver and spleen, palmar erythema, asterixis, testicular atrophy, or physical wasting, among others.

The most common causes of chronic hepatitis are alcoholic liver disease and hepatitis C infection.[24] A diagnosis of liver disease should warrant an investigation for chronic alcohol use, substance abuse, exposure to toxic materials, or history of blood transfusions. Viral hepatitis (hepatitis A, B, C, D) is most often diagnosed on serologic testing, and treatment is only for symptom relief. Hepatitis A is most commonly associated with acute hepatitis, whereas hepatitis B and C usually develop into chronic disease.

Patients with cirrhosis and end-stage liver diseases should be adequately investigated for other organ diseases such as hepatic encephalopathy, pleural effusions, hepatopulmonary syndrome, hepatorenal syndrome, portal hypertension, cirrhotic cardiomyopathy, and coagulation disorders.[25] These groups of patients are not recommended for outpatient sedation, although local anesthetic techniques can be used after conferring with a physician. In cases of severe cirrhosis, oxygenation must be monitored because of the possibility of portal hypertension causing shunting and elevating the diaphragm, leading to decreased functional residual capacity.

Anesthetic Management

Preoperative

- A review of symptoms of liver disease should include fatigue, malaise, nausea, vomiting, hematemesis, pruritus, jaundice, easy bleeding or bruising, hemorrhagic diathesis, abdominal distention, behavioral changes, or altered mental status.
- If a patient has a remote history of hepatitis but no active signs or symptoms of liver disease, outpatient sedation can be considered without further workup.[24]
- Risk stratification for patients with liver disease is best accomplished using the Child-Pugh score (**Table 14**), evaluating the patient's current condition, and through consultation with patient's physician.
- In patients with chronic disease and/or history of bleeding, it is recommend to obtain a baseline complete blood count (CBC) and coagulation profile (prothrombin time, partial thromboplastin time, international normalized

ratio), as this will assist in surgical workup as well.[24]
- Consider proceeding with surgery in Child-Pugh Class A patients after consultation with the patient's physician regarding office-based anesthesia and surgery. The remainder of patients with Child-Pugh Class B, C, and advanced liver disease are better served in a hospital setting.

Perioperative

- In liver disease, there is a decreased ability to metabolize drugs, leading to a lower anesthetic requirement and a longer half-life of drug.
- In general, benzodiazepines require a longer recovery, as they are metabolized by cytochrome P450 enzymes.
  - Single doses of midazolam may be acceptable but should be used cautiously, as some studies suggest it can be less effective[26]
- Propofol is metabolized by the liver through conjugation to glucuronide and sulfate, as well as undergoing extrahepatic metabolism through the lungs.[25]
  - Chronic liver disease has been reported to have no significant alteration in the pharmacokinetic profile of propofol[25]
- Ketamine should be avoided because of concerns for the buildup of secondary metabolites and reduced elimination.[25]
- Most opioids undergo hepatic metabolism.
  - Morphine, oxycodone, and meperidine have prolonged elimination half-lives and active metabolites, and should be avoided in outpatient sedation in this patient population[25]

Table 14
Child-Pugh scoring system

Sign of Hepatic Dysfunction	1 Point	2 Points	3 Points
Encephalopathy	None	Grade I–II	Grade III–IV
Ascites	Absent	Mild	Severe
Bilirubin (mg/dL)	<2	2–3	>3
Albumin (g/dL)	>3.5	2.8–3.5	<2.8
International normalized ratio	<1.7	1.7–2.2	>2.2

Points	Class
5–6	A
7–9	B
10–15	C

Data from Hevesi ZG, Hannaman M. Diseases of the liver and biliary tract. In: Hines RL, Marschall KE, editors. Stoelting's anesthesia and co-existing disease. 6th edition. Philadelphia: Elsevier Saunders; 2012. p. 274–86.

○ Fentanyl is well tolerated and does not have a significantly prolonged half-life[26]
- Modern volatile anesthetics tend to have a low hepatic metabolism and appear to be a good alternative.
  ○ This includes the use of nitrous oxide, which has minimal metabolism within human tissues[25]
- Most amide local anesthetics are metabolized by the liver; however, articaine is an alternative, as it has plasma esterase-based clearance.[17]

GASTROESOPHAGEAL REFLUX DISEASE
Background

The primary cause of GERD is a decrease in resting tone of the lower esophageal sphincter. A reflux of gastric contents into the esophagus causes retrosternal discomfort commonly known as heartburn. The gastric content can also reach the pharynx, causing coughing, pharyngitis, morning hoarseness, and so forth. More than one-third of healthy adults experience reflux at least once a month.[27]

Patients with GERD are at increased risk for aspiration. Common complications include esophagitis, esophageal stricture, laryngitis, bronchitis, bronchospasm, pneumonia, and pulmonary fibrosis.

Treatment modalities include use of H2-antagonists and proton-pump inhibitors (PPIs), which aim to increase gastric pH. Often patients self-medicate using of over-the-counter antacids, which can cause rebound gastric acid production if stopped acutely, leading to worsened symptoms.

Anesthetic Management

Preoperative

- Include in the history and physical examination questions regarding any history of heartburn.
- Poor compliance or frequent as-needed dosing suggests poor control of the disease process.
- Determine the presence of other comorbidities, such as obesity, pregnancy, or diabetes, which could further increase the risk of aspiration.
- Continue home medications on the morning of surgery.

Perioperative

- Confirm fasting status using ASA guidelines (**Table 15**).
  ○ Anecdotally, consider extending fasting 1 to 2 hours if the patient carries higher risk.

Table 15
Recommend fasting guidelines for adults

Ingested Material	Minimum Fasting Period (h)
Clear liquids	2
Breast milk	4
Infant formula	6
Nonhuman milk	6
Light meal	6
Heavy meal	8

Examples of clear liquid include water, fruit juices without pulp, clear tea, and black coffee. With nonhuman milk, similar to solids, consider the amount ingested when making a decision. Light meal consists of toast and clear liquids. Fatty foods considerably delay gastric emptying time.

Data from American Society of Anesthesiologists Committee. Practice guidelines for preoperative fasting and the use of pharmacologic agents to reduce the risk of pulmonary aspiration: application to healthy patients undergoing elective procedures: an updated report by the American Society of Anesthesiologists Committee on Standards and Practice Parameters. Anesthesiology 2011;114(3):495–511.

- There is no evidence for the routine use of pharmacologic therapy to decrease aspiration risk in otherwise healthy individuals.[28,29]
- For high-risk patients (diabetic, obese, pregnant), consider nonparticulate sodium citrate and a gastrokinetic agent such as metoclopramide.[30]
- Avoid supine or Trendelenburg positions.
- If considering premedication for a high-risk GERD patient, H2-blockers or PPIs are effective choices.[30]
  ○ H2-blockers: ranitidine or famotidine should be given at least 1 hour before planned procedure
  ○ PPI should be administered orally the night before in addition to the morning of the procedure

COCAINE ABUSE
Background

Cocaine is an indirectly acting sympathomimetic amine that works by blocking presynaptic uptake of norepinephrine and dopamine, increasing their levels in the synapse. It can be administered by multiple routes such as transmucosal, inhalation, and intravenous. Cocaine is metabolized by plasma cholinesterases within 2 hours of administration.[31]

Acute administration causes coronary vasospasm, which can precipitate myocardial ischemia, myocardial infarction, ventricular dysrhythmias, hypertension, tachycardia, seizures, and hyperthermia. The use of cocaine can sensitize a patient for myocardial ischemia and hypertension for as long as 6 weeks after discontinuation.[31] Chronic cocaine abuse can lead to nasal septal erosion, depression, paranoid delusions, headaches, seizures, hyperpyrexia, lung damage, and pulmonary edema.

Anesthetic Management

Preoperative

- Determine last use of cocaine and severity of use.
  - Be wary, as many patients are not truthful regarding substance abuse
- Consider a 12-lead ECG if there is concern regarding recent use or if the patient's history suggests cardiac disease.
- Urine testing can be done; however, this can detect cocaine and its metabolites for up to 6 days or even 10 days for chronic users.[32]
- At present there is no consensus on the timing of treatment. Anecdotally, 8 hours is sufficient for general anesthesia if the patient is stable.[32]
  - For office anesthesia, consider waiting 24 hours or consider treatment in a hospital setting

Perioperative

- Be prepared to handle hypertension or cardiac dysrhythmias.
  - Avoid use of β1-selective β-blockers, as there is concern for unopposed α stimulation[31]
  - Consider the use of labetalol or adding an α-blocker
- Benzodiazepines, opioids, and propofol are considered safe.
- Do not use ketamine, as it is an indirect sympathomimetic and could further worsen cardiac symptoms.
- Monitor use of local anesthetics containing epinephrine, as there is potential for dysrhythmic effects with both agents in conjunction.

EXOGENOUS STEROIDS
Background

The exogenous administration of glucocorticoids results in secondary adrenal insufficiency as in the adrenal glands innate secretion is repressed via the hypothalamic-pituitary axis (HPA). Cortisol is responsible for approximately 95% of the adrenal glands' glucocorticoid activity, and participates in far-ranging processes from carbohydrate and protein metabolism and fatty acid mobilization to electrolyte and water balance, in addition to modulating inflammatory response.[21] Daily estimates of cortisol production range from the equivalent of 15 to 25 mg/d of hydrocortisone to 5 to 7 mg/d prednisone.[21] In response to surgery, the level of cortisol production increases from 2 to 10 times that of baseline.[33–35]

Under similar surgical stress stimuli, patients who have adrenal suppression produce less cortisol than those who are not suppressed.[35] Manifestations of adrenal crisis include dehydration, hypotension, and shock. However, as most exogenous steroids are glucocorticoid, the mineralocorticoid aldosterone functions remain intact. Therefore symptoms associated with exogenous steroid adrenal insufficiency are often less severe: hypoglycemia, weakness, gastrointestinal complaints, and evolving hypotension.

Clinical factors associated with activation of the HPA and adrenal insufficiency/crisis consist of length and extent of surgery, type and depth of anesthesia, perioperative pain control, and infections.[21] The use of appropriate local anesthesia, postoperative analgesics, and good sedation all have been shown to control increases in cortisol production.[33,36–38]

Patients taking less than 5 mg/d prednisone in a morning dose for any length of time do not demonstrate clinically significant HPA suppression.[21] Any patient who has received the equivalent or greater than 20 mg/d prednisone for more than 3 weeks within the past year is assumed to have adrenal suppression.[21] However, the onset of adrenal suppression can occur as early as 1 week after commencing corticosteroid therapy.[39] Doses between 5 and 20 mg prednisone equivalent for longer than 3 weeks may harbor HPA suppression. Patients who receive more than 2 g/d of topical steroids or more than 1.5 mg/d beclomethasone equivalent of inhaled steroids on a long-term basis may also be suppressed.[33] The recovery of normal adrenal function can take from 2 days to 9 months, depending on dosage and length of administration.[35]

Of note, the majority of research into which levels of steroid administration lead to adrenal insufficiency has been based on patient response to biochemical testing of the HPA (corticotropin stimulation testing, among others). However, the results of these tests are not necessarily predictive of surgical or anesthetic outcomes.[35] Hence clinical recommendations are probably based on data that are overly sensitive and inclusive, thus the consideration to provide a "stress dose" is likely based on the low risks and minimal side effects of additional steroids.[40,41]

Anesthetic Management

Preoperative

- Perform a history and physical examination to determine why a patient is taking steroids, and at what doses and for what period of time.
  - The underlying disease should be evaluated for its stability and potential to affect treatment
  - Evaluate the patient for any side effects they may have experienced
- Be aware of various steroids and equivalents (**Table 16**) in considering which patients may be suppressed.

Perioperative

- Three popular management strategies for perioperative steroid coverage during surgical and dental care are available in the literature.
  - The most common is doubling the morning dose on the day of surgery
  - Administration can be based on the physiologic glucocorticoid production rate associated with the amount of stress a given procedure is likely to produce.[39] Surgeries are categorized into minor, moderate, and major surgical stresses, which are associated with a daily goal of hydrocortisone administration[33]
  - There may be no need for additional coverage as long as the patient has received the baseline dose
    - Although patients may experience lower cortisol levels than would otherwise be generated for a given surgical procedure/stress level, there appears to be little clinical significance[40–42]

- Ultimately the risk and negative side effects of short-term glucocorticoid coverage in the amounts suggested is low in comparison with the possibility of adrenal crisis during or as a result of an outpatient procedure.
- Practitioners should use their clinical judgment to assess for a need for coverage beyond the patient's baseline dose.

EPILEPSY/SEIZURES

Background

The diagnosis of epilepsy represents a broad grouping of neurologic disorders that can be further classified based on the etiology, age at onset, and seizure type, among others. In general, seizures result from excessive neuronal discharge from the brain and can be the result of multiple causes, all of which do not result in a diagnosis of epilepsy. Accordingly the diagnosis of epilepsy can represent a spectrum of disorders, many of which are associated with syndromes or metabolic/structural disorders that have far-reaching consequences outside the implications of seizures.

Epilepsy has its highest incidence in the very young and the elderly.[43,44] Although 10% of the population will experience one seizure in 80 years of life, only around 0.4% to 0.7% of the population is currently diagnosed with epilepsy, and there is an overall 3% lifetime prevalence.[45]

Epileptic seizures can be divided into generalized and focal seizures. Generalized seizures result in bilateral and generalized electroencephalographic abnormalities, whereas focal seizures are a result of abnormal neuronal networks that are initially localized within one hemisphere and, often, one area of the brain.[46]

Symptoms of seizures can be very broad-ranging across auditory, motor, and sensory boundaries. Signs can range from simply staring off into space or clenching the jaw to convulsing on the floor.

Status epilepticus is an emergency situation that can result in patients who have previously diagnosed seizures and those who do not. It has been defined as a single seizure lasting more than 5 minutes or a series of seizures whereby consciousness is not recovered.[43] Its occurrence has a similar bimodal distribution, occurring in both the very young and very old.

First-line therapy for epileptics is usually pharmaceutical and comes from a group of medications called antiepileptic drugs (AED). If monotherapy fails, further drug combinations are considered. These medications seem to work via increasing neuronal inhibition or decreasing

Table 16
Steroid equivalents

Name	Glucocorticoid Potency	Duration of Action ($t_{1/2}$ in hours)
Cortisone acetate	0.8	8
Hydrocortisone	1	8
Prednisone	3.5–5	16–36
Prednisolone	4	16–36
Methylprednisolone	5–7.5	18–40
Triamcinolone	5	12–36
Dexamethasone	25–80	36–54
Betamethasone	25–30	36–54

excitability. Therapy is usually divided between treatment of generalized and focal therapy, although there are medications that are effective for both.

- Common first-line therapy for generalized seizures includes valproate, lamotrigine, phenytoin, phenobarbital, and ethosuximide.[44]
- Common first-line therapy for focal seizures includes phenytoin, carbamazepine, and valproate.[45]

Anesthetic Management

Preoperative

- History and physical examination.
  - Determine current control of seizure activity
  - Type, frequency, and duration of seizures
  - Time period the patient has been seizure free
- Consider hospital-based procedures for patients in whom seizure control is questionable. Such patients can include:
  - Newly diagnosed patient
  - Patient has changed medication regimen
  - Candidate for, or recipient of, vagal nerve stimulators
  - Patient has history of status epilepticus
- All antiepileptic medications should be continued without interruption of dosing schedules.
  - Low AED levels are one of the leading causes of seizures in epileptics[43]

Perioperative

- Benzodiazepines are safe, and have been shown to have a protective effect through dose-dependent anticonvulsant activity at the γ-aminobutyric acid A receptors.[47]
  - Flumazenil, a benzodiazepine reversal agent, should be limited to emergencies with epileptic patients, as its use is known to lower the seizure threshold and can elicit seizures[48,49]
- Opioids such as fentanyl and morphine can be used, but caution is suggested because in animal models they can increase seizure thresholds but become proconvulsant at higher doses.[50–52]
  - Meperidine has a strong association with seizure activity and should be avoided in epileptic patients[53]
- Propofol appears to raise the seizure threshold and to have a dose-dependent anticonvulsant effect, both alone and in combination with opioids in laboratory settings.[54,55]

- Propofol has been found to have a greater effect than methohexital at raising the seizure threshold and shortening seizure duration.[56]
- Ketamine has been reported to have anticonvulsant effects at doses used for sedation/anesthesia, but may have proconvulsant properties at lower doses.[57]
- Barbiturates are known to increase the seizure threshold and have been established for treating status epilepticus; however, it has been suggested that methohexital appears to have the least protective effect of this class[58] and has been known to activate epileptic foci.[59]
- Nitrous oxide has been suggested to provoke seizures in animal models, but this has not been demonstrated in humans.[59,60]
  - Given its widespread use and the rare reporting of it invoking seizure activity, nitrous oxide it is unlikely to provoke them when used alone
- As hypoglycemia can produce seizures, it may be warranted to use intravenous fluids that include glucose/dextrose.
  - Hypoglycemia should also be ruled out in any patient found to be experiencing seizure-like symptoms during sedation, as this is often readily correctable

CHRONIC KIDNEY DISEASE
Background

Chronic kidney disease (CKD) is a progressive and irreversible decline in renal function.[61] It is most commonly caused by diabetic nephropathy followed by hypertensive nephrosclerosis. Progression of chronic renal failure is characterized by a steady decrease in glomerular filtration rate (GFR), which is normally at least 90 mL/min without evidence of disease. As glomerular filtration decreases, patients begin to experience the systemic effects of the accumulated nitrogenous waste normally filtered by the kidney. Patients are said to have CKD once GFR drops below 60 mL/min for 3 months or longer. Patients with a GFR of 40 to 60 mL/min are generally asymptomatic, but if filtration drops low enough (<25 mL/min) it can result in uremia/uremic syndrome. Once filtration drops below 15 mL/min, patients are said to have end-stage renal disease (ESRD) and are dependent on dialysis. The manifestations of CKD are broad, as a result of the many systems of the body affected (**Box 5**).

Systemic manifestations that must be considered with regard to outpatient sedation include anemia, which is associated with CKD progression as a result of decreased erythropoietin production.[61–63]

Box 5
Manifestations of chronic kidney disease

Electrolyte imbalances

Hyperkalemia

Hyperphosphatemia

Hypocalcemia

Metabolic acidosis

Unpredictable status of intravascular fluid volume

Anemia

Increased cardiac output

Rightward shift of oxyhemoglobin dissociation curve

Uremic coagulopathy

Increased bleeding time

Platelet dysfunction

Neurologic changes

Autonomic dysfunction

Encephalopathy

Peripheral neuropathy

Cardiovascular changes

CHF

Dyslipidemia

Systemic hypertension

Renal osteodystrophy

Pruritus

Data from Holt N. Renal disease. Chapter 17. In: Hines RL, Marschall KE, editors. Stoelting's anesthesia and co-existing disease. 6th edition. Philadelphia: Saunders; 2012. p. 334–56.

In addition, multiple electrolyte abnormalities may precipitate cardiac arrhythmias and can lead to decreased protein binding of certain drugs.[61,63]

CKD has a profound effect on the cardiovascular system, significantly increasing cardiac morbidity and mortality.[63] Physiologically, one of the most important effects is increased cardiac output to maintain oxygen delivery in the presence of anemia.[61,62] Furthermore, sodium retention, induced abnormalities of the renin-angiotensin system, and dysfunction of the sympathetic nervous system result in arterial hypertension.[61] Accelerated CAD is intimately linked with CKD, and more than 70% of patients with ESRD have CHF and/or ischemic disease.[61,63]

Initially, treatment is focused on lifestyle modification and control of the underlying disease

process that leads to CKD. With progression, patients often receive an ACE inhibitor or ARB. Anemia can be treated effectively with erythropoietin. Once a patient's GFR begins to drop below 30 mL/min, discussion of transplantation or dialysis begins.

Anesthetic Management

Preoperative

- Assessment of CKD and ESRD revolves around the control and management of a patient's disease by ascertaining any symptoms of disease, as listed in **Box 5**.
  - ○ Evaluate the patient for cardiac and respiratory dysfunction, including evidence of fluid overload or CHF
  - ○ Routine laboratory work such as a CBC and basic metabolic panel should be obtained to evaluate for anemia and electrolyte imbalances
  - ○ If concerned for cardiac dysrhythmias, obtain an ECG and check electrolytes (specifically potassium)
- If the patient is on dialysis, ascertain the dialysis schedule. Often patients receive dialysis at least 3 days a week.
  - ○ Patients on dialysis should be scheduled for dialysis on the day before sedation and the day after
  - ○ Check for AV fistulas in the upper extremities; such extremities should be avoided for placement of blood pressure cuff and intravenous administration
- In general, because of the significant comorbidities associated with CKD, a consultation with the nephrologist is necessary before embarking on outpatient sedation.
  - ○ Recommendations on any perioperative modifications, general medical status, and scheduling modifications should be reviewed

Perioperative

- Anesthetics used must be carefully selected to avoid active metabolites and overdosing for renally eliminated drugs.
  - ○ Propofol is not significantly affected by renal impairment and is safe for use in reduced doses[62,63]
  - ○ Barbiturates, similarly, have unchanged pharmacokinetics but may have increased free barbiturate circulation because of decreased protein binding[61]
  - ○ Ketamine is minimally altered by CKD. However, it is known to have active

metabolites and has potential for accumulation. Be wary of its sympathomimetic effects, as CKD patients often have underlying cardiac disease
- o Benzodiazepines are metabolized in the liver but are eliminated renally
  - Diazepam has active metabolites and should be avoided
  - Short-acting midazolam in reduced dosage can be acceptable
  - Oral variants for presedation anxiolysis should be avoided, as they are unable to be titrated and could easily lead to oversedation
- o Common opioids in sedation are generally inactivated by the liver or by plasma esterases, and are safe in reduced dosage (fentanyl, alfentanil, remifentanil)[61]
  - Fentanyl is safe in reduced doses but approximately 7% is excreted unchanged by the kidneys, suggesting a potential for accumulation[62,63]
  - Meperidine and morphine have significant active metabolites, and can accumulate
- o Atropine and glycopyrrolate are eliminated by up to 50% in urine and have the potential for accumulation, therefore use in reduced doses if administration is necessary
- o Nitrous oxide is safe for this population, but administration is recommended at less than 50% to allow sufficient additional oxygen in the presence of anemia[62]
- Fluid administration should be carefully monitored; 250 mL is usually sufficient for short procedures.
  - o Lactated Ringer should be avoided, as it contains potassium (4 mEq/L)[61]
  - o Use of 5% dextrose or normal saline (0.9% NaCl) is preferable[61–63]
- Patients with CKD can often be volume overloaded; however, patients who receive dialysis can often be volume depleted as a result of aggressive therapy.
  - o Hypotension can be managed with judicious administration of fluid
- Moderate conscious sedation with good local anesthesia is recommended to limit exacerbation of cardiac or respiratory systems and to limit overall drug exposure/accumulation.
- There are no contraindications to the use of local anesthetics in patients with renal disease. However, dosages should be kept to a minimum owing to potential accumulation.

DEPRESSION
Background

Major depressive disorder is the most common psychiatric disorder, currently affecting between 2% and 4% of the population.[31,64] Physiologically, depression is thought to result from a decrease in serotonin and norepinephrine (NE) within the brain. However, the mechanism behind this deficiency and the resulting changes remain controversial.

The mainstay of treatment consists of pharmacotherapy and psychotherapy; however, some patients may benefit from electroconvulsive therapy. Pharmacotherapy for depression revolves around the modification of catecholamine or serotonin levels in the central nervous system.[31] Common antidepressants (**Table 17**) can be categorized by their mechanism of action, as follows: selective serotonin reuptake inhibitor (SSRI), monoamine oxidase (MAO) inhibitor, tricyclic antidepressant (TCA), and atypical antidepressant.

Serotonin syndrome is a potentially life-threatening reaction resulting from elevated levels of serotonin, usually caused by the interactions between multiple drugs that affect the production, release, or metabolism of serotonin. It is characterized by autonomic hyperactivity, neuromuscular abnormalities, and changes in mental status leading to tachycardia, hyperthermia, hypertension, mydriasis, diaphoresis, tremor/clonus, agitation, and delirium.[65,66] This potentially fatal syndrome can be caused by interactions between the common antidepressant classes (MAO inhibitors, SSRIs, TCAs) with medications used in outpatient sedation such as fentanyl, codeine, meperidine, ondansetron, and metoclopramide.[31,65]

Anesthetic Assessment

Preoperative

- Depression is usually not a contraindication for sedation; however, the medications used to treat the patient can interact with and potentiate medications commonly used.
- Laboratory tests or forms of test are not generally required for patients being treated for depression.
- A preoperative interview should ascertain the following:
  - o How long the patient has been on treatment
  - o Has the patient recently switched medications
  - o Does the patient take the medication as scheduled
  - o History of any side effects of the medication

Table 17
Antidepressant medications

Drug Class Generic Name	Mechanism of Action	Adverse Effects
Selective Serotonin Reuptake Inhibitors Fluoxetine Paroxetine Sertraline Citalopram Escitalopram Fluvoxamine	Block reuptake of serotonin from synaptic cleft	Few adrenergic, cholinergic, histaminergic, or dopaminergic effects[31] Associated with discontinuation syndrome and serotonin syndrome
Tricyclic Antidepressants Amitriptyline Nortriptyline Imipramine Trimipramine Doxepin Clomipramine Desipramine Nortriptyline Protriptyline	Block reuptake of serotonin and norepinephrine from synaptic cleft	Anticholinergic effects[31,66] (dry mouth, blurry vision, constipation, urinary retention, increased body temperature) Sedation Postural hypertension Discontinuation syndrome
Monoamine Oxidase Inhibitors Phenelzine Tranylcypromine Isocarboxazid Selegiline	Prevent breakdown of catecholamines and serotonin	Hypertension with sympathomimetics Orthostatic hypotension Sedation Serotonin syndrome

- Any interactions with other medications the patient has experienced
- Does medication cause drowsiness or sedation
- Patients who have been taking TCAs and MAO inhibitors should be queried for a history of palpitations, known arrhythmias, or orthostatic hypotension/syncopal episodes.
  - Avoid ketamine, ephedrine, and meperidine with TCAs and MAO inhibitors
  - Use local anesthetics containing epinephrine with caution
- Patients with a positive history for arrhythmias or postural hypotension/syncope may require an ECG and/or medical consult before sedation.

Perioperative

- Perioperative management is based around awareness of a patient's current regimen and any recent changes that have occurred.
- Most potential issues in this patient population come from drug interactions, which are listed in the aforementioned drug classes.
- Anesthetic agents should be titrated to effect, as most antidepressants produce some level

of sedation at baseline and the effects with sedatives can be synergistic.
  - Benzodiazepines and opioids should be administered in smaller doses to gauge response
- There is evidence that patients treated chronically with SSRIs or TCAs may potentiate the effects of propofol on NE and serotonin reuptake at the synapse, propagating its systemic effects and potentially causing disproportionate interaction.[67]

THYROID DISEASES
Background

Hypothyroidism

Hypothyroidism is more common in women than in men, and affects approximately 10% of adults older than 65 years.[21] Primary hypothyroidism can be a result of autoimmune disease such as Hashimoto thyroiditis or radioiodine therapy, whereas secondary hypothyroidism is the result of a dysfunctional pituitary axis.

The signs and symptoms of hypothyroidism are consistent with the far-reaching metabolic effects on the body. Symptoms include fatigue, cold intolerance, sleepiness, weight gain, deepening or hoarseness of the voice, and muscle aches.

Common signs consist of bradycardia in the resting range of 60 to 80 beats/min (compared with a normal range of 72–84), dry skin, coarse or brittle hair, edema (especially periorbital), and difficulty with memory and concentration.[21,68,69]

Physiologically, hypothyroidism is associated with decreased stroke volume and heart rate, resulting in decreased cardiac output. Peripheral vascular resistance is increased, and if left untreated can lead to reduced myocardial contractility, impaired baroreceptor function, decreased maximal breathing capacity, and decreased ventilatory response to hypercarbia and hypoxia.[21,68,70–72] Patients with hypothyroidism can be sensitive to anesthetics and medications because of decreased cardiac output, abnormal baroreceptor function, decreased hepatic metabolism, and decreased renal excretion.[21]

Levothyroxine (Levo-T4) is acceptable therapy for restoring levels of T3 and T4 for most patients, and consistent therapy can reverse or mitigate many of the systemic effects of hypothyroidism.

Hyperthyroidism

The overall incidence of hyperthyroidism in the United States is thought to be between 0.05% and 1.3%, and may be as high as 3% in patients older than 80 years.[68,73] The majority of cases are subclinical in presentation.[68,73] Usual causes include Graves disease, multinodular goiter, thyroid adenoma, or excessive exogenous thyroid hormones.

Common symptoms of hyperthyroidism consist of nervousness, fatigue, weakness, palpitations, heat intolerance, excessive sweating, dyspnea, diarrhea, insomnia, poor concentration, and oligomenorrhea. Signs consist of weight loss, hair loss, tachycardia, warm moist skin, hyperkinesis, exophthalmos, lid lag, emotional liability, hyperactive tendon reflexes, and, commonly, thyroid enlargement.[21,68]

Physiologically, hyperthyroidism is associated with hyperdynamic cardiac functioning, possibly due to an increased number of β receptors. The result is tachycardia, increased cardiac output, and profound hypertension.[21,72] In addition, disturbances in cardiac rhythm are frequent, with sinus tachycardia being the most common, but with a significantly increased occurrence of atrial fibrillation.[21,68,72,74]

Thyroid storm is a life-threatening exacerbation of hyperthyroidism and is a true medical emergency. Thyroid storm has been associated with administration of anesthesia and more commonly with the postanesthesia recovery period, and should be considered highly in the differential diagnosis of extreme anxiety, fever, tachycardia, cardiovascular instability, and prolonged recovery.

Treatment commonly consists of antithyroid medications such as methimazole and Propylthiouracil, which inhibit the synthesis of thyroid hormones. Symptoms are often controlled with a β-blocker such as propranolol, which controls the anxiety, tachycardia, and palpitations but also reduces the conversion of T4 to T3. Surgical treatments can include radioactive iodine and thyroidectomy. Patients can be left hypothyroid from both thyroidectomy and radioactive iodine treatment, depending on the extent of the gland removed or destroyed.

Anesthetic Management

Preoperative

- Patients with untreated, uncontrolled, or recently diagnosed thyroid disease are not candidates for outpatient sedation,[75] and warrant prompt medical evaluation.
  - Patients with diagnosed or suspected of having hypothyroidism or hyperthyroidism should be questioned regarding the degree of severity and the ability to control the condition
- Emergent surgery should take place with the collaboration of a dedicated anesthesia team.
- Patients who have recently begun treatment for hypothyroidism may see rapid improvement in many symptoms; however, physiologically they may not have returned to normal, so consider delaying procedures.
  - For example, decreased myocardial function and ventilatory drive takes 3 to 6 months to return to normal after treatment is initiated[21]
- Be cautious of patients with goiters, as there is a potential for airway obstruction and increased difficulty with intubation.
  - Patients may have persistent voice changes after surgery, owing to continued edema or paralysis of the vocal cords
- Laboratory studies are not usually necessary in well-controlled patients who are followed regularly by their physicians.
- Consider ECG and medical clearance in patients with arrhythmias including atrial fibrillation, as this can represent refractory hyperthyroidism.

Perioperative
Hypothyroidism
- Patients with hypothyroidism have increased sensitivity to anesthetics.[21]
  - Carefully titrate anesthetics to prevent excessive sedation

- Hypothyroid patients have a hypodynamic cardiovascular system, which can be unmasked by surgical stress and/or the cardiovascular depressant effects of anesthetic agents.[21]
  - The cardiovascular effects of hypothyroidism are generally reversed once patients are rendered euthyroid[72,76]
- There is evidence to suggest that patients rendered with subclinical hypothyroidism after treatment may have significant acceleration of cardiovascular disease.[77,78]
  - Treat this patient population as having CAD
- Avoid ketamine, atropine, and other medications that can increase the demand on the heart.
- Patients should maintain their perioperative dosing schedule, including morning doses even while NPO.

Hyperthyroidism

- Patients who have been euthyroid for at least 6 to 8 weeks have no contraindication for anesthesia.[21]
  - Those receiving propranolol should continue to receive their scheduled dose
- Persistent signs of increased adrenergic activity beyond that normally associated with surgery and the selected anesthetic technique can be managed with β-blockers such as propranolol, esmolol, metoprolol, and atenolol,[21] but should signal the termination of the surgery.
- Intraoperative hypotension can be managed with fluids, a decreased level of anesthesia, and phenylephrine if necessary.
- Avoid anticholinergic medications such as atropine and glycopyrrolate, as these drugs can precipitate a tachycardia and alter heat regulation.[21]
- Sympathetic nervous system stimulants such as ketamine, ephedrine, and epinephrine should be avoided.[21]
- There are no studies concerning local anesthesia with epinephrine in hyperthyroid patients; however, consider avoiding epinephrine in untreated or poorly controlled patients.
- Nitrous oxide, opioids, and benzodiazepines are generally considered safe for administration.[21]

OPIOID TOLERANCE AND ABUSE
Background

Opioid abuse rarely develops from the treatment of immediate postoperative surgical pain. Often, abuse of these drugs is due to their euphoric and analgesic effects.[31] Common routes of administration of opioids are oral, subcutaneous injection, or intravenous injection. Problems from opioid abuse include hepatitis, cellulitis, endocarditis, septic thrombophlebitis, malnutrition, AIDS, and transverse myelitis, among others.[31] Tolerance can develop to the analgesic, sedative, and euphoric effects of opioids, requiring higher concentrations of the drug. However, side effects such as miosis or constipation always remain. Often the tolerance to opioids can lead to opioid-induced hyperalgesia. The magnitude of the phenomenon of clinical opioid tolerance is controversial.[79]

Although withdrawal is rarely life threatening, one must watch out for symptoms in the postoperative setting. Withdrawal symptoms can include sympathetic overactivity (diaphoresis, mydriasis, hypertension, and tachycardia), lacrimation, piloerection, tremors, insomnia, abdominal cramps, and/or muscle spasms. Opioid dependence is often treated with methadone, levomethadyl, or buprenorphine (Subutex). Buprenorphine can be combined with the antagonist naloxone (Suboxone), which prevents patients from dissolving the tablets and using the drugs intravenously.

Anesthetic Management

Preoperative

- Patients on preoperative opioids or methadone should continue their prescribed dosages throughout the preoperative period.[79]
- A thorough history and physical examination should be obtained, specifically targeting any complications secondary to opioid abuse.

Perioperative

- Avoid any opioid agonist-antagonist or partial antagonist drugs, owing to concern for developing acute withdrawal.[31]
- Patients may have exaggerated postoperative pain, which needs to be managed.
  - Continue home dosages of methadone or opioids
  - Add appropriate narcotics and analgesics (nonsteroidal anti-inflammatory agents) for postoperative pain control
  - Give good local anesthetic and consider long-acting local anesthetics
  - Do not attempt to wean these patients during the perioperative period
  - Continue perioperative and postoperative pain adjuncts such as antidepressants or antianxiety medications[79]

- Benzodiazepines appear to be safe, and likely useful for amnesia and anxiolysis.[31]
- Ketamine can be a good choice, owing to the analgesia and effect on amnesia being nonopioid.[79]
- Propofol is also safe for amnesia; however, this patient subgroup can be cross-tolerant to central nervous system depressants.[31]
- Be wary of using intravenous opioids, as owing to tolerance patients may require excessive amounts, which can reach the level of unwanted effects such as respiratory depression.
- The pain specialist should be available for assistance during postoperative management.

REFERENCES

1. Matei V, Sami Haddadin A. Systemic and pulmonary arterial hypertension. In: Hines RL, Marschall KE, editors. Stoelting's anesthesia and co-existing disease. 6th edition. Philadelphia: Elsevier Saunders; 2012. p. 104–19.
2. Garg J, Messerli AW, Bakris GL. Evaluation and treatment of patients with systemic hypertension. Circulation 2002;105:2458–61.
3. Mizuno J, Kato S, Sato T, et al. Pre-anesthesia systolic blood pressure increases with age regardless of sex. J Anesth 2012;26(4):496–502.
4. Akhtar S. Ischemic heart disease. In: Hines RL, Marschall KE, editors. Stoelting's anesthesia and co-existing disease. 6th edition. Philadelphia: Elsevier Saunders; 2012. p. 1–30.
5. Servin FS. Is it time to re-evaluate the routines about stopping/keeping platelet inhibitors in conjunction to ambulatory surgery? Curr Opin Anaesthesiol 2010;23:691–6.
6. Fleisher LA, Beckman JA, Brown KA, et al. ACC/AHA 2007 guidelines on perioperative cardiovascular evaluation and care for noncardiac surgery: a report of the American College of Cardiology/American Heart Association Task Force on Practice Guidelines (Writing Committee to Revise the 2002 Guidelines on Perioperative Cardiovascular Evaluation for Noncardiac Surgery): developed in collaboration with the American Society of Echocardiography, American Society of Nuclear Cardiology, Heart Rhythm Society, Society of Cardiovascular Anesthesiologists, Society for Cardiovascular Angiography and Interventions, Society for Vascular Medicine and Biology, and Society for Vascular Surgery. Circulation 2007;116(17):e418–99.
7. Van Diermen DE, Aartman IH, Baart JA, et al. Dental management of patients using antithrombotic drugs: critical appraisal of existing guidelines. Oral Surg Oral Med Oral Pathol Oral Radiol Endod 2009;107:616–24.
8. Herrera A. Valvular heart disease. In: Hines RL, Marschall KE, editors. Stoelting's anesthesia and co-existing disease. 6th edition. Philadelphia: Elsevier Saunders; 2012. p. 31–47.
9. Wilson W, Taubert KA, Gewitz M, et al. Prevention of infective endocarditis: guidelines from the American Heart Association: a guideline from the American Heart Association Rheumatic Fever, Endocarditis, and Kawasaki Disease Committee, Council on Cardiovascular Disease in the Young, and the Council on Clinical Cardiology, Council on Cardiovascular Surgery and Anesthesia, and the Quality of Care and Outcomes Research Interdisciplinary Working Group. Circulation 2007;116(15):1736–54.
10. Popescu WM. Heart failure and cardiomyopathies. In: Hines RL, Marschall KE, editors. Stoelting's anesthesia and co-existing disease. 6th edition. Philadelphia: Elsevier Saunders; 2012. p. 120–43.
11. Becker DE. Preoperative medical evaluation: part 1: general principles and cardiovascular considerations. Anesth Prog 2009;56:92–103.
12. Watson KT. Abnormalities of cardiac conduction and cardiac rhythm. In: Hines RL, Marschall KE, editors. Stoelting's anesthesia and co-existing disease. 6th edition. Philadelphia: Elsevier Saunders; 2012. p. 73–103.
13. American Society of Anesthesiologists Task Force on Perioperative Management of Patients with Cardiac Rhythm Management Devices. Practice advisory for the perioperative management of patients with cardiac rhythm management devices: pacemakers and implantable cardioverter-defibrillators: a report by the American Society of Anesthesiologists Task Force on Perioperative Management of Patients with Cardiac Rhythm Management Devices. Anesthesiology 2005;103:186–98.
14. Joshi GP. Perioperative management of outpatients with implantable cardioverter defibrillators. Curr Opin Anaesthesiol 2009;22(6):701–4.
15. Al-Ruzzeh S, Kurup V. Respiratory diseases. In: Hines RL, Marschall KE, editors. Stoelting's anesthesia and co-existing disease. 6th edition. Philadelphia: Elsevier Saunders; 2012. p. 181–217.
16. Dones F, Foresta G, Russotto V. Update on perioperative management of the child with asthma. Pediatr Rep 2012;4(2):e19.
17. Becker DE. Preoperative medical evaluation: part 2: pulmonary, endocrine, renal, and miscellaneous considerations. Anesth Prog 2009;56:135–45.
18. Joshi GP, Ankichetty SP, Gan TJ, et al. Special article: society for ambulatory anesthesia consensus statement on preoperative selection of adult patients with obstructive sleep apnea scheduled for ambulatory surgery. Anesth Analg 2012;115(5):1060–8.

19. Susarla SM, Abramson ZR, Dodson TB, et al. Cephalometric measurement of upper airway length correlates with the presence and severity of obstructive sleep apnea. J Oral Maxillofac Surg 2010;68:2846–55.

20. Ankichetty S, Chung F. Considerations for patients with obstructive sleep apnea undergoing ambulatory surgery. Curr Opin Anaesthesiol 2011;24(6): 605–11.

21. Wall RT III. Endocrine disease. Chapter 19. In: Hines RL, Marschall KE, editors. Stoelting's anesthesia and co-existing disease. 6th edition. Philadelphia: Elsevier Saunders; 2012. p. 376–406.

22. Joshi GP, Chung F, Vann MA, et al. Society for Ambulatory Anesthesia consensus statement on perioperative blood glucose management in diabetic patients undergoing ambulatory surgery. Anesth Analg 2010;111(6):1378–87.

23. Candiotti K, Sharma S, Shankar R. Obesity, obstructive sleep apnoea, and diabetes mellitus: anaesthetic implications. Br J Anaesth 2009; 103(Suppl 1):i23–30.

24. Hevesi ZG, Hannaman M. Diseases of the liver and biliary tract. In: Hines RL, Marschall KE, editors. Stoelting's anesthesia and co-existing disease. 6th edition. Philadelphia: Elsevier Saunders; 2012. p. 274–86.

25. Hoetzel A, Ryan H, Scmidth R. Anesthetic considerations for the patient with liver disease. Curr Opin Anaesthesiol 2012;25:340–7.

26. Bamji N, Cohen LB. Endoscopic sedation of patients with chronic liver disease. Clin Liver Dis 2010;14(2):185–94.

27. Tantawy H, Mysaljek T. Diseases of the gastrointestinal system. In: Hines RL, Marschall KE, editors. Stoelting's anesthesia and co-existing disease. 6th edition. Philadelphia: Elsevier Saunders; 2012. p. 287–304.

28. American Society of Anesthesiologists Committee. Practice guidelines for preoperative fasting and the use of pharmacologic agents to reduce the risk of pulmonary aspiration: application to healthy patients undergoing elective procedures: an updated report by the American Society of Anesthesiologists Committee on Standards and Practice Parameters. Anesthesiology 2011;114(3):495–511.

29. Albright BE, Popescu WM. Nutritional diseases: obesity and malnutrition. In: Hines RL, Marschall KE, editors. Stoelting's anesthesia and co-existing disease. 6th edition. Philadelphia: Elsevier Saunders; 2012. p. 314–34.

30. Ng A, Smith G. Gastroesophageal reflux and aspiration of gastric contents in anesthetic practice. Anesth Analg 2001;93(2):494–513.

31. Hines RL, Marschall KE. Psychiatric disease, substance abuse, and drug overdose. Chapter 25. In: Hines RL, Marschall KE, editors. Stoelting's anesthesia and co-existing disease. 6th edition. Philadelphia: Elsevier Saunders; 2012. p. 533–57.

32. Granite EL, Farber NJ, Adler P. Parameters for treatment of cocaine-positive patients. J Oral Maxillofac Surg 2007;65(10):1984–9.

33. Miller CS, Little JW, Falace DA. Supplemental corticosteroids for dental patients with adrenal insufficiency: reconsideration of the problem. J Am Dent Assoc 2001;132(11):1570–9.

34. Marik PE, Varon J. Requirement of perioperative stress doses of corticosteroids: a systematic review of the literature. Arch Surg 2008;143(12): 1222–6.

35. Yong SL, Marik P, Esposito M, et al. Supplemental perioperative steroids for surgical patients with adrenal insufficiency. Cochrane Database Syst Rev 2009;(4):CD005367.

36. Shannon I, Isbell G, Prigmore J, et al. Stress in dental patients, II: the serum free 17-hydroxycorticosteroid response in routinely appointed patients undergoing simple exodontias. Oral Surg Oral Med Oral Pathol 1962;15:1142–6.

37. Banks P. The adreno-cortical response to oral surgery. Br J Oral Surg 1970;8:32–44.

38. Desborough JP. The stress response to trauma and surgery. Br J Anaesth 2000;85:109–17.

39. Salem M, Tainsh R, Bromberg J, et al. Perioperative glucocorticoid coverage: a reassessment 42 years after emergence of a problem. Ann Surg 1994;4: 416–25.

40. Glowniak J, Loriaux D. A double-blind study of perioperative steroid requirements in secondary adrenal insufficiency. Surgery 1997;121:123–9.

41. Thomason JM, Girdler NM, Kendall-Taylor P, et al. An investigation into the need for supplementary steroids in organ transplant patients undergoing gingival surgery: a double-blind, split-mouth, crossover study. J Clin Periodontol 1999;26(9): 577–82.

42. Udelsman R, Ramp J, Gallucci WT, et al. Adaptation during surgical stress. A reevaluation of the role of glucocorticoids. J Clin Invest 1986;77(4): 1377–81.

43. Knake S, Hamer HM, Rosenow F. Status epilepticus: a critical review. Epilepsy Behav 2009;15(1): 10–4.

44. Perks A, Cheema S, Mohanraj R. Anaesthesia and epilepsy. Br J Anaesth 2012;108(4):562–71.

45. Nair D. Neurology: epilepsy. Section 10. In: Carey WD, editor. Cleveland clinic: current clinical medicine. 2nd edition. Philadelphia: Saunders/ Elsevier; 2010. p. 883–7.

46. Berg AT, Berkovic SF, Brodie MJ, et al. Revised terminology and concepts for organization of seizures

and epilepsies: report of the ILAE Commission on Classification and Terminology, 2005-2009. Epilepsia 2010;51(4):676–85.

47. Dhir A, Rogawski MA. Role of neurosteroids in the anticonvulsant activity of midazolam. Br J Pharmacol 2012;165(8):2684–91.

48. Auta J, Costa E, Davis JM, et al. Imidazenil: an antagonist of the sedative but not the anticonvulsant action of diazepam. Neuropharmacology 2005;49(3):425–9.

49. Yi J, Torres J, Azner Y, et al. Flumazenil pretreatment in benzodiazepine-free patients: a novel method for managing declining ECT seizure quality. J ECT 2012;28(3):185–9.

50. Frey HH. Interactions between morphine-like analgesics and anticonvulsant drugs. Pharmacol Toxicol 1987;60(3):210–3.

51. Czuczwar SJ, Frey HH. Effect of morphine and morphine-like analgesics on susceptibility to seizures in mice. Neuropharmacology 1986;25(5):465–9.

52. Lauretti GR, Ahmad I, Pleuvry BJ. The activity of opioid analgesics in seizure models utilizing N-methyl-DL-aspartic acid, kainic acid, bicuculline and pentylenetetrazole. Neuropharmacology 1994;33(2):155–60.

53. Yillar DO, Akkan AG, Akcasu A, et al. The effect of oral and subcutaneous meperidine on the maximal electroshock seizure (MES) in mice. J Basic Clin Physiol Pharmacol 2009;20:159–68.

54. Ahmad I, Pleuvry BJ. Interactions between opioid drugs and propofol in laboratory models of seizures. Br J Anaesth 1995;74(3):311–4.

55. Galvin GM, Jelinek GA. Midazolam: an effective intravenous agent for seizure control. Arch Emerg Med 1987;4(3):169–72.

56. Vaidya PV, Anderson EL, Bobb A, et al. A within-subject comparison of propofol and methohexital anesthesia for electroconvulsive therapy. J ECT 2012;28(1):14–9.

57. Myslobodsky MS, Golovchinsky V, Mintz M. Ketamine: convulsant or anti-convulsant? Pharmacol Biochem Behav 1981;14:27–33.

58. Taylor S. Electroconvulsive therapy: a review of history, patient selection, technique, and medication management. South Med J 2007;100(5):494–8.

59. Pasternak JJ, Laier WL Jr. Diseases affecting the brain. Chapter 10. In: Hines RL, Marschall KE, editors. Stoelting's anesthesia and co-existing disease. 6th edition. Philadelphia: Saunders; 2012. p. 218–54.

60. Patsalos PN, Perucca E. Clinically important drug interactions in epilepsy: general features and interaction between antiepileptic drugs. Lancet Neurol 2003;2:347–56.

61. Morgan GE Jr, Mikhail MS, Murray MJ. Anesthesia for patients with renal disease. Chapter 32. In: Morgan GE Jr, Mikhail MS, Murray MJ, editors. Clinical anesthesiology. 4th edition. New York: McGraw-Hill; 2006.

62. Holt N. Renal disease. Chapter 17. In: Hines RL, Marschall KE, editors. Stoelting's anesthesia and co-existing disease. 6th edition. Philadelphia: Saunders; 2012. p. 334–56.

63. Trainor D, Borthwick E, Ferguson A. Perioperative management of the hemodialysis patient. Semin Dial 2011;24(3):314–26.

64. Maurizio F, Cassano P. Mood disorders: major depressive disorder and dysthymic disorder. Chapter 29. In: Stern TA, Rosenbaum JF, Maurizio F, et al, editors. Massachusetts General Hospital comprehensive clinical psychiatry. Philadelphia: Mosby; 2008.

65. Ward MC, Garlow S. Mood and anxiety disorders. Chapter 225. In: McKean SC, Ross JJ, Dressler DD, et al, editors. Principles and practice of hospital medicine. New York: McGraw-Hill; 2012. p. 1875–89.

66. Schellander R, Donnerer J. Antidepressants: clinically relevant drug interactions to be considered. Pharmacology 2010;86(4):203–15.

67. Zhao Y, Sun L. Antidepressants modulate the in vitro inhibitory effects of propofol and ketamine on norepinephrine and serotonin transporter function. J Clin Neurosci 2008;15(11):1264–9.

68. Skugor M, Fleseriu M. Endocrinology: hypothyroidism and hyperthyroidism. Section 4. In: Carey WD, editor. Cleveland Clinic: current clinical medicine. 2nd edition. Philadelphia: Saunders/Elsevier; 2010. p. 416–9.

69. Klein I, Ojamaa K. Thyroid hormone and the cardiovascular system. N Engl J Med 2001;344(7):501–9.

70. Fazio S, Palmieri EA, Lombardi G, et al. Effects of thyroid hormone on the cardiovascular system. Recent Prog Horm Res 2004;59:31–50.

71. Dörr M, Völzke H. Cardiovascular morbidity and mortality in thyroid dysfunction. Minerva Endocrinol 2005;30(4):199–216.

72. Klein I, Danzi S. Thyroid disease and the heart. Circulation 2007;116:1725–35.

73. Schraga ED. Hyperthyroidism, thyroid storm, and Graves disease. 2006. Available at: http://www.emedicine.com/emerg/topic269.htm. Accessed November 21, 2012.

74. Cappola AR, Fried LP, Arnold AM, et al. Thyroid status, cardiovascular risk, and mortality in older adults. JAMA 2006;295(9):1033–41.

75. Murkin JM. Anesthesia and hypothyroidism: a review of thyroxine physiology, pharmacology, and anesthetic implications. Anesth Analg 1982;61(4):371–83.

76. Palmieri EA, Fazio S, Lombardi G, et al. Subclinical hypothyroidism and cardiovascular risk: a reason to treat? Treat Endocrinol 2004;3(4):233–44.

77. Becker C. Hypothyroidism and atherosclerotic heart disease: pathogenesis, medical management, and the role of coronary artery bypass surgery. Endocr Rev 1985;6(3):432–40.

78. Ochs N, Auer R, Bauer DC, et al. Meta-analysis: subclinical thyroid dysfunction and the risk for coronary heart disease and mortality. Ann Intern Med 2008;148(11):832–45.

79. Gordon D, Intrurrisi CE, Greensmith JE, et al. Perioperative pain management in the opioid-tolerant individual. J Pain 2008;9(5):383–7.

Pharmacology of Intravenous Sedative/Anesthetic Medications Used in Oral Surgery

Joseph A. Giovannitti Jr, DMD

KEYWORDS

- Total intravenous anesthesia (TIVA) • Pharmacology of sedative/anesthetic drugs
- Emergence delirium • Dental sedation

KEY POINTS

- Total intravenous anesthesia (TIVA) is a technique whose time has come because of the advent of ultra–short-acting drugs and computerized infusion technology.
- Patients may be sedated to any desired level, maintained there for indefinite periods, and recovered to near baseline within minutes.
- Future trends in TIVA may include patient-controlled sedation, whereby patients sedate themselves with an infusion device similar to those used for postoperative analgesia.
- The future may also bring titration of sedatives to target blood levels, leading to more precise dosing and greater efficiency.

INTRODUCTION

Patients have historically been considered to be in a state of general anesthesia when the following parameters were met: unconsciousness, analgesia, amnesia, immobility, and attenuation of the autonomic response to noxious stimulation. This was, and is, accomplished easily by the inhalation of potent halogenated hydrocarbons such as isoflurane, sevoflurane, and desflurane. In the past, when inhalational anesthesia was not desired or was contraindicated, a balanced technique was advocated using various intravenous drugs to achieve the desired level of anesthesia. The evolution of total intravenous anesthesia (TIVA) began when Stanley Drummond-Jackson, using methohexital in the UK, and Adrian Hubbell, using sodium pentothal in the United States, first used incremental boluses of these drugs to produce unconsciousness for dental surgery. These introductions were followed by the introduction of intravenous drug combinations to produce sedation by Niels Jorgensen, Leonard Monheim, and C. Richard Bennett. With the advent of designer medications and sophisticated computer-aided technologies and monitoring, TIVA has come into its own. During TIVA, each individual agent is typically selected for its ability to achieve a particular parameter of general anesthesia. Drugs such as propofol are used to induce and maintain unconsciousness, opioids are used for analgesia, benzodiazepines are selected for their amnestic qualities, and muscle relaxants produce immobility. The classic induction agents, thiopental and methohexital, have been largely supplanted by propofol as the primary agent for the production and maintenance of unconsciousness. Adjunctive agents such as fentanyl,

Department of Dental Anesthesiology, Center for Patients with Special Needs, University of Pittsburgh School of Dental Medicine, 3501 Terrace Street, G-89 Salk Hall, Pittsburgh, PA 15261, USA
E-mail address: jag74@pitt.edu

Oral Maxillofacial Surg Clin N Am 25 (2013) 439–451
http://dx.doi.org/10.1016/j.coms.2013.03.004

oralmaxsurgery.theclinics.com

remifentanil, midazolam, ketamine, and dexmedetomidine are used for analgesia, amnesia, immobility, and attenuation of the autonomic stress response. This article highlights these drugs, explores the rationale for their use, and discusses their clinical usefulness in an office-based setting.

THIOPENTAL

Thiopental is an ultra–short-acting thiobarbiturate first introduced into clinical practice by Dr Ralph Waters in 1934 (**Fig. 1**). Its use ushered in the age of intravenous anesthesia. It is the prototypical intravenous induction agent against which all others are compared. Although currently no longer being manufactured, it is necessary to understand its pharmacology to understand the rationale for the use of induction agents and their evolution into drugs that are now used for induction and maintenance of anesthesia via continuous infusion techniques. Until it was supplanted by propofol in popularity and usefulness, thiopental was the standard intravenous induction agent for general anesthesia for years. Despite its widespread use, it had detractors. After the attack on Pearl Harbor, thiopental was maligned as "the ideal form of euthanasia in war surgery"[1] because of its propensity to produce cardiovascular collapse in extremely hypovolemic patients. More recently, thiopental was part of the regimen for lethal injection executions in the United States. Hospira (Lake Forest, IL), the sole manufacturer of thiopental, removed the drug from the market when the government of Italy (where thiopental was produced) demanded that Hospira guarantee that thiopental would not be used for lethal injection. This development prompted the company to halt manufacture of the drug.[2]

Mechanism of Action

Many of the pharmacologic effects of barbiturates closely resemble the effects of benzodiazepines. Barbiturates enhance gamma-aminobutyric acid (GABA)–activated chloride ion channel opening by acting at specific barbiturate binding sites on the $GABA_A$ receptor complex, leading to hyperpolarization and decreased neuronal firing.[3] Barbiturates also act directly on the chloride channel,

not requiring the presence of GABA. These actions produce what is known as barbiturate anesthesia and may explain the lower margin of safety and steeper dose-response curve relative to benzodiazepines.

Pharmacologic Effects

Thiopental rapidly achieves therapeutic plasma concentrations and can induce unconsciousness within 15 to 30 seconds. After a single intravenous induction dose of 4 mg/kg, the clinical duration of effect is between 20 and 30 minutes. Because thiopental is highly lipid soluble, it has the ability to enter tissues at a rate proportional to blood flow. The vessel-rich group, which includes the brain, receives the highest proportion of the cardiac output relative to body mass (**Fig. 2**). Thus it achieves the highest concentration of thiopental following intravenous injection, and its effects are exerted almost immediately. Redistribution to the more poorly perfused tissues such as muscle, and later fat, results in a rapid decline in the concentration of the drug, which terminates the effect. Because the drug accumulates in fatty tissue, especially after repeated administration or continuous infusion, the clinical duration and recovery time may be prolonged in obese patients.

Cardiovascular Effects

Peripheral vasodilation is the primary effect of an induction dose of thiopental. This dose is usually accompanied by a reflex increase in heart rate. Mean arterial pressure may be unchanged or slightly diminished. Further myocardial depression occurs with higher doses, and blood pressure may decrease precipitously. Hypovolemic patients are especially susceptible to profound hypotension and cardiovascular collapse.

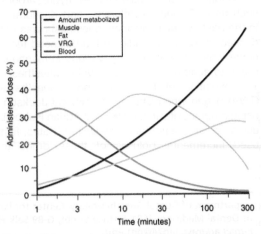

Fig. 2. Thiopental distribution in different tissues. VRG, vessel rich group.

Thiopental Sodium
$C_{11}H_{17}N_2NaO_2S$

Fig. 1. Thiopental, the prototypical induction agent.

Respiratory Effects

Thiopental produces dose-dependent respiratory depression via decreased minute ventilation. Both tidal volume and respiratory rate are decreased, and apnea ensues, especially in the presence of other respiratory-depressant drugs. Airway reflex activity may be increased with a predisposition to coughing and laryngospasm.

Other Effects

Thiopental is an anticonvulsant and can be used to treat patients with status epilepticus. It also reduces cerebral blood flow, intracranial pressure, and cerebral metabolic rate. It is hyperalgesic, and patients may exhibit heightened responses to pain stimulation. Analgesics must be given concurrently with barbiturates to ensure adequate increase of the pain threshold. Thiopental is highly alkaline and care must be taken to ensure that the drug is only given intravenously. Extravasation into the tissues may result in tissue necrosis, and intra-arterial injection results in severe vasospasm. Thiopental also releases histamine, which may produce hives, urticaria, edema, and bronchospasm. An interesting, but common, effect of thiopental is the perception of a garlic or onion taste after the drug has been administered.

Contraindications

Patients with chronic obstructive lung disease or difficult airway predictors are adversely affected after thiopental administration. Thiopental produces profound hypotension and circulatory collapse in patients with cardiac instability or hemorrhagic shock. Because thiopental releases histamine, it is contraindicated in patients with status asthmaticus and in patients with poorly controlled asthma. Barbiturates are absolutely contraindicated in cases of acute intermittent porphyria. They stimulate the formation of D-aminolevulinic acid synthetase, leading to the accumulation of porphyrins and porphyrin precursors, and an acute exacerbation of the disease.

METHOHEXITAL

Methohexital is an ultra–short-acting oxybarbiturate similar in effect to thiopental, but approximately 2.5 times as potent and much shorter acting. An induction dose of 1 to 2 mg/kg rapidly produces unconsciousness for 5 to 7 minutes. Rapid redistribution is responsible for its abrupt termination of action. Advantages compared with thiopental include a more rapid recovery and clearance, no histamine release, less accumulation and saturation of peripheral tissues, and a more favorable context-sensitive half-time, making it suitable for maintenance of anesthesia via continuous infusion. An infusion of 50 to 150 µg/kg/min for a short-duration procedure lasting 60 minutes or less produces a recovery comparable with a similar propofol infusion. Thus, methohexital is more suitable for outpatient procedures than thiopental. The major disadvantage of methohexital is the frequency of excitatory phenomena such as coughing, hiccoughing, tremors and twitching, heightened airway reflexes, and laryngospasm. Methohexital is also associated with pain on injection and phlebitis. Despite these adverse effects, methohexital was the mainstay of anesthesia for oral surgery for decades, given either as a full induction dose or as an incremental bolus to deepen the level of sedation as needed. Methohexital has been supplanted by propofol for dental sedation and anesthesia. However, with the frequent drug shortages, it benefits the practitioner to become familiar with this drug if and when a backup medication becomes necessary.

PROPOFOL

Propofol is a 2,6-diisopropylphenol anesthetic drug available in several generic forms and the brand name Diprivan (APP Pharmaceuticals, Schaumberg, IL). Propofol is the most commonly used intravenous anesthetic, producing unconsciousness within 40 seconds after a single induction dose of 2 to 2.5 mg/kg, followed by a rapid recovery with minimal postoperative confusion. It is formulated in an oil-in-water emulsion containing soybean oil, glycerol, and egg lecithin and has a characteristic milky white appearance. This preparation has the potential to become a culture medium for bacterial growth, so any unused portion must be discarded 6 hours after puncturing the vial to prevent sepsis.

Mechanism of Action

Propofol is an N-methyl-D-aspartate (NMDA) receptor inhibitor and an agonist at the β_1 subunit of the GABA$_A$ receptor. Its termination of activity is similar to thiopental in that it is rapidly redistributed (distribution half-life 2–4 minutes), resulting in rapid recovery following induction or maintenance doses. It is metabolized in the liver (elimination half-life 3–12 hours), but the clearance of propofol exceeds liver blood flow, suggesting some extrahepatic metabolism. Other effects of propofol include pain on injection, amnesia, and possibly some antiemetic effects. It has a favorable context-sensitive half-time, which makes it ideal for maintenance of deep sedation or general anesthesia via continuous infusion.

Cardiovascular Effects

Propofol has some cardiovascular effects, specifically a reduction in stroke volume and peripheral vasodilation that may produce a significant decrease in systemic blood pressure. There is no compensatory increase in heart rate, as seen with thiopental. It therefore should be used with caution in the elderly or hypovolemic patient, or those with limited cardiac reserve.

Respiratory Effects

Propofol is a potent respiratory depressant, producing a significant reduction in tidal volume and apnea in 30% of patients following an induction dose. Unlike thiopental, propofol does not release histamine and may be used safely in asthmatic patients. Propofol does not promote airway hyperactivity, making patients less susceptible to laryngospasm compared with thiopental and methohexital. Propofol is useful in deepening sedation levels to aid in the management of laryngospasm.

Other Effects

Propofol is known for its amnestic and antiemetic properties. Propofol acts as an antiemetic during administration and may be helpful in the intraoperative management of patients with a significant history of postoperative nausea and vomiting. It is also useful as a treatment modality for patients who are actively nauseated in the immediate recovery period.

Propofol causes pain during injection, which can vary from mild to severe. The drug irritates the venous intima and activates the kallikrein-kinin system to increase bradykinin production. Pain on injection may be attenuated by slowly injecting the drug into a large vein, rapidly flushing with intravenous fluid, and the prior administration of intravenous lidocaine. However, to be effective, lidocaine should be held for a time within the vein before being released into the systemic circulation. Injecting lidocaine while the tourniquet is still applied, waiting for a few minutes, and then releasing the tourniquet before the administration of propofol may accomplish this.

Propofol infusion syndrome has been reported in critically ill patients undergoing prolonged sedation with propofol. Its features include rhabdomyolysis, severe metabolic acidosis, and renal and cardiac failure.[4] It has most often appeared in pediatric patients, but has also more recently been reported in adults. Propofol infusion syndrome is a multifactorial process with critical neurologic or inflammatory illnesses and prolonged propofol infusions as initiating factors, and concomitant catecholamine and glucocorticoid administration as triggering factors. The syndrome may manifest with infusions of more than 5 mg/kg/h for a period of more than 48 hours.

There has been concern that propofol should not be used in patients with egg allergy because of its formulation containing egg lecithin. The package insert for Diprivan states that the drug "is contraindicated in patients with allergies to eggs, egg products, soybeans or soy products."[5] However, a review of allergic reactions during anesthesia by Hepner and Castells[6] reveals that the incidence of propofol allergy during anesthesia is 1:60,000, and the cause is likely to be the presence of isopropyl groups and/or phenols, not egg or soy allergies. In addition, most patients with egg allergy are allergic to the protein, ovalbumin, found in egg whites. Egg lecithin, found in egg yolks, has a low allergic potential and its formulation in propofol is highly purified. Lizaso and colleagues[7] reported that skin-prick and intradermal testing with propofol and its lipid vehicle were negative in 25 patients with documented egg allergy. Current evidence suggests that patients with an egg allergy are no more likely to develop anaphylaxis than the nonallergic population when exposed to propofol.

ETOMIDATE

Etomidate is a short-acting intravenous anesthetic, chemically unrelated to other intravenous induction agents. It is similar pharmacokinetically to thiopental, but with less respiratory depression and minimal cardiovascular effect. Therefore, it is used primarily for induction of anesthesia (0.2–0.6 mg/kg) in patients in whom hypotension cannot be tolerated. It maintains hemodynamic stability and does not release histamine, making it the drug of choice for induction of anesthesia in hypovolemic patients or those with cardiopulmonary compromise. A severe side effect is the inhibition of steroidogenesis, making it unsuitable for prolonged maintenance administration. This effect may even occur following induction doses, which could potentially impair the patient's ability to respond appropriately to stress. The potential for this side effect severely limits the routine use of etomidate. Other disruptive effects of etomidate include a high incidence of nausea and vomiting, pain and phlebitis on injection, hiccough, and disruptive myoclonic movements.

OPIOIDS

Thomas Sydenham, a physician deemed the English Hippocrates, once profoundly asserted that, "Among the remedies which it has pleased Almighty God to give to man to relieve his sufferings, none is so universal and so efficacious as opium." Opioids have the ability to relieve pain, produce sedation and euphoria, alter the mood, attenuate the cardiovascular stress response, and coincidentally produce profound respiratory depression. The primary site of opioid activity occurs in the central nervous system (CNS) and the gut. Since 1973, it has been known that the activation of opioid-specific receptors in these areas is responsible for the pharmacologic actions of opioids (**Box 1**). The CNS effects include analgesia and sedation, changes in mood, and mental clouding. Opioids attenuate all types of pain regardless of origin or intensity, increase the pain threshold, and alter the affective response to pain. Gastrointestinal (GI) effects include decreased GI motility, which may produce constipation and delayed gastric emptying. This effect could potentially alter the patient's nil-by-mouth status. Opioids stimulate the chemoreceptor trigger zone and may produce nausea and vomiting. Esophageal sphincter tone is reduced, which may lead to vomiting and aspiration during anesthesia. Opioids may also increase biliary duct pressure and sphincter of Oddi tone and produce severe epigastric or abdominal pain in susceptible individuals.

Cardiovascular Effects

Opioids are generally accepted to promote cardiovascular and hemodynamic stability and are important in attenuating the cardiovascular response to surgical stress. A μ-receptor–mediated modulation of the hypothalamic-pituitary-adrenal axis reduces may prevent adrenocorticotropic hormone release, resulting in decreased sympathetic tone.[8] Opioids may also act directly on the vagal nuclei and inhibit the SA-node to produce bradycardia in most cases. These effects may produce hypotension in some individuals. Histamine-releasing opioids such as morphine and meperidine may also produce postural hypotensive changes secondary to peripheral vasodilation.

Respiratory Effects

Opioids are primary and continuous depressants of respiration through a direct and dose-dependent depression of the medullary respiratory center. Respiratory rate is slowed more in proportion to decreases in tidal volume. The net effect is a significant reduction in minute ventilation. Opioids obtund the respiratory center's hypercapnic response, diminishing the patient's drive to breathe as carbon dioxide levels increase. Thus, opioid-sensitive patients, or those receiving high doses, may become apneic even while conscious, but may breathe on command. Respiratory depression with opioids may be further enhanced by the administration of high doses, the concomitant administration of other CNS-depressant drugs, and in sensitive patients such as the elderly or those with severe renal disease.

Opioids depress upper airway reflexes and may be valuable in reducing the coughing spasms sometimes seen during the sedation of patients with reactive airway disease. They also may be helpful in attenuating laryngeal and bronchoconstrictive reflexes.

Other Effects

In addition to the effects of GI immobility and nausea and vomiting mentioned earlier, opioids exert a variety of ancillary effects. For example, opioids alone have minimal effect on intracranial pressure, but, in instances of closed head injury or with severe opioid-induced respiratory

---

Box 1
Opioid receptors and their actions

- μ1
  - Analgesia (supraspinal, spinal)
  - Miosis
  - Urinary retention
  - Nausea and vomiting
  - Pruritus
- μ2
  - Sedation
  - Respiratory depression
  - GI motility decrease
- σ
  - Dysphoria
  - Psychotomimesis
- δ
  - Analgesia (supraspinal, spinal)
  - Alterations of affective behavior
- κ
  - Analgesia (supraspinal, spinal)
  - Sedation
  - GI motility decrease
  - Psychotomimesis

The primary site of opioid activity is in the CNS and bowel.

depression, intracranial pressure increases with hypercapnia.

All opioids are capable of increasing skeletal muscle tone; however, this phenomenon is most often associated with the rapid administration of high doses of fentanyl, sufentanil, and remifentanil. Chest wall rigidity results in decreased lung compliance, decreased functional residual capacity, and vocal cord closure, which makes ventilation difficult and increases the risk of hypoxemia. Chest wall rigidity should be immediately recognized, and, if ventilation is difficult, muscle relaxation or reversal should be considered. The concomitant administration of benzodiazepines may help prevent rigidity.

A clinical sign of opioid use is pupillary constriction. This effect is mediated through the Edinger-Westphal nucleus of the occulomotor nerve, and is pathognomonic of their use. However, opioids do not increase intraocular pressure, and can prevent increases in intraocular pressure during intubation.[9]

Allergic reactions to opioids are rare. Most allergiclike reactions to opioids are related to the histamine-releasing drugs such as morphine and meperidine. Typical wheal and flare reactions may be noticed, especially along the vein as the drug travels centrally. Dilation of cutaneous blood vessels in the face, neck, and thorax is common, producing flushing and redness that may mimic an allergic response. Histamine release is also associated with pruritus; however, non–histamine-releasing opioids can produce itching as well. Facial itching is common and can be severe enough to be disruptive to dental surgery. The mechanism of facial itching is not known, but mediation through μ-receptors has been proposed.[10]

MORPHINE

Morphine is the prototypical opioid with which all other opioids are compared (**Table 1**). Once an integral part of a sedation regimen for prolonged procedures, morphine has no application in modern TIVA procedures. Its main usefulness is

in acute pain management. Although a dose of 10 mg (0.1 mg/kg) provides optimal pain relief, the dose should be titrated intravenously to effect following anesthesia in the immediate postoperative period. The onset of morphine is slow: 5 to 10 minutes following intravenous administration and up to 20 minutes following intramuscular injection. It produces analgesia, euphoria, and sedation lasting from 2 to 4 hours. Its use may be limited by side effects such as histamine release, postural hypotension, and nausea and vomiting.

MEPERIDINE

Meperidine is the prototype of the phenylpiperidine series of opioids, which includes fentanyl, sufentanil, alfentanil, and remifentanil (**Fig. 3**). For years meperidine was the mainstay of intravenous sedation regimens for procedures of all durations. It has a more rapid onset than morphine, within 3 minutes following intravenous administration, making it more easily titratable than morphine. It is 10 times less potent than morphine, producing sedation and analgesia lasting 45 to 90 minutes. Meperidine was first investigated as an atropine-like agent and is unique among opioids in that it may produce tachycardia and drying of secretions. It also releases histamine, and may produce orthostatic hypotension with rapid position change. Severe asthma is a relative contraindication. Other side effects include dysphoria, especially in the absence of pain, and nausea and vomiting. Meperidine is associated with increased neuronal activity that may result in CNS excitation. Its metabolite, normeperidine, is twice as potent as meperidine in producing CNS excitation and convulsions. Meperidine is contraindicated in patients taking monoamine oxidase inhibitors because concentrations of normeperidine are increased with these drugs.

Although meperidine is still used on a limited basis for dental sedation, its main use is currently in the management of postanesthetic shivering. Opioids in general reduce thermoregulation thresholds similarly to potent inhalational agents.

Table 1
Comparative effects of commonly used opioids in oral surgery

	Meperidine	Morphine	Fentanyl	Sufentanil	Alfentanil	Remifentanil
Comparative potency	0.1	1	75–125	500–1000	10–25	250
Peak Effect (min)	5–7	20–30	3–5	3–5	1.5–2	1.5–2
Duration (h)	2–3	3–4	0.5–1	0.5–1	0.2–0.3	0.1–0.2
Half-life (h)	3–4	2–4	1.5–6	2.5–3	1–2	0.15–0.3

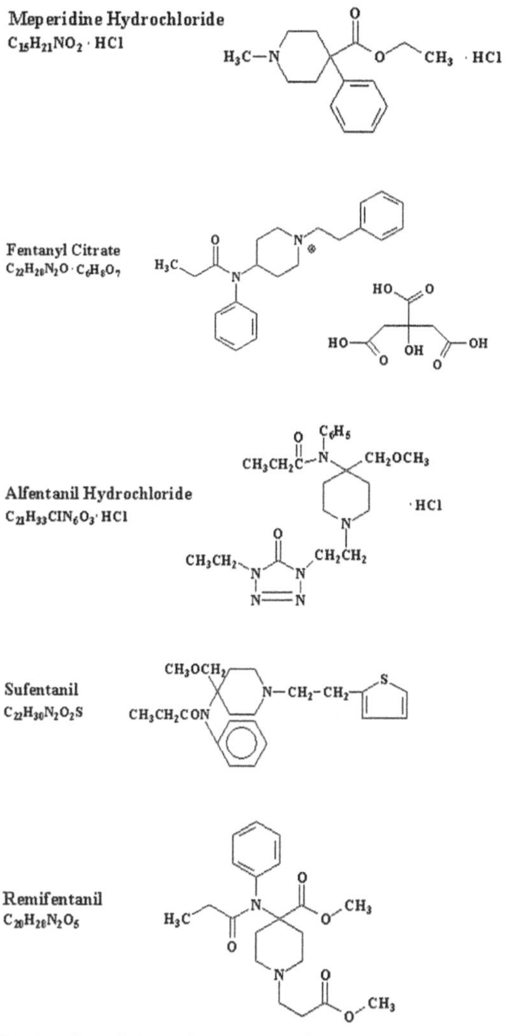

Meperidine Hydrochloride
$C_{15}H_{21}NO_2 \cdot HCl$

Fentanyl Citrate
$C_{22}H_{28}N_2O \cdot C_6H_8O_7$

Alfentanil Hydrochloride
$C_{21}H_{33}ClN_6O_3 \cdot HCl$

Sufentanil
$C_{22}H_{30}N_2O_2S$

Remifentanil
$C_{20}H_{28}N_2O_5$

Fig. 3. Phenylpiperidine series of opioids.

However, meperidine is unique in that it can terminate shivering in 70% to 80% of cases. The exact mechanism is unknown, but may be related to a κ-receptor–mediated reduction in the shivering threshold and to α_2b-receptor agonism.[11]

FENTANYL

Fentanyl is the most popular and useful opioid in anesthesia today. It is used in every situation from moderate dental sedation to cardiothoracic surgery. It is approximately 100 times more potent than morphine, and has a rapid onset and short duration. It produces excellent analgesia and is useful during induction of anesthesia to provide background sedation and to attenuate the systemic effects of intubation. Fentanyl provides cardiovascular stability, but may produce bradycardia. It produces profound dose-dependent respiratory

depression. Fentanyl may be difficult to titrate to effect because it produces little or no euphoria. There is a tendency to overshoot the goal if the clinician waits to see a clinical effect from fentanyl. Thus, dosing should be done on an empiric basis.

SUFENTANIL

Sufentanil is an ultrapotent opioid with a similar profile to fentanyl, but 10 times as potent. It may be used readily as a substitute for fentanyl, with 10 μg of sufentanil being equivalent to 100 μg of fentanyl. Its context-sensitive half-time is favorable enough to permit its use as a continuous infusion agent during TIVA.

ALFENTANIL

Alfentanil is 10 times less potent than fentanyl, with 1000 μg of alfentanil being equivalent to 100 μg of fentanyl. It also has a similar clinical profile to fentanyl and may be used in lieu of fentanyl in a sedation regimen. Alfentanil also has a context-sensitive half-time compatible with a continuous infusion technique.

REMIFENTANIL

Remifentanil is an ultra–short-acting opioid that is 2.5 times as potent as fentanyl and is ideally suited for continuous infusion techniques. It is unique in that it contains ester linkages, which are hydrolyzed in the plasma by nonspecific esterases that profoundly limit its duration of action. Its short context-sensitive half-time results in recovery within minutes, even after hours of infusion. It is primarily used for maintenance of deep sedation in doses of 0.05 to 0.1 μg/kg/min, or general anesthesia in doses of 0.05 to 2.0 μg/kg/min. It may also be used for the induction of general anesthesia in bolus doses of 1 μg/kg. Combined with propofol, this dosing regimen can produce excellent intubating conditions without the need for muscle relaxants.

BENZODIAZEPINES

Benzodiazepines form the basis of sedative drugs and techniques because of their selectivity of effect and high margin of safety (**Fig. 4**). Benzodiazepines exert their effect at the GABA-receptor complex to produce the clinical effects of anxiolysis, sedation, amnesia, anticonvulsant activity, and skeletal muscle relaxation. Benzodiazepine receptors are linked to a specific GABA-receptor subtype, the $GABA_A$ receptor. Binding at the $GABA_A$ receptor facilitates GABA-activated membrane hyperpolarization by enhancing chloride ion

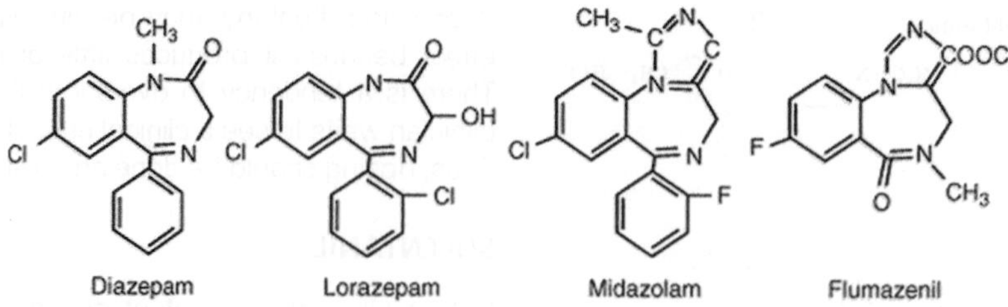

Diazepam   Lorazepam   Midazolam   Flumazenil

Fig. 4. Typical benzodiazepines and their reversal agent have similar chemical structures.

influx through the chloride channel associated with the macromolecular receptor complex.

Cardiovascular Effects

Benzodiazepines exert little effect on cardiovascular parameters in therapeutic doses. Excessive doses and concomitant use with other sedatives may result in cardiovascular system depression. Benzodiazepines are useful in attenuating the cardiovascular stress response.

Respiratory Effects

Benzodiazepines have little effect on the respiratory system, but can cause respiratory depression in a dose-dependent manner, or when administered in conjunction with other CNS-depressant drugs. Midazolam has been associated with respiratory depression and apnea, and clinically significant respiratory depression can occur when combined with opioids.[12]

Other Effects

Paradoxic reactions to benzodiazepines have been seen in all patients, but most notably in the elderly and pediatric populations. These reactions, also described as idiosyncratic, are manifested as excitement, agitation and confusion, irritability, rage, and hostility. The cause for these unusual reactions is not well known, but may be likened to the disinhibitory effects sometimes seen with alcohol. Caution should be exercised when administering benzodiazepines to these groups.

Diazepam has been associated with pain on injection and an increased incidence of phlebitis following intravenous administration. This effect is caused by its formulation in a propylene glycol solvent that is irritating to veins. Phlebitis is more likely to occur when using hand veins and with repeated injections. Patients who are smokers, the elderly, and those taking oral contraceptives are most likely to develop phlebitis. At the height of its popularity, diazepam-induced phlebitis was a leading cause of anesthetic-related lawsuits.

Benzodiazepines are contraindicated in pregnancy and are classified as pregnancy category D, except for triazolam, which is pregnancy category X.[13] If sedation or anesthesia is to be considered during pregnancy, benzodiazepines should be avoided. Except for lorazepam and oxazepam, benzodiazepines are also found in the breast milk of lactating mothers, which could result in the unwanted sedation of the infant. If benzodiazepines are to be used as part of a sedative or anesthetic regimen in these patients, the risk may be decreased by administering the medication immediately after the mother feeds the infant, or during periods in which the infant is asleep for long periods. A safer alternative would be to have the mother self-express and store the milk for later use before procedure, and self-express and discard the milk for 3 to 4 half-lives of the drug following the procedure.

Aside from the drug interactions involving other CNS depressants, interactions involving the cytochrome P450 (CYP) enzyme system are the most significant. Benzodiazepines are biotransformed in the liver by the CYP3A4 isoenzymes. Drugs such as rifampin and carbamazepine induce these enzymes in the liver and gut, reducing the bioavailability of various benzodiazepines by up to 96%.[14] Triazolam is so effectively metabolized in the gut by these induced enzymes that its bioavailability is reduced to only 12% of normal.[15] The clinical implications of this include loss of seizure control, and reduced or lack of effectiveness of benzodiazepines.

Drugs including calcium channel blockers, azole antifungals, macrolide antibiotics, protease inhibitors, and selective serotonin reuptake inhibitors inhibit the CYP3A4 isoenzymes. Thus, coadministration of benzodiazepines in patients taking these agents could result in increased bioavailability with significant augmentation and prolongation of their effects. Patients taking any of these drugs may exhibit extreme oversedation and respiratory depression.

DIAZEPAM

Diazepam is the prototypical benzodiazepine that is noted for excellent anxiolysis and sedation of moderate duration. It was the mainstay of most enteral and parenteral sedation regimens for years, and is still used occasionally for this purpose. However, its many drawbacks have caused it to be supplanted by newer agents, such as midazolam and triazolam. Diazepam is a water-insoluble drug that is formulated with propylene glycol for injection. This formulation makes it unsuitable for effective intramuscular injection because of poor absorption. Propylene glycol is also known to contribute to pain on injection, venous irritation, and thrombophlebitis. Diazepam has 3 active metabolites: oxazepam, nordiazepam, and desmethyldiazepam. Their half-lives range from 22 to 100 hours, which may account for residual hangover effects sometimes seen after diazepam administration.

MIDAZOLAM

Midazolam is the benzodiazepine of choice for TIVA because of its water solubility and excellent sedative, anxiolytic, and amnestic effects. It has a short elimination half-life (2.5 hours) and lacks significant active metabolites. Midazolam can be counted on to produce reliable antegrade amnesia, attenuate the cardiovascular response to stress, and suppress the psychotomimetic effects of ketamine. Unlike diazepam, it is well absorbed intramuscularly and does not cause pain on injection or venous irritation. Its effects may be intensified in the presence of CYP3A4 inhibitors. Midazolam is also available as an oral elixir, which is an effective premedicant in doses of 0.5 to 1.0 mg/kg (maximum 20 mg) for pediatric and special-needs populations.

ADJUNCTIVE AGENTS
Ketamine

Ketamine is a water-soluble phencyclidine derivative first synthesized in 1963. It produces a characteristic dissociative state characterized by profound analgesia, amnesia, and catalepsy. Its racemic form, containing equal amounts of its dextro and levo isomers, is used clinically. Its high degree of lipid solubility enables it to enter the CNS rapidly. Ketamine is thought to produce its unique clinical state by inducing dissociation between the thalamnoneocortical and limbic systems, thus preventing the higher centers from perceiving visual, auditory, and painful stimuli.[16] The result is a cataleptic state manifested by a vacant stare, glassy eyes, and horizontal nystagmus. Patients may appear to be removed or detached from their physical beings, but may still respond to command when ketamine has been administered in a low dose. These effects are caused by the binding of ketamine to NMDA receptors in the CNS.

Peak plasma concentrations of ketamine are achieved in about 1 minute after intravenous administration and in about 5 minutes following intramuscular administration. The pharmacokinetic profile of ketamine is similar in both adults and children, conforming to a classic 2-compartment model. Termination of activity occurs through slow redistribution to the peripheral compartment. Thus, the clinical effects of ketamine begin to wane in about 15 minutes after intravenous administration and in about 30 to 120 minutes following intramuscular injection. The elimination half-life of ketamine is 2 to 3 hours in adults, but children metabolize the drug more rapidly.

Cardiovascular effects

Ketamine exerts sympathomimetic effects on the cardiovascular system, resulting in mild to moderate increases in blood pressure, heart rate, and cardiac output. Coronary perfusion increases along with myocardial oxygen consumption. Ketamine is therefore relatively contraindicated in patients with uncontrolled hypertension, arteriosclerotic heart disease, and severe congestive heart failure. Hypertensive responses to ketamine may be exaggerated by rapid intravenous bolus injection and may be minimized by slow administration of low-dose ketamine.

Respiratory effects

Ketamine preserves spontaneous respiration and enhances the muscular tone of the upper airway. Protective airway reflexes are preserved. Respiratory depression is rarely associated with ketamine administration, although it may occur after rapid intravenous bolus injection or with the concomitant use of opioids. Ketamine is a bronchodilator, decreasing airway resistance by direct smooth muscle dilation, increased circulating catecholamines, and inhibition of vagal outflow. The effect of ketamine on ventilation is clinically insignificant, although the carbon dioxide response curve is shifted to the right. The slope of the curve remains unchanged, indicating that hypercarbic respiratory stimulation remains intact but may require a slightly higher $Paco_2$ for a ventilatory response. Ketamine stimulates salivary and tracheobronchial secretions that may induce laryngospasm. These effects can be adequately controlled by the concomitant administration of an antisialogue. Although laryngospasm is a possible side effect of ketamine administration and is potentially life threatening, a literature review conducted by Green and Johnson[17] revealed only 2 cases of laryngospasm in 11,589 pediatric patients who required intubation. Because upper airway protective reflexes remain intact, there seems to be minimal risk of the aspiration of gastric contents. In the 20 years of ketamine use studied by Green and Johnson,[17] only 2 cases of aspiration were found.

Neuromuscular effects

Ketamine produces skeletal muscle hypertonicity and rigidity, which may interfere with dental procedures because of inability to open the mouth. This phenomenon seems to be dose related, and increasing the ketamine dose or the addition of other sedative agents alleviates this problem. Random movement unrelated to surgical or painful stimuli often occurs with ketamine administration. This random movement may be mistaken for an inadequate sedation level when it is unrelated to the dental procedure. Myoclonus, twitching and jerking movements, are common following ketamine administration. When these movements have been extensive, they have been mistaken for seizure activity. However, ketamine has been shown to have anticonvulsive properties and has been used without complication in patients with seizure problems. Ketamine also causes an increase in intracranial pressure by producing cerebral vasodilation and increased perfusion pressure. It is therefore relatively contraindicated in patients with serious head trauma, hydrocephalus, and intracranial lesions. In addition, ataxia and dizziness may persist for up to 4 hours following ketamine administration. Therefore, rapid independent ambulation is not recommended following the use of ketamine.

Emergence phenomenon

Psychic reactions associated with ketamine may result from the disconnection of external stimuli from higher cerebral function. The incidence of psychic phenomena with ketamine has been reported to be between 0% and 50% in adults and 0% and 10% in children.[17] These experiences have been described as detachment, floating or bodily suspension, out-of-body experiences, and strange thoughts or dreams. Factors that may place patients at increased risk for these reactions may include age greater than 10 years, female gender, rapid intravenous administration of high doses, and personality disorders. Not all psychic responses to ketamine are unpleasant. Blankstein and Anderson,[18] in a comparison of low-dose ketamine with methohexital in adults undergoing oral surgery, found that ketamine was not associated with unpleasant dreaming, whereas some subjects given methohexital experienced horrifying dreams. The psychotomimetic effects of

ketamine seem to be readily attenuated with the adjunctive administration of benzodiazepines or propofol. As discussed later, dexmedetomidine may be useful in preventing or attenuating emergence delirium associated with ketamine.

A possible cause for concern with ketamine use is nausea and vomiting. Although reports indicate that the incidence of nausea and vomiting may be from 0% to 43%, the incidence in pediatric patients is less than 10%. When vomiting does occur, it usually occurs late in the recovery phase or when the patient becomes ambulatory. At this juncture, the patient is alert and the airway may be cleared without assistance.

Clinical use

Sedation with ketamine may be induced either intravenously or intramuscularly. An intramuscular induction dose of 2 to 4 mg/kg of ketamine is useful in gaining behavioral control of unruly pediatric patients or patients with special needs. Intraoperative maintenance may be achieved with either a continuous infusion at a rate of 50 μg/kg/min, or by intermittent boluses of 5 to 20 mg as needed. Midazolam may be administered in 1-mg increments to provide background sedation and to control possible psychotomimetic effects. An antisialogogue may be needed to control the excessive secretions sometimes seen with ketamine.

Ketamine may be combined with propofol in a single syringe (ketofol) and administered by continuous infusion for procedural sedation. Kramer and colleagues[19] compared the combination of propofol-remifentanil with propofol-ketamine for third molar surgery. The concentration of 10 mg/mL of propofol and 2.5 μg/mL of ketamine produced sedation hemodynamic stability, and respiratory stability that was comparable with the concentration of 10 mg/mL of propofol and 5 μg/mL of remifentanil. However, the combination of propofol and ketamine was associated with longer emergence and recovery times, which could limit its usefulness in third molar surgery.

Dexmedetomidine

Dexmedetomidine is a highly selective α_2-agonist similar to clonidine but with a greater affinity for the α_2-receptor. Alpha$_2$-receptors are located in the peripheral vasculature and produce vasoconstriction when activated. However, their primary site of action in the sympathetic nervous system is at the adrenergic neural endplate where they initiate a negative feedback loop that modulates the release of norepinephrine. This feedback results in an attenuation of the sympathetic stress response. Alpha$_2$-receptors are also found in the CNS in the locus ceruleus and the spinal column.

Activation of these areas results in anxiolysis, sedation, and analgesia.

Stimulation of α_2-receptors in the dorsal horn of the spinal column inhibits nociceptive neurons and reduces the release of substance P. Although there is some evidence for supraspinal and peripheral sites of action for dexmedetomidine, it is thought that the spinal mechanism produces most of the drug's analgesic action.[20,21] Dexmedetomidine is rapidly redistributed, with an elimination half-life of 6 minutes and an elimination half-life of 2 hours.

Cardiovascular effects

Dexmedetomidine produces a significant reduction in heart rate, systemic vascular resistance, and systolic blood pressure.[22] These effects aid in modulating the stress response, which may be particularly useful in patients with systemic hypertension and/or myocardial ischemia who could respond adversely to surgical stressors. Dexmedetomidine promotes stability and may protect against radical fluctuations in cardiovascular parameters intraoperatively.

Dexmedetomidine loses its α_2-receptor selectivity as the dose is increased by intravenous bolus injection or rapid infusion. This loss results in an initial increase in blood pressure and concomitant decrease in heart rate, which normalizes within 15 minutes, followed by a further reduction in blood pressure.[20,22]

Respiratory effects

A major advantage of dexmedetomidine compared with other anesthetic drugs is its minimal effect on the respiratory system. In patients with poor airways, obesity, and/or limited range of motion, dexmedetomidine produces excellent sedation without compromising the airway or depressing respiration.

Clinical use

Dexmedetomidine is a useful adjunct for procedural sedation, either via bolus injection or continuous infusion. A bolus injection of 0.25 μg/kg to 0.5 μg/kg given slowly in divided doses, to avoid a transient increase in blood pressure, produces a noticeable quieting or mellowing effect without respiratory depression. As an alternative, sedation may be induced by a continuous infusion of dexmedetomidine, 1 μg/kg over 10 minutes, followed by a maintenance infusion of 0.2 μg/kg/h to 0.7 μg/kg/h. Dexmedetomidine has been shown to decrease the requirement for the coadministration of propofol, opioids, and benzodiazepines.[23,24]

Emergence delirium can be a significant problem following outpatient anesthesia because of the potential for serious disruption of the office, the potential for serious disruption of the office, damage to instruments and equipment, and injury to the patient or office personnel. Delirium is described as a disturbance of consciousness, characterized by the acute onset of impaired cognitive functioning, significantly impairing a patient's ability to process and store information. Pediatric patients, patients with special needs, and the elderly are particularly prone to emergence delirium following anesthesia, especially when benzodiazepines and potent inhalational agents are used. Patients who develop delirium are more likely to have poor outcomes when hospitalized, including increased length of stay, the need for subsequent institutionalization, and higher mortality. Cognitive impairment has been reported to negatively affect key outcome indicators such as removal from the ventilator, pneumonia, and total length of hospital stay.[25]

Dexmedetomidine has been studied to assess its efficacy in reducing the occurrence of emergence delirium. Riker and colleagues[26] compared the efficacy of dexmedetomidine with midazolam for the maintenance of mechanically ventilated patients, and also examined the incidence of delirium in those patients. Although the two drugs produced comparable levels of sedation, dexmedetomidine significantly reduced the incidence of delirium, 54% versus 75% for midazolam. In addition, the duration of delirium was reduced by 48% in the dexmedetomidine group. Patients treated with dexmedetomidine had a statistically significant greater ability to communicate and to cooperate than those treated with midazolam.

Pandharipande and colleagues[27] compared the efficacy and incidence of delirium of dexmedetomidine and lorazepam in mechanically ventilated intensive care patients. Lorazepam has been recommended by the Society of Critical Care Medicine for the sustained sedation of mechanically ventilated patients in the intensive care unit. However, it has been proposed that the GABA effects of lorazepam and other benzodiazepines may alter levels of potentially deliriogenic neurotransmitters, with negative consequences. Compared with the lorazepam group, the dexmedetomidine group had a lower prevalence of coma (63% vs 92%), fewer days with delirium (3 vs 7 days), and the 12-month time to death was 363 days versus 188 days.

Emergence delirium is also common in children recovering from deep sedation and general anesthesia. Shukry and colleagues[28] studied 2 groups of children between the ages of 1 and 10 years receiving general anesthesia with sevoflurane. One study group received an infusion of dexmedetomidine and the other received saline. The dexmedetomidine group had an emergence delirium incidence of 26% versus 60% for the saline group. Another study investigated the incidence of emergence delirium in children receiving general anesthesia for a nonsurgical procedure.[29] One group received an infusion of dexmedetomidine after induction of anesthesia and the other group received a placebo infusion. The children who received dexmedetomidine had a 4.8% incidence of delirium compared with 47.6% for the placebo group.

Dexmedetomidine may be used either prophylactically or emergently for the prevention or control of emergence delirium. In patients who are deemed at risk for emergence delirium, 0.25 µg/kg of dexmedetomidine may be slowly injected intravenously during the maintenance phase of anesthesia. Should emergence delirium occur, another 0.25 µg/kg may be administered. In cases in which prophylaxis has not been administered, emergence delirium may be controlled with the intravenous administration of 0.5 µg/kg of dexmedetomidine.

SUMMARY

TIVA is a technique whose time has come because of the advent of ultra–short-acting drugs and computerized infusion technology. Patients may be sedated to any desired level, maintained there for indefinite periods, and recovered to near baseline within minutes, which gives the operator extreme, moment-to-moment control of the anesthetic and improves patient outcomes. Future trends in TIVA may include patient-controlled sedation, whereby patients sedate themselves with an infusion device similar to those used for postoperative analgesia. It seems that, of the drugs currently available, a remifentanil/propofol combination would be suitable. The future may also bring titration of sedatives to target blood levels, leading to more precise dosing and greater efficiency.

This article provides an overview of historical and current sedative agents available to the dentist anesthetist. The discussion is intended to provide the surgeon with rational choices for sedation and the individualization of drug selection for each patient.

REFERENCES

1. Halford F. A critique of intravenous anaesthesia in war surgery. Anesthesiology 1943;4:67–9.
2. ASA statement on sodium thiopental's removal from the market. 2011. Available at: www.asahq.org/For-the-Public-and-Media/Press-Room/ASA-News/ASA-State. Accessed July 19, 2012.
3. MacDonald RL, Olsen RW. GABA$_A$ receptor channels. Annu Rev Neurosci 1994;17:569–602.
4. Vasile B, Rasulo F, Candiani A, et al. The pathophysiology of propofol infusion syndrome: a simple name for a complex syndrome. Intensive Care Med 2003;29:1417–25.
5. Diprivan [package insert]. Schaumberg (IL): APP Pharmaceuticals; 2011.
6. Harper DL, Castells MC. Anaphylaxis during the perioperative period. Anesth Analg 2003;97:1381–95.
7. Lizaso Bacaicoa MT, Acero Sainz S, Alvarez Puebla MJ, et al. Cutaneous response to Diprivan (propofol) and intralipid in patients with leguminous and egg allergy. Rev Esp Alergol Immunol Clin 1998;13:153–7.
8. Delitala G, Trainer PJ, Oliva O, et al. Opioid peptide and alpha-adrenoreceptor pathways in the regulation of the pituitary-adrenal axis in man. J Endocrinol 1994;141:163–8.
9. Ng HP, Chen FG, Yeoung SM, et al. Effect of remifentanil compared with fentanyl on intraocular pressure after succinylcholine and tracheal intubation. Br J Anaesth 2000;85:785–7.
10. Ko MC, Naughton NN. An experimental itch model in monkeys: characterization of intrathecal morphine-induced scratching and nociception. Anesthesiology 2000;92:795–805.
11. Kranke P, Eberhart LH, Roewer N, et al. Pharmacological treatment of postoperative shivering: a quantitative systematic review of randomized controlled trials. Anesth Analg 2002;94:453–60.
12. Dionne RA, Yagiela JA, Moore PA, et al. Comparing efficacy and safety of four intravenous sedation regimens in dental outpatients. J Am Dent Assoc 2001;132:740–51.
13. Moore PA. Selecting drugs for the pregnant dental patient. J Am Dent Assoc 1998;129:1281–6.
14. Backman JT, Olkkola KT, Neuvonen PJ. Rifampin drastically reduces plasma concentrations and effects of oral midazolam. Clin Pharmacol Ther 1996;59:7–13.
15. Villikka K, Kivisto KT, Backman JT, et al. Triazolam is ineffective in patients taking rifampin. Clin Pharmacol Ther 1997;61:8–14.
16. Giovannitti JA. Dental anesthesia and pediatric dentistry. Anesth Prog 1995;42:95–9.
17. Green SM, Johnson NE. Ketamine sedation for pediatric procedures: part 2, review and implications. Ann Emerg Med 1990;19:1033–46.
18. Blankstein KC, Anderson JA. A double blind comparison of low dose intravenous ketamine and methohexital in adults. J Oral Maxillofac Surg 1991;49:468–75.
19. Kramer KJ, Ganzberg S, Prior S, et al. Comparison of propofol-remifentanil versus propofol-ketamine deep sedation for third molar surgery. Anesth Prog 2012;59:107–17.

20. Virtanen R, Savola JM, Saano V, et al. Characterization of the selectivity, specificity and potency of medetomidine as an α_2-adrenoceptor agonist. Eur J Pharmacol 1988;150:9–14.

21. Jaakola ML, Salonen M, Lehtinen R, et al. The analgesic action of dexmedetomidine-a novel alpha2-adrenoceptor agonist in healthy volunteers. Pain 1991;46:281–5.

22. Dyck JB, Maze M, Haack C, et al. The pharmacokinetics and hemodynamic effects of intravenous and intramuscular dexmedetomidine hydrochloride in adult human volunteers. Anesthesiology 1993; 78:813–20.

23. Aantaa RE, Kanto JH, Scheinin M, et al. Dexmedetomidine premedication for minor gynecologic surgery. Anesth Analg 1990;70:407–13.

24. Aantaa RE, Kanto JH, Scheinin M, et al. Dexmedetomidine, an alpha2-adrenoceptor agonist, reduces anesthetic requirements for patients undergoing minor gynecologic surgery. Anesthesiology 1990; 73:230–5.

25. Ely EW, Shintani A, Truman B, et al. Delirium as a predictor of mortality in mechanically ventilated patients in the intensive care unit. JAMA 2004;291: 1753–62.

26. Riker RR, Shehabi Y, Bokesch PM, et al. Dexmedetomidine vs. midazolam for sedation of critically ill patients: a randomized trial. JAMA 2009;301: 489–99.

27. Pandharipande PP, Pun BT, Herr DL, et al. Effect of sedation with dexmedetomidine vs. lorazepam on acute brain dysfunction in mechanically ventilated patients: the MENDS randomized controlled trial. JAMA 2007;298:2644–53.

28. Shukry M, Mathison C, Kalarickel P, et al. Does dexmedetomidine prevent emergence delirium in children after sevoflurane-based general anesthesia? Paediatr Anaesth 2005;15:1098–104.

29. Isik B, Arslan M, Tunga AD, et al. Dexmedetomidine decreases emergence agitation in pediatric patients after sevoflurane anesthesia without surgery. Paediatr Anaesth 2006;16:748–53.

Pharmacology of Local Anesthetics Used in Oral Surgery

Joseph A. Giovannitti Jr, DMD[a],*,
Morton B. Rosenberg, DMD[b,c], James C. Phero, DMD[d]

KEYWORDS

- Local anesthetics • Pharmacology • Complications and reasons for failure • Future trends

KEY POINTS

- Local anesthesia remains the foundation of pain control in dentistry especially when combined with moderate-deep sedation for invasive and painful procedures in the contemporary oral and maxillo-facial surgical model.
- Local anesthetics remain the safest and most effective drugs in medicine and dentistry to relieve intraoperative and postoperative pain.
- It is only with a thorough understanding of pharmacology and anatomy that clinicians have the basic clinical foundation to enhance the care of patients.

INTRODUCTION

The ability to provide safe, effective local anesthesia is the cornerstone of clinical oral surgical practice. Like any regional anesthetic technique, the use and effectiveness depend on patient considerations, the extent and duration of the procedure, choice of drug and technique, and the skill and experience of the practitioner. Every clinician should be aware of his or her skill limitations, and the limitations of the contemplated technique and agent. These factors must be clearly understood preoperatively to enhance the chance of success. The administration of local anesthetics is often complicated by the existence of multifactorial psychological considerations associated with the delivery of dental care. It is imperative for health care professionals to understand and appreciate these issues to properly implement perioperative behavioral or pharmacologic management strategies to reduce fear and anxiety to acceptable levels. These considerations are discussed elsewhere in this issue. This article focuses on the pharmacology and clinical application of local anesthetics used in dentistry. A thorough knowledge of these agents gives the surgeon the ability to individualize care to meet the specific surgical and anesthetic needs of the patient. A discussion of the anatomy and routine injection techniques is not included in this article because it is assumed that the reader already has an expert's command of these subjects.

As with any anesthetic, medical, dental, or surgical procedure, a careful and thorough preoperative evaluation must be conducted before selection of technique and agents. This should include, but not be limited to, a review of the

[a] Department of Dental Anesthesiology, Center for Patients with Special Needs, University of Pittsburgh School of Dental Medicine, 3501 Terrace Street, G-89 Salk Hall, Pittsburgh, PA 15261, USA; [b] Division of Anesthesia and Pain Control, Tufts Medical Center, Tufts University School of Dental Medicine, 1 Kneeland Street, Boston, MA 02111, USA; [c] Department of Anesthesiology, Tufts University School of Medicine, 1 Kneeland Street, Boston, MA 02111, USA; [d] Department of Anesthesiology, College of Medicine (UCCOM), University of Cincinnati Academic Health Center, PO Box 670764, 234 Goodman Street, Cincinnati, OH 45267–0764, USA
* Corresponding author.
E-mail address: jag74@pitt.edu

Oral Maxillofacial Surg Clin N Am 25 (2013) 453–465
http://dx.doi.org/10.1016/j.coms.2013.03.003
1042-3699/13/$ – see front matter © 2013 Elsevier Inc. All rights reserved.

medical history with special emphasis on past anesthetic experiences, a focused physical examination, determination of physical risk, and the potential for adverse drug interactions. The patient's weight and body mass index are also important considerations. Without this information and practitioner knowledge base, a reasonable and rational anesthesia plan cannot be successfully formulated.

HISTORY

The next major advance in pain control, after the introduction of inhaled nitrous oxide and ether, was the isolation of cocaine by Niemann in 1859. At the suggestion of Sigmund Freud, Karl Koller began using topical cocaine for ophthalmologic procedures in 1884. In that same year, the famous surgeon William Halstead began his experiments with the application of cocaine to peripheral nerves to produce a conduction blockade. Using the newly available hypodermic needle and syringe, he performed the first peripheral nerve block, successfully anesthetizing the inferior alveolar nerve. It was apparent that cocaine-induced anesthesia was short acting, so Corning actually advocated the use of a tourniquet to retard the absorption of the drug and prolong the effect. In 1903, Heinrich Braun suggested the addition of epinephrine to act as a "chemical" tourniquet to prolong duration. Because of the transient effect of cocaine and its addictive potential, the search was intensified for a more effective and less toxic anesthetic. Alfred Einhorn introduced a cocaine analog, procaine, in 1904. Procaine remained the sole local anesthetic in dentistry until 1948, when lidocaine was introduced by Nils Lofgren. Lidocaine is an aminoamide local anesthetic with improved efficacy and duration, and less toxicity than procaine. It has become the gold standard for local anesthetics in dentistry against which all others are compared. Other amide local anesthetics followed: mepivacaine in 1960, prilocaine in 1965, bupivacaine in 1983, and articaine in 2000.

Another major event in the history of local anesthesia in dentistry was the invention of the dental syringe and cartridge by Harvey Cook in 1920. Before this development, powdered local anesthetics had to be mixed in solution and then drawn into a syringe for administration. An Army medic, Cook based his design on the bolt-action rifle and cartridges in use during World War I. Later, his Cook-Waite laboratories developed the disposable sterile needle, which reduced infection and needle breakage. A review of historical developments in local anesthesia is found in **Table 1**.

Table 1
History of local anesthesia

Date	Individual/Company	Event
1859	Niemann	Isolation of cocaine
1884	Koller	Cocaine topical anesthesia
1884	Halstead	Cocaine regional anesthesia
1885	Corning	Tourniquet to retard absorption
1903	Braun	Epinephrine as a chemical tourniquet
1904	Einhorn	Synthesis of procaine
1905	Braun	Clinical use of procaine
1920	Cook Laboratories	Anesthetic syringe and cartridge
1943	Lofgren	Synthesis of lidocaine
1947	Novocol	Dental aspirating syringe
1948	Astra	Lidocaine for dentistry
1959	Cook-Waite	Sterile disposable needle

PHARMACOLOGY

Local anesthetics reversibly block conduction along a nerve distal to the site of application. They are generally classified according to their chemical structure, rate of onset, potency, and duration of action. Chemically, they are either aminoesters or aminoamides (ie, an aromatic, lipophilic ring connected to a hydrophilic amine group by an intermediate chain containing either an ester or amide linkage) (**Fig. 1**). Ester local anesthetics are not available in dental cartridges primarily because of lack of efficacy, the potential

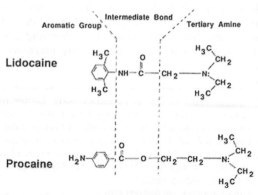

Fig. 1. Lidocaine is the prototypical aminoamide. Procaine is the prototypical aminoester.

for allergenicity, and the advantages of newer aminoamides.

Mechanism of Action

Normal depolarization causes conformational changes in the nerve membrane that allow for the passage of sodium ions through specified channels resulting in the propagation of the action potential along the nerve. Local anesthetics bind to specific sites within the sodium channels, preventing these conformational changes, and thus impair conduction. As more receptors are occupied, there is a progressive reduction in the rate and degree of depolarization until conduction fails.

Franz and Perry[1] noted that nerve conduction was disrupted when a critical length of the nerve was exposed to a local anesthetic. The size of the nerve fiber was not a factor. However, because conduction along myelinated nerves occurs from one node of Ranvier to another (ie, saltatory conduction), a longer critical length is required for exposure to local anesthetics for a block to occur. This results in a differential sensitivity of nerve fibers to the effects of local anesthetics based on their size. Because larger-diameter myelinated fibers have a greater internodal distance than smaller myelinated fibers, there is a differential sensitivity to the effects of local anesthetics based on the diameter of the nerve fiber. Smaller nerve fibers, either myelinated or unmyelinated, typically transmit pain and proprioceptive impulses, whereas larger myelinated fibers carry motor impulses. Thus, when local anesthetics are applied to a nerve trunk, there is a sequence of disappearance of sensations based on the differential sensitivity of the nerves involved. Typically, pain fibers are blocked first, followed by temperature, touch, pressure, and motor function.

The differential sensitivity of nerves to local anesthetics is also influenced by the frequency of impulses along the nerve fiber. Higher-frequency impulses make more sodium channels available to exposure by local anesthetics, and these fibers are blocked faster than slower frequency fibers. This is known as use-dependent block, and is clinically significant in that pain impulses are of higher frequency than motor impulses. Thus, pain impulses are blocked preferentially and more rapidly.

Clinical onset and recovery characteristics are determined by the organization of nerve trunks themselves. Because the local anesthetic diffuses through the nerve bundle, the outer or mantle axons are affected first. Because the drug diffuses into the core, the structures innervated by these axons are affected later. In the case of the inferior alveolar nerve, proximal structures are innervated by the mantle fibers and distal structures are innervated by the core. The onset of an inferior alveolar nerve block is therefore proximal to distal, molars to incisors and lower lip. Recovery is also proximal to distal, with the lip being the last to recover from the block.

Ionization

The degree of ionization after a local anesthetic is injected determines its rate of onset. After the acidic local anesthetic solution is injected it is buffered by the body and dissociates into an uncharged base and a cationic form. The uncharged base form diffuses through the nerve membrane. The amount of base form depends on the pKa of the local anesthetic and the pH of the tissue. The closer the anesthetic's pKa is to the tissue pH, the more base form is available for diffusion, resulting in a faster onset. Local anesthetics with the lowest pKa values have the fastest rate of onset (**Table 2**). When inflammation is present, tissue pH becomes more acidic and local anesthesia is more difficult to achieve.

Lipid Solubility and Protein Binding

The aromatic ring of the local anesthetic molecule determines its lipid solubility. Because nerve membranes are primarily lipid, the drugs with the greatest lipid affinity demonstrate the greatest potency. The protein-binding properties of local anesthetics determine their duration of action. Sodium channels and receptor sites are largely protein and highly protein-bound molecules attach securely to the active site. Additionally, protein binding creates a reservoir of drug that can be made available as the unbound drug is removed from the active site by vascular uptake. A higher percentage of protein binding means a longer duration of action (**Table 3**).

Systemic Effects

Local anesthetics impair conduction in all neural tissues at the site of injection, but with particular

Table 2
Ionization properties of local anesthetics

Drug	pKa	% Base Form at pH 7.4	Onset of Action (min)
Mepivacaine	7.7	33	2–4
Articaine	7.8	29	2–4
Lidocaine	7.9	25	2–4
Prilocaine	7.9	25	2–4
Bupivacaine	8.1	17	5–8

Table 3
Protein-binding properties

Drug	Protein Binding (%)	Duration
Lidocaine	65	Moderate
Mepivacaine	75	Moderate
Bupivacaine	95	Long

affinity for those in the cardiovascular and central nervous systems. In the central nervous system, neuronal excitation occurs as local anesthetic concentrations rise rapidly. This is counterintuitive because local anesthetics block conduction. It is postulated that inhibitory pathways are affected first, allowing excitatory pathways to manifest themselves. Local anesthetics are also known to affect potassium channels, which may in itself produce neural excitation.[2] Patients may experience agitation, disorientation, dizziness, tinnitus, involuntary muscle activity, or frank seizures when local anesthetics are given higher than maximum recommended doses or injected directly into the vasculature.

All local anesthetics inhibit cardiac conduction. In therapeutic doses lidocaine prolongs the refractory period in the myocardial conduction system and is useful in preventing or controlling ventricular dysrhythmias. In toxic doses, local anesthetics diminish myocardial contractility and conduction resulting in reduced cardiac output and systemic hypotension. Cardiovascular system collapse is the end result of local anesthetic-induced cardiac toxicity.

Although hypoxia associated with seizure activity likely contributes to the cardiac toxicity of other local anesthetics, bupivacaine is known to be directly cardiotoxic. The high lipid solubility of bupivacaine compared with other local anesthetics contributes to its increased potential for cardiac toxicity. Additionally, bupivacaine preparations contain dextrorotatory and levorotatory enantiomers. Cardiac toxicity is primarily associated with the dextrorotatory enantiomer.[3] The inhibition of myocardial potassium channels also contributes to its toxicity. In obstetric anesthesia it is known that high concentrations or volumes of systemic bupivacaine can cause instantaneous cardiovascular system collapse that is resistant to usual resuscitative measures. Methods for the reversal of this complication are discussed later in this article. Fortunately, the doses of bupivacaine used in dentistry are far below that of other medical major nerve blocks, making this type of cardiac toxicity highly unlikely.

Finally, local anesthetics have varying effects on the peripheral vasculature. Most local anesthetics are vasodilators to varying degrees. Lidocaine, bupivacaine, and articaine are combined with epinephrine to enhance the duration and efficacy of the nerve block, whereas mepivacaine, prilocaine, and ropivacaine are not as profound vasodilators and may be used as plain solutions. Cocaine is unique in that it causes vasoconstriction by inhibiting the reuptake of norepinephrine into the adrenergic nerve end plates. For this reason, cocaine potentiates the effects of added vasoconstrictors and may produce a severe drug interaction leading to malignant hypertension, stroke, myocardial infarction, and death. Because of these profound vasoconstrictor effects and other associated issues, injectable cocaine preparations are not used in dentistry.

Metabolism and Excretion

Ester local anesthetics are hydrolyzed in the plasma by pseudocholinesterase into para-aminobenzoic acid and other derivatives. These derivatives undergo further biodegradation in the liver, and a small amount of the drug is eliminated unchanged. Patients with pseudocholinesterase deficiencies are at an increased risk for toxicity from ester local anesthetics. Para-aminobenzoic acid has allergic potential and has been implicated in the development of allergic reactions to esters, such as procaine and tetracaine, and to amide solutions containing methylparaben as an antimicrobial. At this point in time, there are no commercially available ester local anesthetics in dental cartridges. Local anesthetics available in dental cartridges are paraben-free, and paraben-free amides are also available in single- or multiple-dose vials. The practitioner must be aware, however, that many multiple-dose vials do contain methylparaben. Bisulfites are also found in local anesthetic solutions containing epinephrine and act as an antioxidant and preservative. When considering allergy testing for local anesthetics, methylparaben and bisulfite free solutions must be used for accurate interpretation.

Amide local anesthetics are metabolized in the liver primarily by CYP3A4 and CYP1A2 isoforms.[4] The rate of metabolism depends on liver blood flow and liver function, so conditions that slow liver blood flow can retard the metabolism of amides and have the potential for increased toxicity. Although still classified an as amide, articaine, by virtue of its ester side-chain, undergoes partial hydrolysis by nonspecific plasma esterases and liver metabolism. Its resultant 25-minute half-life is much shorter than other amide local anesthetics, thus reducing its toxic potential. Pseudocholinesterase deficiency does not add to the toxicity of articaine.

Certain metabolites of local anesthetics may have activity unrelated to their clinical intent. Monoethylglycinexylidide, a metabolite of lidocaine, may produce sedation and drowsiness after lidocaine administration. Ortho-toluidine, a metabolite of prilocaine, has been implicated in the development of methemoglobinemia.

LOCAL ANESTHETICS

Although any available local anesthetic solution acceptable for neural blockade in other parts of the body may be used for regional anesthesia of the head and neck, only five agents are currently available in cartridge form for dentistry (**Table 4**). As in other types of neural blockade, the choice of anesthetic agent, amount, type, and concentration of vasoconstrictor is based on many factors, such as physical status, age and weight of the patient, duration of the procedure, the need for hemostasis, and practitioner bias. Local anesthesia toxicity is a concern where large volumes of concentrated local anesthetic are used. Toxicity is avoided by using the lowest concentration of local anesthetic that produces the required block, calculating the maximum volume of solution that each patient may receive in advance of the injection, injecting slowly, and always aspirating before injection. This is especially true in the pediatric, severely compromised, and geriatric patients where drug toxicity can become a life-threatening complication if maximum doses are not strictly adhered (**Table 5**).

Local anesthetics are supplied in single-dose glass cartridges containing either 1.7 or 1.8 mL, depending on the origin of manufacture. Cartridges manufactured in Canada and Europe contain 1.7 mL of solution, whereas cartridges manufactured in the United States contain 1.8 mL of solution. This discrepancy matters little in determining the ultimate dose administered, and traditionally the 1.8-mL volume is used to calculate the administered dose and the maximum recommended dose. Cartridges of a plain local anesthetic solution contain the hydrochloride salt of the local anesthetic and distilled water. Cartridges containing a vasoconstrictor also contain epinephrine or levonordefrin, sodium metabisulfite, and citric acid. These latter act to stabilize the vasoconstrictor and prevent oxidative breakdown.

Lidocaine

Lidocaine is the most commonly used dental local anesthetic in the United States, and has become the gold standard against which all other dental local anesthetics are compared. Although lidocaine is supplied in dental cartridges as a 2% plain solution, it is rarely used because of its relative ineffectiveness and short duration. Lidocaine 2% combined with a vasoconstrictor in a 1:100,000 concentration provides reliable and profound pulpal anesthesia for approximately 60 minutes with a duration of soft tissue anesthesia ranging from 3 to 5 hours.[5] Lidocaine is also supplied as a 2% solution with 1:50,000 epinephrine. Although this concentration may be useful to provide surgical hemostasis by local infiltration, its routine use for primary operative or surgical anesthesia should be avoided because of the possibility of an acute epinephrine reaction, which may often manifest as hypertension or tachycardia in susceptible patients.

Mepivacaine

Mepivacaine is very similar to lidocaine in its efficacy, onset, and duration. It is supplied in dental cartridges as a 2% solution with 1:20,000 levonordefrin and as a 3% plain solution. It is effective as a plain solution because of its weaker vasodilator properties. This gives the plain solution practical use for short-duration procedures or for use in patients where vasoconstrictors would be contraindicated. Mepivacaine 3% plain solution is a popular alternative for patients in whom epinephrine may be contraindicated.

Prilocaine

Prilocaine is somewhat less potent than lidocaine and so is supplied in a higher concentration. It is available as a plain 4% solution, or as a 4% solution with 1:200,000 epinephrine. It is similar in duration and efficacy as lidocaine and its plain and lowered concentration of vasoconstrictor are useful for procedures of short duration or when the amount of vasoconstrictor should be minimized. Prilocaine has been implicated in a higher incidence of paresthesia associated with nerve

Table 4
Local anesthetics available in dental cartridges

Drug	Preparation
Lidocaine 2%	1:50,000 epinephrine
	1:100,000 epinephrine
Mepivacaine 3%	Plain (no vasoconstrictor)
Mepivacaine 2%	1:20,000 levonordefrin
Prilocaine 4%	Plain
	1:200,000 epinephrine
Articaine 4%	1:100,000 epinephrine
	1:200,000 epinephrine
Bupivacaine 0.5%	1:200,000 epinephrine

Table 5
Maximum local anesthetic dose for adult and pediatric patients (based on weight)

Weight (kg)	Weight (lb)	Lidocaine 2% 1:100,000 Epinephrine Maximum Cartridges	Articaine[a] 4% 1:100,000 or 1:200,000 Epinephrine Maximum Cartridges	Mepivacaine 3% Plain Maximum Cartridges	Mepivacaine 2% 1:20,000 Levonordefrin Maximum Cartridges	Prilocaine 4% Plain 1:200,000 Epinephrine Maximum Cartridges	Bupivacaine[b] 0.5% 1:100,000 Epinephrine Maximum Cartridges
10	22	1.9	NR	1.2	1.8	1.1	NR
15	33	2.9	NR	1.8	2.8	1.7	NR
20	44	3.9	NR	2.4	3.7	2.2	NR
25	55	4.9	2.4	3.1	4.6	2.8	NR
30	66	5.8	2.9	3.7	5.5	3.3	NR
35	77	6.8	3.4	4.3	6.4	3.9	NR
40	88	7.8	3.9	4.9	7.3	4.4	NR
45	99	8.8	4.4	5.5	8.3	5.0	6.6
50	110	9.7	4.9	6.1	9.2	5.6	7.3
55	121	10.7	5.3	6.7	10.1	6.1	8.1
60	132	11.1	5.8	7.3	11.0	6.7	8.8
65	143	11.1	6.3	7.4	11.1	7.2	9.5
≥70	≥154	11.1	6.9	7.4	11.1	8.3	10.0

Drug	Cartridges/10 kg	Maximum Cartridges	Maximum Cartridges for the Cardiovascular-impaired Patient
2% Lidocaine 1:100,000 epinephrine	2	11.1	1–2
4% Articaine 1:100,000 epinephrine	1	6.9	1–2
4% Articaine 1:200,000 epinephrine	1	6.9	2–4
3% Mepivacaine plain	1.2	7.4	7.4
2% Mepivacaine 1:20,000 levonordefrin	1.8	11.1	1–2
4% Prilocaine plain	1.1	8.3	7.8
4% Prilocaine 1:200,000 epinephrine	1.1	8.3	2–4

Abbreviation: NR, not recommended.
[a] Articaine is *not* recommended for children younger than 4 years old.
[b] Bupivacaine is *not* recommended for children younger than 12 years old.

block injections compared with lidocaine.[6] Its potential to induce methemoglobinemia also may limit its use.

Articaine

Articaine is the newest local anesthetic available in dental cartridges, introduced in 1976 in Europe and in 2000 in the United States. Articaine with epinephrine has a similar clinical profile as lidocaine, mepivacaine, and prilocaine with vasoconstrictors.[7] It is available in dental cartridges as a 4% solution containing either epinephrine in 1:100,000 or 1:200,000 concentrations. The lower concentration of epinephrine is useful when the total amount of vasoconstrictor should be reduced. A major advantage of articaine is that its half-life is significantly reduced because of hydrolysis of its ester side-chain by nonspecific plasma esterases. This reduces its toxic potential. Its 4% concentration has been implicated as a causative factor in the development of paresthesia after nerve block injections.[7] Articaine seems to be more effective for infiltration techniques in the maxilla and mandible than other local anesthetics.[8]

Bupivacaine

Bupivacaine is similar chemically to mepivacaine, but is much more lipid soluble and thus more potent. It is much more cardiotoxic than other local anesthetics because of the activity of its dextrorotary enantiomer on cardiac tissue. Its pKa value is much higher than other drugs in this class, resulting in a clinically significant slower onset time. Its high lipid solubility renders it unsuitable for maxillary infiltration injection because its diffusion is retarded by sequestration in mucosal tissues. Bupivacaine is available in dental cartridges as a 0.5% solution with 1:200,000 epinephrine. Bupivacaine is primarily used in dentistry to produce long-acting soft tissue anesthesia lasting 8 hours or more after oral surgical procedures. Combined with appropriate postoperative analgesics and anti-inflammatory drugs, bupivacaine plays an important role in reducing pain in the postoperative period.

VASOCONSTRICTORS

Vasoconstrictors are used to prolong the duration of anesthetic effect, decrease the rate of absorption of local anesthetics, and decrease localized bleeding at the site of administration. Profound α-adrenergic agonism significantly reduces blood flow at the injection site, causing retention of the local anesthetic in the vicinity of the neuronal tissue. The most pronounced effect is to increase the duration of intermediate-acting local anesthetics in the maxilla and mandible.

The two vasoconstrictors available in dental cartridges are epinephrine and levonordefrin. Epinephrine is available in three concentrations: (1) 5 µg/mL (1:200,000); (2) 10 µg/mL (1:100,000); and (3) 20 µg/mL (1:50,000). A standard dental cartridge with 1:100,000 epinephrine contains 18 µg of epinephrine. Levonordefrin is found only in dental cartridges containing mepivacaine in a concentration of 50 µg/mL (1:20,000). A standard dental cartridge with 1:20,000 levonordefrin contains 90 µg of levonordefrin. Although levonordefrin is a weaker adrenergic agonist than epinephrine, the 1:20,000 concentration is five times greater than the standard concentration of epinephrine. Levonordefrin also has a preponderance of α-adrenergic effects relative to its β-adrenergic stimulation. This could create a potential drug interaction resulting in significant hypertension when administered to patients taking nonselective β-blocking drugs.[9] The mucosa of the oral cavity is highly vascularized, and the systemic uptake of vasoconstrictors following intraoral injection may be rapid. A single dental cartridge of lidocaine 2% with 1:100,000 epinephrine can double the resting epinephrine titer within minutes.[10,11] Furthermore, the intraoral administration of eight dental cartridges of a 1:100,000 epinephrine solution may produce plasma epinephrine concentrations equivalent to

those present during heavy exercise.[12] Sung and colleagues[13] demonstrated that a slow infusion of epinephrine produced a significant incidence of chest pain and ST-segment depression in patients with coronary artery disease. It is therefore important to limit the amount of vasoconstrictor-containing local anesthetic solutions in patients with severe anxiety or cardiovascular disease. As a general rule, the minimum possible amount of vasoconstrictor should be used. Caution should also be exercised in patients taking nonspecific β-adrenergic blockers, adrenergic neuron blockers, tricyclic antidepressants, phenothiazine derivatives, and cocaine.

USE IN PEDIATRICS

Local anesthetics are important in the dental care of children and are safe and effective. However, pediatric patients are easily susceptible to local anesthetic toxicity if care is not taken to calculate the correct dosage before administration. All children and small adults should be weighed before establishing the maximum amount of local anesthetic that can be administered safely. Calculations of the maximum recommended local anesthetic dose are based on weight and patient acuity. Although some authors[14] have made no dose modifications on a milligram per kilogram basis, the American Academy of Pediatric Dentistry has developed a *Guideline on Use of Local Anesthetics for Pediatric Dental Patients* with dosage recommendations for the safe use of local anesthetics in pediatric patients.[15] Specifically, the dosages of lidocaine and mepivacaine have been significantly reduced compared with the recommended adult doses. The maximum recommended dose of these two drugs is 4.4 mg/kg. Thus, for a 20-kg child, the maximum dose of lidocaine is 88 mg, or 2.4 cartridges of the drug. Articaine, which has a lower toxic potential, may be given in a dose up to 7 mg/kg. The same 20-kg child could therefore receive 140 mg, or 1.9 cartridges of articaine. Bupivacaine is not used in the pediatric patient because of the prolonged duration of action and the potential for self-mutilation.

Although lip and cheek biting might be minimized by the administration of phentolamine mesylate (OraVerse; Novalor Pharmaceuticals, San Diego, CA) at the end of a procedure, this may not be practical for oral surgical procedures in which the rapid onset of postoperative pain is a major concern, but could be of use in the pediatric or special needs patient.

In a landmark paper, Goodson and Moore[16] demonstrated that life-threatening toxic local anesthetic reactions occurred with higher frequency in pediatric patients undergoing sedation that included opioids. Care should be taken during pediatric sedation to use the minimally effective dose of opioid and local anesthetic. The use of oral midazolam as a premedicant combined with nitrous oxide–oxygen is a viable sedation technique, as is the use of short-acting opioids, such as remifentanil.

COMPLICATIONS AND REASONS FOR FAILURE
Paresthesia

One of the most devastating localized complications after any intraoral injection is the occurrence of prolonged paresthesia in any of the trigeminal nerve distributions. Most typically it is associated with the inferior alveolar and especially lingual nerves, and may result from direct mechanical needle trauma, hemorrhage, extraneural or intraneural edema, or chemical neurotoxicity of the local anesthetic drug itself. The altered sensation is usually transient and resolves spontaneously within days, weeks, or months. In rare instances, the damage can be of long duration or permanent. Haas and Lennon[6] conducted a long-term retrospective study examining the incidence of paresthesia associated with local anesthesia. They reported that paresthesia was more frequent with 4% prilocaine and 4% articaine relative to the frequency of use. They reported an incidence of 1 in 500,000 for prilocaine and articaine, and an incidence of 1 in 1.2 million for other local anesthetics. Although it is possible that the drugs themselves could be neurotoxic, it seems more likely that the 4% concentration is the determining factor. The surgeon should carefully weigh the benefit/risk ratio when considering the use of articaine or any other 4% local anesthetic solution for a mandibular block injection.

Muscle Trismus

Muscle trismus can also be a sequela of a mandibular block. Limitation of muscular function after an intraoral injection may be caused by hematoma formation, direct muscle injury secondary to needle trauma, localized muscle necrosis secondary to the anesthetic drug or vasoconstrictor, infection in a fascial space, or the introduction of a foreign body. The treatment of intraoral trismus may include nonsteroidal anti-inflammatory agents, saline mouth rinses, antibiotics, and physical therapy.

Hematoma

Formation of a hematoma is the result of direct needle trauma to a blood vessel, and is most likely to occur after a posterior superior alveolar nerve block and greater palatine canal and high tuberosity approaches to the maxillary nerve. Signs and symptoms of hematoma include rapid swelling, a sensation of fullness in the area, facial asymmetry, and mild trismus. Management of a hematoma includes patient reassurance and application of ice to the affected area on the day of injury, followed in 24 hours by application of heat. When indicated, posttreatment antibiotics may also be necessary.

Mucosal Irritation

This may be produced by several different causes. Topical anesthetics, when applied to the mucosa for extended periods, may compromise the capillary integrity of the underlying tissue and produce irritation. The injection of excessive volumes of local anesthetics with vasoconstrictors under pressure into tightly attached tissue may produce localized tissue ischemia and ulceration. The taut tissue overlying the hard palate is the most frequent location of this complication. High-pressure injection techniques, such as the periodontal ligament and intraosseous injections, have been reported to produce irritation and even necrosis of the interdental papilla, with exposure of the underlying bone. Self-inflicted injuries, such as cheek, lip, and tongue biting, are common causes of mucosal irritation after local anesthesia in children and occasionally in adults.

Infection

Although it is an extremely rare complication of local anesthesia with the use of sterile, single-use needles and cartridges, infection may result from injection into or through an infected area; the use of the same cartridge or needle in more than one patient (a major breech in patient safety); and multiple uses of the same needle in the same patient. Preparing the injection site with an antiseptic agent before injection may reduce the amount of bacteria at the site, but it is inconclusive as to whether this action prevents infection from intraoral needle injections.

Needle Breakage

Needle breakage is a rare occurrence during intraoral injection. The advent of the single-use, disposable needles coupled with high-quality manufacturing techniques have minimized this problem. However, unexpected patient movement, excessive lateral force by the operator, manufacturing defects, intentional overbending of needles, and use of 30-gauge needles have all been implicated in needle breakage. Needles are most susceptible to breakage at the needle-hub interface and should never be inserted to this level because the needle is not easily retrieved and must be recovered surgically.

Reasons for Failure

With an understanding of the anatomic foundations of clinical techniques and the correct choice of local anesthetic agent, the success rate for neural blockade of the dentition and soft tissue of the oral cavity is very high. The most common cause of a failed injection is improper identification of appropriate anatomic landmarks or a patient exhibiting anatomic variations.

Inappropriate needle selection may also contribute to failure. A needle that is too long or too short, coupled with uncertainty about the required depth of penetration, could lead to failure or breakage. The selection of a thin needle for certain injections may result in deflection as it passes through mucosa, muscle, and soft tissue away from the intended path of insertion. For this reason, a 25-gauge needle is preferable to a 27- or 30-gauge needle for intraoral injections. Occasionally, patients may experience some subjective signs of anesthesia but may not be able to withstand instrumentation without pain. This may be caused in part by injection of an inadequate volume of anesthetic solution or not waiting long enough for the action of the local anesthetic to penetrate the neural sheath. Increasing the volume of injected solution often remedies this problem. Increasing volume may also be of benefit in patients with anatomic variations. Patients who continually respond to vibration and pressure sensations despite profound local anesthesia probably require sedation or general anesthesia for complete comfort.

Cross-innervation from the contralateral side especially in procedures in and around the midline or from other less common neural elements must always be considered. In the mandible, variant branches of the inferior alveolar nerve may leave the nerve before it enters the mandibular foramen. These branches are not blocked by the conventional inferior alveolar nerve block. A more superiorly oriented injection may be necessary for success in a case such as this. The mylohyoid nerve, which supplies sensory and motor function to the mylohyoid muscle and anterior belly of the digastric, may enter the mandible on the lingual side by a foramen in the bicuspid region. This occurs in about 10% of patients and may provide sensory innervation to the incisor teeth. Again, an apparently successful conventional inferior alveolar block does not affect this nerve, and a higher injection or lingual infiltration may be necessary.

Finally, when the previously mentioned causes for failed anesthesia have been ruled out, the possibility of alternative innervation should be considered. Variant nerves may exist that supply structures not usually associated with them. This can occur in patients with an extremely high palate and long alveolar process. The nasopalatine nerve may exchange fibers with the anterior superior alveolar nerve, and contribute to the innervation of the incisor teeth. The long buccal nerve, although a branch of the third division of the trigeminal nerve, may innervate the buccal soft tissue in the maxillary molar area.

Occasionally, the pharyngeal plexus of nerves, which normally supply the pharynx, may supply impacted mandibular third molars. Very rarely the cutaneous coli nerve, a branch of the cervical plexus, may enter the mandible on the inner surface of the lingual cortical plate and provide accessory innervation to the mandibular teeth.

Another possible cause for failed local anesthesia is the presence of tissue inflammation. Because inflammation increases tissue blood flow, the systemic absorption of local anesthetic solutions is usually increased. Inflammation may also modify the activity of peripheral nerves by lowering the response threshold, changing the protein structure of the nerve, or enhancing conduction. Most significantly, inflammation lowers the tissue pH and creates an acidic environment. Lowered tissue pH significantly reduces the ability of local anesthetic drugs to block nervous tissue, and may render them ineffective. Injecting through areas of active inflammation is to be avoided and blocks more proximal to the lesion are advised.

UPDATES AND FUTURE TRENDS

This section updates changes in current practices and looks at possible future local anesthetic modalities and research possibilities. It serves to illustrate that nothing in medicine and dentistry is ever static. Who could have imagined a few years ago that local anesthetic effects could be shortened or reversed, or that major toxic reactions could be treated successfully? There is hope that advances in basic research will translate into clinical practice.

Reversal

One of the effects of local anesthetics that may be at best annoying, and at worst injurious, is the prolonged duration of soft tissue anesthesia beyond the therapeutic need. Prolonged numbness may result in difficulty with eating, drinking, speaking, and inadvertent cheek, lip, and tongue biting. Prolonged numbness is also a major cause of anxiety and severe behavioral problems in pediatric and special needs patients. Dentists have tried to decrease the duration by using infiltration instead of nerve block injections whenever possible, by using local anesthetics without vasoconstrictors and alternative techniques, such as intraligamentary injections with limited success. Recently, phentolamine mesylate (OraVerse) has been introduced to reduce the duration of dental anesthetics. Phentolamine is a nonselective α-adrenergic blocking agent that was initially used to treat hypertension. Clinically, when injected into the anesthetic site, it produces a localized vasodilation. It is postulated that the injection of phentolamine into an area awash with local anesthetic would result in an accelerated clearance of the local anesthetic from the submucosal tissue and thus shorten the duration of effect. Hersh and colleagues[17] studied the effects of phentolamine on the duration of soft tissue anesthesia in adolescents and adults. There was an 85-minute reduction in the median time to recovery of normal lip sensation compared with control subjects. Tavares and colleagues[18] studied the effects of phentolamine in pediatric patients aged 4 to 11 years. There was greater than a 55% reduction in the median time to return to normal lip sensation, and a 60% reduction in the median time to return of normal tongue sensation compared with control subjects. No cardiovascular or other side effects were evident in either adult or pediatric patient groups. Phentolamine was determined to be safe and well-tolerated in adults and children. Studies are currently underway to determine the safety and efficacy of phentolamine in children younger than the age of 4. Phentolamine is supplied in a cartridge that fits into a standard dental syringe. The drug is injected directly into the same area, in the same volume as the original local anesthetic solution.

Lipid Emulsions and the Treatment of Toxicity

Bupivacaine is known to cause rapid and resistant cardiac toxicity when administered rapidly in high concentrations and volumes. In 1998, Weinberg and colleagues[19] demonstrated that the doses and serum concentrations of bupivacaine required for cardiac toxicity in rats were increased when the rats were pretreated with a lipid emulsion (Intralipid; Fresenius Kabi, Uppsala, Sweden). It is postulated that a "lipid sink" is created, which reduces the serum concentration by removing bupivacaine from the sites of action in the myocardium and reversing the bupivacaine-induced cardiac toxicity. There have been several case reports of the successful use of Intralipid to reverse the cardiac toxicity of local anesthetics.[20,21] Treatment of local anesthetic toxicity with lipid emulsions has become so successful that it is now a part of the Advanced Cardiac Life Support Guidelines for the treatment of local anesthetic toxicity.[22]

Buffering

Local anesthetics containing vasoconstrictors are acidic solutions, which when injected, dissociate into an uncharged base form and a cationic form. The uncharged base diffuses into the nerve where it dissociates again to occupy sodium channels. It has been theorized that buffering the anesthetic solution to raise its pH should increase the amount of base form available for diffusion into the nerve. This would result in a faster onset with better efficacy compared with standard vasoconstrictor-containing solutions. The carbonation of the anesthetic may also diminish pain on injection and increase the depth of anesthesia by concentrating the local anesthetic molecules by iontrapping. Several authors have reported an increased rate of onset and intensity of peripheral nerve blocks with buffered local anesthetics.[23,24] A recent study, however, failed to confirm a faster onset, greater success, or less pain with buffered versus standard lidocaine with epinephrine for inferior alveolar nerve block.[25] Buffering of local anesthetic solutions in dentistry has always been hampered by the decrease in shelf-life of the solutions and the difficulty of buffering the drug in a dental cartridge. OnPharma, Inc. (Los Gatos, CA) has developed a mixing pen device that enables the dentist to remove a set volume of local anesthetic from a dental cartridge immediately before injection and replace it with the same volume of sodium bicarbonate. This technique makes buffering easier and more available, but more studies are needed to confirm its benefits for routine dental or surgical procedures.

Mannitol

In a further attempt to increase the efficacy of local anesthetics, the osmotic diuretic mannitol has been added to local anesthetic solutions to increase diffusion. Mannitol's principle use is to reduce the risk of perioperative renal failure, help chemotherapeutic agents cross the blood-brain barrier, and treat cerebral edema. The perineural sheath surrounding the nerve trunk acts as a diffusional barrier for local anesthetics. This may lead to incomplete blockade, as is sometimes seen with blocks of the inferior alveolar nerve. The addition of this hyperosmolar solution can shrink the perineural sheath and allow the anesthetic to penetrate more readily.[26] Mannitol has been shown to be effective in opening the perineural membrane.[27]

Wolf and colleagues[28] examined the effect of the addition of mannitol to lidocaine 2% with 1:100,000 epinephrine compared with a mannitol-free solution for an inferior alveolar nerve block. They were able to demonstrate that the addition of mannitol significantly improved the effectiveness of the block. Although the results are promising, this technique is still in its experimental phase.

Extended-release Bupivacaine

Long-lasting postoperative pain control is an important issue after extensive oral surgical procedures. Traditional postoperative opioid prescriptions, although somewhat effective, have been associated with adverse effects, abuse, and over-prescribing. A multimodal approach to pain control improves postoperative pain outcomes. This approach combines different modalities targeting different pain mechanisms. For example, a patient may be given preoperative oral nonsteroidal anti-inflammatory agents, intravenous sedation, or general anesthesia in which opioids or ketamine are used; intraoral injection of long-acting local anesthetics; perioperative steroids; and intravenous ketorolac or acetaminophen. Recently, a new drug delivery system has been introduced that may have future application in oral surgery. Pacira Pharmaceuticals (Parsippany, NJ) has received Food and Drug Administration approval for a bupivacaine liposome injectable suspension marketed as Exparel. Bupivacaine is encapsulated in DepoFoam (Pacira Pharmaceuticals), an extended-release liposomal drug delivery technology. DepoFoam is a microscopic, spherical honey-combed structure with internal chambers filled with encapsulated bupivacaine. After injection, the drug is released over time as the particles erode. In a study evaluating this extended-release bupivacaine delivery system for pain control after hemorrhoidectomy, Gorfine and coworkers[29] showed a 30% reduction in pain 72 hours postoperatively compared with placebo. They also noted a reduction in the amount of rescue medication (morphine) needed for breakthrough pain. Extended-release bupivacaine offers exciting possibilities for the future of postoperative pain control in oral surgery.

Intranasal Tetracaine

It has been reported that there is a 33% failure rate when anesthetizing the maxillary central incisor with the anterior superior alveolar block.[30] When the nasopalatine nerve was blocked in addition, the success rate reached 100%. A 2:1 relationship was demonstrated between the anterior superior alveolar nerve and the nasopalatine nerve for central incisor innervation. It is known that fibers of the

superior alveolar plexus occasionally join the nasopalatine nerve just below the nasal floor and travel with the nasopalatine nerve to reach the central incisor.[31] Physicians and oral surgeons have long applied topical local anesthetics to the nasal cavity. Noorily and coworkers[32] compared the effects of cocaine, lidocaine, and tetracaine on nasal mucosa and determined that tetracaine produced superior long-lasting nasal anesthesia. Because tetracaine is hydrolyzed by pseudocholinesterase, toxic reactions, if any, would be brief. Because tetracaine is capable of producing profound nasal anesthesia it might also be effective in anesthetizing branches of the anterior superior alveolar and nasopalatine nerves. Currently, there is ongoing interest in evaluating the efficacy of an intranasal tetracaine spray to act as a functional dental anesthetic for maxillary anterior teeth.

Ropivacaine

Ropivacaine was approved for clinical use in 1996. Structurally related to mepivacaine and bupivacaine, it was found to have low toxicity, a long duration, and selectivity for nerve fibers responsible for pain transmission. Ropivacaine seems to have a 70% to 75% greater margin of safety than bupivacaine.[33] Cardiac toxicity is reduced because it contains only the S-enantiomer, whereas bupivacaine is a racemic mixture. El-Sharrawy and Yagiela[34] compared various concentrations of ropivacaine for use as an injectable local anesthetic for inferior alveolar nerve block. The 0.25% and 0.375% solutions had a slow onset and produced poor surgical conditions. The 0.5% and 0.75% concentrations had a rapid onset and produced good surgical conditions lasting more than 3 hours. Although the pKa values are equal, ropivacaine had a much faster onset than bupivacaine because of weaker binding to extraneural and submucosal tissues. This allows for more rapid diffusion to the site of action. The long duration is attributed to ropivacaine's inherent vasoconstrictive properties. Further studies in dental models evaluated the efficacy of a plain 0.75% solution of ropivacaine compared with one containing epinephrine.[35] The addition of epinephrine did not improve the quality or duration of effect, so the addition of a vasoconstrictor is not necessary for the use of ropivacaine in dentistry. Additionally, ropivacaine has proved successful for third molar surgery and for maxillary infiltration anesthesia.[36,37] At this time, the main disadvantage to the routine use of ropivacaine in dentistry is that it is not available in dental cartridges. Otherwise, it has advantages over bupivacaine in that it is more rapid-acting, does not require a vasoconstrictor, and produces less central nervous system and cardiac toxicity. Ropivacaine would be a welcome addition to the dental local anesthetic armamentarium. Consideration should be given to its manufacture and availability for dentistry.[38]

New Local Anesthetic Formulations

The adverse effects of vasoconstrictors in patients with significant cardiovascular system impairments are a real issue whenever the risks or benefits of a particular local anesthetic are considered. Although plain solutions are valuable, readministration may be necessary to augment the duration and effect. Prilocaine and articaine are available in reduced vasoconstrictor concentrations (1:200,000 epinephrine), but there is some concern about an increased incidence of paresthesia with mandibular block anesthesia with these 4% solutions. The potential advantages of ropivacaine as a plain solution are clear, but cost and availability are factors. The efficacy of lidocaine with 1:200,000 epinephrine has been compared with lidocaine with 1:100,000 epinephrine, and no clinical difference was detected in success or failure between these two concentrations.[39] Articaine 4% with 1:400,000 epinephrine was shown to be adequate for pain control and hemostasis during dental treatment, although decreasing its duration of action.[40] With the combination of an aging population, increasing medical complexity, wide spectrum of drug interactions, and medical and surgical advances, the application of local anesthesia is not static, but dynamic. Newer drugs and techniques continue to impact the ability to treat patients safely and effectively.

SUMMARY

Local anesthesia remains the foundation of pain control in dentistry especially when combined with moderate-deep sedation for invasive and painful procedures in the contemporary oral and maxillofacial surgical model. Dentistry has never had the choice of local anesthetic drugs and techniques that can be tailored to individual patients and procedures as are available today. Local anesthetics remain the safest and most effective drugs in medicine and dentistry to relieve intraoperative and postoperative pain. It is only with a thorough understanding of pharmacology and anatomy that clinicians have the basic clinical foundation to enhance the care of patients.

REFERENCES

1. Franz DN, Perry RS. Mechanisms for differential block among single myelinated and nonmyelinated axons by procaine. J Physiol 1974;236:193–210.

2. Kindler CH, Paul M, Zou H, et al. Amide local anesthetics potently inhibit the human tandem pore domain background K$^+$ channel TASK-2 (KCNK5). J Pharmacol Exp Ther 2003;306:84–92.

3. Tsuchiya H, Ueno T, Mizogami M. Stereostructure-based differences in the interactions of cardiotoxic local anesthetics with cholesterol-containing biomimetic membranes. Bioorg Med Chem 2011;19:3410–5.

4. Yagiela JA. Local Anesthetics. In: Yagiela JA, Dowd FJ, Johnson BS, et al, editors. Pharmacology and therapeutics for dentistry. 6th edition. St Louis (MO): Mosby Elsevier; 2010. p. 256.

5. American Dental Association. 2002 survey of dental practice: characteristics of dentists in prive practice & their patients. Chicago: American Dental Association; 2002.

6. Haas DA, Lennon D. A 21 year retrospective study of reports of paresthesia following local anesthetic administration. J Can Dent Assoc 1995;61:319–30.

7. Malamed SF, Gagnon S, Leblanc D. Efficacy of articaine: a new amide local anesthetic. J Am Dent Assoc 2000;131(5):635–42.

8. Abdulwahab M, Boynes S, Moore P, et al. The efficacy of six local anesthetic formulations used for posterior mandibular buccal infiltration anesthesia. J Am Dent Assoc 2009;140:1018–24.

9. Mito RS, Yagiela JA. Hypertensive response to levonordefrin in a patient receiving propranolol: report of a case. J Am Dent Assoc 1988;116:55–7.

10. Cryer PE. Physiology and pathophysiology of the human sympathoadrenal neuroendocrine system. N Engl J Med 1980;303(8):436–44.

11. Bennett CR. Monheim's local anesthesia and pain control in dental practice. 7th edition. St Louis (MO): Mosby; 1984.

12. Cioffi GA, Chernow B, Glahn RP, et al. The hemodynamic and plasma catecholamine responses to routine restorative dental care. J Am Dent Assoc 1985;111(1):67–70.

13. Sung BH, Wilson MF, Robinson C, et al. Mechanisms of myocardial ischemia induced by epinephrine: comparison with exercise-induced ischemia. Psychosom Med 1988;50:381–93.

14. Finder RL, Moore PA. Adverse drug reactions to local anesthesia. Dent Clin North Am 2002;46:747–57.

15. AAPD Guideline on Use of Local Anesthetics for Pediatric Dental Patients. Adopted 2005, Revised 2009. Available at: http://www.aapd.org/media/Policies_Guidelines/G_LocalAnesthesia.pdf. Accessed July 16, 2012.

16. Goodson JM, Moore PA. Life-threatening reactions after pedodontic sedation: an assessment of narcotic, local anesthetic, and antiemetic drug interaction. J Am Dent Assoc 1983;107:239–45.

17. Hersh EV, Moore PA, Papas AS, et al. Reversal of soft-tissue local anesthesia with phentolamine

mesylate in adolescents and adults. J Am Dent Assoc 2008;139:1080–93.

18. Tavares M, Goodson JM, Studen-Pavlovich D, et al. Reversal of soft-tissue local anesthesia with phentolamine mesylate in pediatric patients. J Am Dent Assoc 2008;139:1095–104.

19. Weinberg GL, VadeBoncouer T, Ramaraju GA, et al. Pretreatment or resuscitation with a lipid infusion shifts the dose-response curve to bupivacaine-induced asystole in rats. Anesthesiology 1998;88: 1071–5.

20. Litz RJ, Popp M, Stehr SN, et al. Successful resuscitation of a patient with ropivacaine-induced asystole after axillary plexus block using lipid infusion. Anaesthesia 2006;61:800–1.

21. Rosenblatt MA, Abel M, Fischer GW, et al. Successful use of a 20% lipid emulsion to resuscitate a patient after a presumed bupivacaine-related cardiac arrest. Anesthesiology 2006;105:217–8.

22. Vanden Hock TL, Morrison LJ, Shuster M, et al. Part 12: cardiac arrest in special situations: 2010 American Heart Association Guidelines for Cardiopulmonary Resuscitation and Emergency Cardiovascular Care. Circulation 2010;122:S843.

23. Galindo A. pH-adjusted local anesthetics: clinical experience. Reg Anesth 1983;8:35–6.

24. Benzon HT, Toleikis JR, Dixit P, et al. Onset intensity of blockade and somatosensory evoked potential changes of the lumbosacral dermatomes after epidural anesthesia with alkalinized lidocaine. Anesth Analg 1993;76:328–32.

25. Whitcomb M, Drum M, Reader A, et al. A prospective, randomized, double-blind study of the anesthetic efficacy of sodium bicarbonate buffered 2% lidocaine with 1:100,000 epinephrine in inferior alveolar nerve blocks. Anesth Prog 2010;57:59–66.

26. Taylor RE. Modification of permeability of frog perineurium to (^{14}C)-sucrose by stretch and hypertonicity. Brain Res 1979;173:503–12.

27. Antonijevic I, Mousa S, Schafer M, et al. Perineural defect and peripheral opioid analgesia in inflammation. J Neurosci 1995;15:165–72.

28. Wolf R, Reader A, Drum M, et al. Mannitol and lidocaine with epinephrine in inferior alveolar nerve blocks: a prospective randomized, single-blind study. Anesth Prog 2011;58:157–65.

29. Gorfine SR, Onel E, Patou G, et al. Bupivacaine extended-release liposome injection for prolonged postsurgical analgesia in patients undergoing hemorrhoidectomy: a multicenter, randomized, double-blind, placebo-controlled trial. Dis Colon Rectum 2011;54:1552–9.

30. Meyer TN, Lemos LL, Nascimento CNM, et al. Effectiveness of nasopalatine nerve block for anesthesia of maxillary central incisors after failure of the anterior superior alveolar nerve block technique. Braz Dent J 2007;18:69–73.

31. Blanton PL, Jeske AH. The key to profound local anesthesia: neuroanatomy. J Am Dent Assoc 2003; 134:753–60.

32. Noorily AD, Noorily SH, Otto RA. Cocaine, lidocaine, tetracaine: which is best for topical nasal anesthesia? Anesth Analg 1995;81:724–7.

33. Reiz S, Haggmark S, Johansson G, et al. Cardiotoxicity of ropivacaine: a new amide local anesthetic agent. Acta Anaesthesiol Scand 1989;33:93–8.

34. El-Sharrawy E, Yagiela JA. Anesthetic efficacy of different ropivacaine concentrations for inferior alveolar nerve block. Anesth Prog 2006;53:3–7.

35. Oliveira NE, Lima Filho NS, Lima EG, et al. Effects of regional anesthesia with ropivacaine on arterial pressure and heart rate in healthy subjects. Eur J Oral Sci 2006;114:27–32.

36. Brkovic BM, Zltkovic D, Jovanovic D, et al. Maxillary infiltration anaesthesia by ropivacaine for upper third molar surgery. Int J Oral Maxillofac Surg 2010;39: 36–41.

37. Krzeminski TF, Gilowski L, Wiench R, et al. Comparison of ropivacaine and lidocaine with epinephrine for infiltration anesthesia in dentistry. A randomized study. Am J Dent 2011;24:305–9.

38. All-Atabakhsh A, Rosenberg MB. Ropivacaine: the next dental local anesthetic? J Mass Dent Soc 2012;61:14–6.

39. Vreeland DL, Reader A, Beck M, et al. An evaluation of volumes and concentrations of lidocaine in human inferior alveolar nerve block. J Endod 1989;15:6–12.

40. Daublander M, Kammerer PW, Willerhausen B, et al. Clinical use of an epinephrine-reduced (1:400,000) articaine solution in short-time dental routine treatments-a multicenter study. Clin Oral Invest 2012;16(4):1289–95.

Pediatric Sedation and Anesthesia for the Oral Surgeon

David W. Todd, DMD, MD, FACD

KEYWORDS

• Pediatric • Sedation • Anesthesia • Oral surgery

KEY POINTS

- The OMS must be familiar with pediatric anesthetic techniques to enable performance of procedures on young patients as a result of complexity of procedures and need to control the surgical field. Even simple surgical procedures require expertise in pediatric anesthetic techniques when general practitioners or pediatric dentists have attempted procedures and found that the child patient is not cooperative with local anesthetic or enteral sedation.
- The OMS must have techniques available to provide pediatric anesthesia that is safe, relatively predictable, and efficient.
- Differences in anatomy and physiology between the adult and pediatric patient, preanesthetic assessment, fasting guidelines, and choices of sedation routes are reviewed, and equipment options for the management of pediatric anesthesia are discussed.

INTRODUCTION

Treating a child who requires the expertise of the oral and maxillofacial surgeon (OMS) can be a simple process when the child is cooperative, has low fear and anxiety, and has no medical problems, and when the procedure is relatively simple. However, even simple procedures can become challenging when the child patient has a high degree of fear and anxiety. The OMS often becomes involved with surgical and anesthetic management when general practitioners or pediatric dentists have attempted simple procedures and have found that the child patient is not cooperative with local anesthetic or enteral sedation. For medically compromised pediatric patients or for those requiring more extensive procedures, the hospital or an ambulatory surgery center (ASC) is the best location to treat these patients, and may be the best choice when the fearful and uncooperative child patient has medical comorbidities. For a variety of

reasons, however, scheduling all children for procedures in the ASC or hospital is not feasible. The OMS must have techniques available to provide pediatric anesthesia that is safe, relatively predictable, and efficient. This article discusses the approach to the pediatric patient and expands on concepts outlined in the American Association of Oral and Maxillofacial Surgeons (AAOMS) *Office Anesthesia Evaluation Manual.*[1] Differences in anatomy and physiology between the adult and pediatric patient, preanesthetic assessment, fasting guidelines, and choices of sedation routes are reviewed, and equipment options for the management of pediatric anesthesia are discussed. Management of pediatric emergencies is discussed elsewhere in this issue. After reflection on these topics the OMS can decide, based on training and experience, the ages of patients, medical comorbidities, and techniques with which they are most comfortable in performing surgery in the office in a safe and effective manner.

Private Practice, 120 Southwestern Drive, Lakewood, NY 14750, USA
E-mail address: drtodd@stny.rr.com

Oral Maxillofacial Surg Clin N Am 25 (2013) 467–478
http://dx.doi.org/10.1016/j.coms.2013.03.009
1042-3699/13/$ – see front matter © 2013 Elsevier Inc. All rights reserved.

oralmaxsurgery.theclinics.com

PSYCHOLOGICAL ASSESSMENT

The assessment of the anxiety of the pediatric patient can be obtained in a variety of ways, and the ability of the OMS to determine this is somewhat dependent on the patient's age. Younger children less than 6 years old are less able to verbalize their concerns and anxiety. In addition, children of this age group are less able to understand the purpose or benefit of the procedure. The parents of the child are an important source of information in describing how much anxiety and potential cooperation are present, and the previous dental or medical care providers can describe their experience with the patient and responses to various previous interventions. The information gathered will affect the options available for the anesthetic plan. Older children are more able to describe their anxiety and fears, and can help make decisions about the anesthetic plan. Although a variety of behavioral techniques are available and are important, often these techniques must be augmented by pharmacologic interventions. It is estimated that 50% to 75% of child patients develop significant anxiety in the perioperative period, consisting of several concerns.[2] Parental presence in the operatory can be considered as an aide to patient management. Most parents feel that they are a great benefit to their children in this setting, although the perspective of the health care providers is that it can be helpful or harmful.[3–5] For procedures under local anesthetic, this author believes that parental presence is beneficial in most cases. If parents do desire to observe their child during induction it is important to explain what they may observe as their child becomes sedated or falls asleep. When intravenous (IV) sedation or general anesthetic is performed, this author has the parent escorted out of the room after initiation of the anesthetic technique, fearing that the parental presence could be a major distraction if treatment of an adverse event has to be initiated.

DIFFERENCES IN PHYSIOLOGY AND ANATOMY

The OMS treating the pediatric anesthetic patient must understand the differences in anatomy and physiology between the adult and the pediatric patient. These differences account for the different equipment required and different responses to anesthetic interventions. Normal vital signs for pediatric patients can be found in a variety of resources such as the American Heart Association (AHA) Pediatric Advanced Life Support (PALS) book[6] or the Broselow tape (**Table 1**).[7] These differences in vital signs normalize toward adult values after about age 12 years. There are important differences in the airway, cardiorespiratory systems, and thermoregulation of pediatric patients. As most OMS are not treating patients younger than 3 or 4 years in the office environment, other organ systems such as the renal, hepatic, hematologic, and endocrine systems, and distribution of body water can be considered similar to those of the adult patient for the purposes of this discussion.[8] In terms of thermoregulation, it is important to understand that pediatric patients have a higher surface area to body weight ratio in comparison with adults, and thus lose heat a greater rate than do adults.[8] Hypothermia is a frequently unrecognized problem in all surgical patients, which in the pediatric patient can result in slower awakening, cardiac instability, and respiratory depression.

Differences in the airway anatomy of the pediatric patient are outlined in **Table 2**. These differences can lead to airway management problems using open airway, mask ventilation, supraglottic airways, and endotracheal intubation. Having the appropriately sized equipment and always having the next possible airway intervention available will minimize the risk of losing the airway. Differences in the respiratory and cardiovascular systems are outlined in **Table 3**.[8–12] The pediatric patient has

Table 1
Sample vital signs for pediatric patients

Age	Heart Rate	Blood Pressure	Respiratory Rate
3 mo to 2 y	100–190		24–40
2–10 y	60–140	100/60	22–34 preschooler 18–30 school-aged
>10 y	60–100	110/60	12–16 adolescent
Definition of hypotension			
Children 1–10 y	<70 + (age in y × 2)		
Children >10 y	<90		

Data from Chamedies L, Samson R, Schexnayder S, et al. Pediatric advanced life support provider manual. Dallas, TX: American Heart Association; 2011.

Table 2
Differences in airway anatomy and consequences

Tongue	Larger in proportion to the oral cavity	More difficult to manipulate More prone to obstruction
Larynx	Higher and more cephalad More anterior	More difficult to visualize More prone to obstruction
Vocal cords	More angulated	More difficult to visualize
Epiglottis	More narrow and angled away from trachea	Backfolding with supraglottic airways more common More difficult to visualize larynx
Lymphoid tissue	Relatively large	Airway more prone to obstruction
Cricoid cartilage	Narrowest portion of the airway	Endotracheal tube can cause injury and edema
Submucosal glands	Greater in number	Possibly increase in airway secretions

an airway that is more prone to collapse, has less compensatory capability during upper airway obstruction, and has less pulmonary reserve. Functional residual capacity (FRC) is the amount of air remaining in the lung after normal expiration, and is significantly lower in the pediatric patient. Pediatric patients have a higher metabolic rate, and this reduced pulmonary reserve leads to shorter safe apnea periods compared with the adult patient. Pediatric patients, especially if very young, have a higher rate of laryngospasm[13] than adult patients, and because of their lack of reserve desaturate rapidly without intervention. Recommended airway interventions for a variety of scenarios are shown in **Table 4**.[14] By age 10 to 12 years, most of these differences in the pediatric airway have developed to adult status. The consequences of the immature cardiovascular system mean that there is less compensatory capability in the pediatric patient. Cardiac output depends on heart rate; bradycardia will predictably cause hypotension, especially in children younger than 3 years, and is a premorbid event unless corrected. Unfortunately, the cardiovascular system will respond to hypoxia with

bradycardia, and has a higher baseline vagal tone. Having the correct dose of a paralytic, atropine, and epinephrine available preoperatively is important in managing the very young pediatric patient.

PREOPERATIVE EVALUATION AND PATIENT SELECTION

The goal of the preoperative evaluation in the healthy pediatric patient is to identify unrecognized medical problems or anatomic problems that will increase risk of surgery and anesthesia (**Fig. 1**).[15] It is interesting that provider-related risk is included in this figure, and that Cote,[16,17] in his review of adverse events in pediatric anesthesia, found that monitoring and resuscitative skills of the provider were more important than the route of administration or drugs used for sedation. For pediatric patients with chronic medical problems, optimizing their condition and anticipating potential complications is the goal of the preoperative evaluation. For very young children, questions should focus on whether prematurity occurred, whether normal

Table 3
Differences in respiratory and cardiovascular system

Cardiovascular system	Dependent on heart rate for cardiac output (CO) CO higher than in adults to meet metabolic demand Cannot compensate well for hypovolemia or fluid overload High parasympathetic tone
Respiratory system	Chest wall more compliant Rib cage more angulated and diaphragm more horizontal Accessory muscles of respiration less well developed Low functional residual capacity expressed on a weight basis Smaller airway cross section making edema and secretions proportionately more significant in airway reduction and increased resistance Fewer number and smaller size of alveoli

Table 4
Airway obstructions: causes and treatment

Causes	Treatment
Anatomic and mechanical airway obstructions	
Inadequate head position	Repositioning/reopening the airway
Poor facemask technique	Oro-/nasopharyngeal airway
Large adenoids/tonsils/obesity	Two-hand/2-person technique
Foreign body, regurgitated gastric contents, blood	Direct laryngoscopy, removal of obstruction, tracheal intubation
Unknown reasons	Supraglottic airway devices
Functional airway obstructions	
Insufficient anesthesia	Deepen anesthesia
Laryngospasm	Muscle paralysis
Opioid-induced muscle rigidity	Muscle paralysis
Bronchospasm	Epinephrine

growth and development milestones have been met, and medical history review has focused on the cardiac and respiratory systems.

Asthma is an important disease process whose incidence has increased dramatically in the pediatric population over the past 20 years. A patient with well-controlled mild asthma is a good candidate for outpatient surgery. Patients with moderate to severe asthma requiring multiple agents for control or who have a history of multiple visits to the emergency room are at increased risk of complications during anesthesia, including intraoperative bronchospasm, hypoxia, desaturation, and laryngospasm. Patients with moderate asthma are often taking an inhaled corticosteroid, a leukotriene inhibitor, and a β2-agonist nebulizer or inhaler. Patients presenting with an inhaled β2-agonist rescue inhaler that is used frequently (3 or more times per week) generally indicate poor control, and should be referred to their primary care doctor for reassessment and likely started on other additional agents. Older pediatric patients will be able to cooperate with peak flow meters, which is the best way to measure the extent of control of their asthma. Those patients obtaining 80% of their predicted peak flow or better are considered

good managers of their asthma, whereas those with 70% to 79% predicted peak flow indicate mild exacerbation for which intervention would be appropriate,[18] with deferral of any planned procedure until better control is demonstrated. Patients with active preoperative wheezing should be deferred until better control can be obtained. Delaying surgery for 6 weeks after an asthma attack is recommended, as FEV_1 (forced expiratory volume in 1 second) remains low for this time frame. A pulse dose of oral steroids can be used to gain control of airway reactivity preoperatively starting either 48 or 24 hours preoperatively, with no taper postoperatively. A typically recommended dose is prednisone, 1 mg/kg.[19] Patients should be continued on their bronchodilator and oral medications on the morning of the surgery.

The issue of upper respiratory infections (URI) in children as it relates to risk in outpatient anesthesia is a frequent topic of concern. Children with a URI have an increased risk of laryngospasm, bronchospasm, coughing, and hypoxia in the perioperative period. Children who live in the northern half of the country experience frequent URI during the winter months, and it is estimated that school-age children have approximately 6 to 8 per year. It is generally accepted that airway reactivity persists for 6 weeks after a URI, leaving very little time between episodes to provide care. Differentiating between a mild and a severe URI becomes important, and Tait and colleagues[20] have outlined these factors in several reviews of the topic (**Table 5**). For a mild URI, it may be possible to proceed without increased risk especially if intubation is not required,[21,22] but for the office practitioner outside the confines of the hospital, where fewer resources are available, it is best to defer. Those patients who

Patient related risk   Procedure related risk

↓   ↓

Perioperative risk

↑   ↑

Anesthesia related risk   Provider related risk

Fig. 1. Preoperative evaluation.

Table 5
Differentiating a mild upper respiratory infection (URI) from severe URI or lower respiratory infection

Mild	Severe
No fever	Fever
No purulent secretions	Purulent secretions
Minimal cough	Cough prominent
Nontoxic appearance	Sick-appearing child

Box 2
Heart murmurs and congenital heart defects

Most systolic murmurs are benign, except pansystolic murmurs, which generally indicate a ventriculoseptal defect

All diastolic murmurs are pathologic

Murmurs that radiate in a pediatric patient are pathologic

present with a mild URI can usually be rescheduled in 1 to 2 weeks. Those with a severe URI should be allowed 4 to 6 weeks of recovery. It is important to understand that seasonal rhinitis is not the same as a URI, and that pneumonia is also not a URI but a lower respiratory tract infection. Tait also reviewed independent risk factors associated with adverse respiratory events that help to make a decision on whether to proceed in the presence of a URI (**Box 1**).

Patients with congenital heart disease are a heterogeneous group of patients who present with diverse pathophysiology. A murmur detected in a pediatric patient who has good exercise tolerance and is asymptomatic is not likely to be pathologic. Pathologic murmurs can usually be grouped with characteristics found in **Box 2**.[23] If there is a question regarding a murmur, it is best to refer the patient to the pediatrician for more thorough assessment. Baseline vital signs, pulse oximetry, and exercise tolerance history are important parameters in helping to assess patients with repaired cardiac defects and to establish which baseline physiologic derangements the patient might have. Exercise tolerance of 4 metabolic equivalents or greater will allow good physiologic tolerance of the stress of procedures and anesthetic techniques. The appropriate history of cardiac interventions and studies, as well as current clinical status, is generally easily obtained

except in emergency situations. Low-risk patients are generally those with patent ductus arteriosus repair and uncomplicated atrial septal defect or ventricular septal defect repair.[24] Office procedures are those with low physiologic stress and minimal blood loss; after consultation with their cardiologist such patients may thus be amenable to office-based anesthesia. High-risk patients would be those with unrepaired defects and significant ventricular dysfunction and shunt-dependent blood flow, and these patients would obviously not be amenable to office-based anesthesia. Inquiry about the need for prophylaxis for subacute bacterial endocarditis would be appropriate for this group of patients.

Obesity in children is an important consideration in preoperative assessment, just as in obese adult patients. Approximately 17% of children are obese, and this percentage has increased dramatically over the past decade.[25] Determination of the extent of obesity is more complex in children, and takes into account sex and age of the patient as well as the height and weight. A body mass index calculator for children is available from the Centers for Disease Control and Prevention.[26] Obese pediatric patients can have the same disturbance in ventilatory mechanics as the obese adult patient, including decreased FRC, tidal volumes that approach closing volumes, and more rapid desaturation than nonobese patients, and can present with hypoxia and hypercarbia and more frequent coughing perioperatively. Obese patients can be expected to have a more complex airway management in comparison with nonobese patients and to present with difficult mask ventilation. Other concerns for the obese pediatric patients include poor IV access, possible delayed gastric emptying time, gastroesophageal reflux disease, diabetes, and obstructive sleep apnea (OSA). Patients with obesity should be given antireflux treatment. Long-standing obesity in pediatric patients can lead to hypertension and left ventricular hypertrophy. In addition, nonalcoholic steatohepatitis and nonalcoholic fatty liver disease are becoming more frequent causes of elevated liver enzymes in obese pediatric patients.[23] OSA is a concern not

Box 1
Independent risk factors for adverse respiratory events in children with active URIs

Use of an endotracheal tube (<5 years old)

History of prematurity

History of reactive airway disease

Parental smoking

Surgery involving the airway

Presence of copious secretions

Nasal congestion

only in obese pediatric patients but is also seen in patients with adenotonsillar hypertrophy and those with Down syndrome. Active questioning should be undertaken to detect this problem in these patients.

Epilepsy is another disease process that is seen with some frequency in pediatric patients. It is important that the type of seizures and frequency of seizures are documented. Performing a check of levels of anticonvulsant medication is unnecessary if there have been no seizures within the last 2 years, there has been no change in dosage, and the patient is compliant with medications. It is recommended to continue antiepileptic medicines on the morning of the surgery. Most anticonvulsant medicines have a long half-life, so missing one dose on the morning of the procedure would not warrant canceling the case if the patient is under good control. All antiepileptic drugs can cause a sedative effect, which is additive to the effects of sedative medications. Whether ketamine consistently produces seizure activity is debatable. Sevoflurane has more epileptic potential than isoflurane, but is thought to be acceptable in patients with seizure disorders.[8] It is important to be aware of medications that increase the risk of seizure (**Table 6**).[27]

The increased incidence of diabetes in the pediatric population has paralleled the increase in childhood obesity. Preoperative assessment of the diabetic patient should ensure that the patient is under good metabolic control. A patient under good metabolic control is a good candidate for outpatient anesthesia for the type of procedures typically performed by an OMS in the office. Ranges of hemoglobin A_{1C} indicating good metabolic control for a variety of ages are as follows: under 5 years of age, 7% to 9%; ages 5 to 13, 6%

to 8.5%; over 13 years of age, 6% to 8%.[28] Blood sugar levels should be between 150 and 250 g/dL. The patient should be scheduled as one of the first cases of the day. Blood sugars are taken preoperatively and postoperatively. Oral medicines should be discontinued on the morning of surgery and short-acting insulins should be held unless needed to control a blood sugar of greater than 250 g/dL. A suggested pathway for patients on long-acting insulin is shown in **Fig. 2**.[28] Despite this recommended pathway, it has been the author's experience that few clinicians provide long-acting insulin on the morning of the procedure and instead use short-acting insulins for the control of blood glucose.

The dose of short-acting insulin necessary to control blood sugar can be calculated using some guidelines. A rough rule of thumb is to provide insulin at a dose of 0.1 U/kg to achieve glycemic control for those patients who normally do not use insulin. A more tailored approach for those who use insulin is to use the "rule of 1500,"[28] which allows for calculation of the change in blood sugar anticipated from 1 unit of insulin. The total daily dose of insulin is divided into 1500. For example, if the patient uses 30 units of insulin daily, then 1500/30 = 50, therefore 1 U of insulin would be expected to lower the blood sugar by 50 g/dL. For patients on an insulin pump and for procedures shorter than 2 hours, it is recommended to maintain basal rate for the procedure and use boluses as needed to achieve glycemic control postoperatively.

The risk of malignant hyperthermia (MH) is higher in the pediatric population than in the adult population. Known triggering agents are succinylcholine and the inhalational anesthetics. The family should be questioned about family history of sudden death during anesthesia, fever during or after anesthesia, history of dark-colored urine after anesthesia, or history of neuromuscular disease such as Duchenne or Becker muscular dystrophy. Since 1994, the routine use of succinylcholine in children has not been recommended by the Food and Drug Administration, but is still acceptable in emergency situations for airway control.[29] The dose of succinylcholine in children is 2 mg/kg IV or 4 mg/kg intramuscular (IM). The OMS needs to understand the risk of MH with triggering agents and to have an appropriate emergency protocol in place to treat such an emergency. The Malignant Hyperthermia Association of the United States is an excellent resource for patients and practitioners regarding this disease process.

Laboratory testing is generally not needed for outpatient procedures. More often a review of recent laboratory values that the pediatrician may have for patients with chronic disease is

Table 6 Selected medications that increase seizure risk in the perioperative period	
Antimicrobials	β-Lactams and related compounds
Anesthetics	meperidine, tramadol (intravenous?), local anesthetics
Immunoregulatory	Cyclosporine, tacrolimus, interferons
Psychotropics	Antidepressants, antipsychotics, lithium
Flumazenil	
Withdrawal from sedative hypnotics	

Evening before surgery, Lantus at dinner or bedtime? → No → full dose of long acting

insulin morning of

Yes

surgery

Hold short acting insulin morning of procedure if BS < 250,

if BS > 250 then use short acting insulin to achieve

BS < 250 according to the "rule of 1500".

Fig. 2. Management of patients taking long acting insulin.

helpful in gaining a better understanding of the control of the disease process. Pregnancy testing should be considered if the patient is sexually active and if the time since the last menstrual period indicates possible pregnancy.

Fasting guidelines for pediatric patients can be remembered using the "8-6-4-2" rule.[23] The rule allows for 8 hours for a solid meal or those with possible delayed gastric emptying, 6 hours for a light meal or formula, 4 hours for breast milk, and 2 hours for clear liquids.

The topic of latex allergy should be reviewed in the medical history form. With increased awareness of this topic over the past 2 decades, manufacturers of medical devices have developed products that are largely latex free. The incidence of contact dermatitis is much more common than true latex anaphylaxis. Children with spina bifida have a high incidence of latex allergy (as much as 71%), and children with history of multiple surgeries (defined as 5 or more) or atopy have a higher incidence of latex allergy compared with those without prior surgical history. Those with a history of true latex allergy should likely be deferred to the hospital setting for management. Avoidance of latex products is the main treatment goal. It is unclear as to whether prophylaxis with H1 and H2 blockers or perioperative steroids is helpful, but these measures continue to be recommended.[30]

APPROACHES TO MANAGEMENT OF THE PEDIATRIC PATIENT

After patient selection and excluding those patients who are not appropriate for an office-based anesthetic, management of pediatric patients depends on the anxiety of patients and their ability to cooperate with initiation of the anesthetic technique. A variety of routes are available and well described in the literature, including the oral, transnasal, rectal, IM, IV, and inhalation routes. Those age ranges whereby the rectal route might be considered generally do not present to the OMS for office-based procedures. Although the transnasal route is available for midazolam and ketamine, the author's experience is that it is not well tolerated by the pediatric patient. It is important to understand that drug dosages and effects in young children are less predictable than those in the adult patient because of differences in physiology, and that the oral and IM routes are less predictable than the IV route (**Table 7**). Younger patients (up to 7 years old) may not cooperate with oral medications. In addition, many patients in the pediatric age group are as fearful of the IV start, as they are of the procedure, so that as a sole technique this is problematic. If the patient has high anxiety regarding the IV start, eutectic mixture of local anesthetic

Table 7 Physiologic differences in children	
Physiologic Characteristic	**Net Effects**
Increased cardiac output to vessel-rich groups	↓ Time to onset of action ↑ Profundity of action
Decreased redistribution because of less fat/muscle mass	↑ Duration of initial drug action ↓ Residual drug effects
Decreased binding by plasma proteins	↑ Increased profundity of action ↓ Decreased residual drug effects
Increased metabolic rate	↓ Duration of drug action
Differences in receptor sensitivity	Variability of dosages needed

(EMLA) cream or amethocaine can be used with nitrous oxide (N_2O_2) to accomplish IV start before proceeding with the IV technique.[12] The strong disadvantage of these topical creams is that they require about an hour of exposure time to be effective. This long time for preparation means that the patient usually has to come an hour earlier than their appointment time to allow application. Alternatively, the OMS can provide a prescription for EMLA cream and directions to the parent as to how and where to apply it. Another method is to combine oral premedication with N_2O_2/O_2 to allow for sedation to accomplish IV start. Oral clonidine, triazolam, ketamine, or midazolam, alone or in combination, are effective for a wide range of ages (**Box 3**) and have an onset time of 20 to 60 minutes. The use of a single agent rather than a combination of agents generally decreases the incidence of adverse events. The author uses clonidine or triazolam as the main oral preoperative medication. Triazolam is used more commonly than clonidine in dentistry, but clonidine has several advantages including minimal respiratory depression, sedation, a sympatholytic effect, postoperative analgesia, and may reduce postoperative nausea and vomiting.[31–34] The disadvantage of the oral route are that there is first-pass metabolism, so that the effect of a given dose has a variable effect, there is delay in onset, and it cannot, of course, be titrated. For patients younger than 12 years, generally the oral premedications are given to the child in the office where monitoring can be performed. Children aged 12 years and older without comorbidities can have premedication of oral triazolam or clonidine at home with the dosages outlined about an hour before the appointment, without fear of respiratory compromise. State regulations vary in permitting oral premedication outside the office environment and should be consulted. Children who are of the age whereby they need to be transported in car seats should not be given oral premedication at home. Use of triazolam and clonidine in this manner is an off-label use of both these medications. If the patient is uncooperative with oral medication or N_2O_2/O_2, the IM route (**Table 8**) becomes another choice, using midazolam or ketamine, or a combination, to allow for initiation of IV start. The IM route is more predictable than the oral route but still must be estimated, and titration is impossible. Although the IM route could be used as the sole sedation technique, when it is used this way larger doses are required and the drug is released slowly, resulting in prolonged recovery times. The author prefers to use a lower IM dose that allows cooperation for initiation of the IV and further titration of medications intravenously. When IM ketamine is used, the 100 mg/mL concentration is preferred to minimize volume at the injection site, rather than the 50 mg/mL concentration. When ketamine is used in IM or IV form, glycopyrrolate is given to decrease oral secretions and help prevent nausea postoperatively. The author prefers glycopyrrolate over atropine as the anticholinergic, as it does not cross the blood-brain barrier and does not contribute to the sedation. Another route is use of inhalation anesthetic if the patient is cooperative. Sevoflurane has become the inhalational anesthetic of choice for pediatric patients because it has rapid induction, a nonirritating odor, and rapid emergence. The face mask is coated with a flavored "chapstick" of the patient's choice to enhance the odor of the induction. It is the author's experience that this choice is tolerated by a wide range of pediatric patients. In all cases where an inhalational induction is performed, an IV is started for emergency preparedness and to enable postoperative medication access, even if the procedure is very short (**Table 9**).[11]

Box 3
Oral doses for triazolam, clonidine, midazolam, and ketamine

Midazolam (2 mg/mL), 0.1 to 0.5 mg/kg to maximum dose of 20 mg

Clonidine (0.1 mg tablets), crushed and dissolved in a few milliliters of Kool-Aid

 50 lb (22.6 kg), (1) 0.1-mg tablet

 75 lb (34 kg), (1½) 0.1-mg tablet

 100 lb (45.3 kg), (2) 0.1-mg tablets

Triazolam (0.125 mg tablets), crushed and dissolved in a few milliliters of Kool-Aid

 40 lb (18.1 kg), (½) 0.125-mg tablet

 60 lb (27.2 kg), (¾) 0.125-mg tablet

 80 lb (36.3 kg), (1) 0.125-mg tablet

Ketamine (50/5 mL), 5 to 10 mg/kg

Table 8
Intramuscular doses for ketamine, midazolam, and glycopyrrolate

Ketamine	0.5 mg/kg, very low dose
	1 mg/kg, low dose
	2–3 mg/kg, moderate dose
Glycopyrrolate	0.01 mg/kg
Midazolam	0.07–0.08 mg/kg

Table 9
Approaches to management of the pediatric patient

Low Anxiety	Local Anesthetic and Parental Reassurance
Mild to moderate anxiety	N_2O_2/O_2 and local anesthetic
	N_2O_2/O_2, and oral premed of oral midazolam and/or clonidine
	N_2O_2/O_2 and sevoflurane or intravenous ketamine, vs propofol and/or fentanyl
Moderate to severe anxiety	Oral premed of oral midazolam/clonidine and then N_2O_2/O_2 and intravenous ketamine, midazolam, propofol, and/or fentanyl or sevoflurane
	If uncooperative with oral medicine, intramuscular ketamine then intravenous medications as above or sevoflurane
	Oral premed as above, then sevoflurane for 3–4 min until intravenous infusion started, then intravenous medications as above
	Oral premed as above, then sevoflurane inhalational anesthetic

Discharge of the pediatric patient from the office after anesthetic should follow discharge criteria such as the Aldrete score, with documentation made part of the anesthetic record. An additional simple question that can be asked is "can the child stay awake continually for 20 minutes when undisturbed?" If a reversal agent is used, the patient needs to be maintained in the office in a monitored fashion for a minimum of 1 hour, and as much as 2 to 3 hours might be required after the reversal agent is used to ensure resedation does not take place. An adult needs to be with the patient after discharge home to monitor the patient for the remainder of the procedure day.

EQUIPMENT FOR MANAGEMENT OF PEDIATRIC ANESTHESIA AND EMERGENCIES

Performance of anesthetic techniques for the pediatric patient requires appropriately sized equipment for airway management and possible emergency management. Appropriately sized face masks, Ambu bags, oral and nasopharyngeal airways, laryngeal mask airways (LMAs), endotracheal tubes, laryngoscope blades, and Magill forceps are required to successfully manage the pediatric airway. Basic management and maneuvers are the same as for the adult patient, and the goals are to provide gas exchange and assure an open airway with chin lift, jaw thrust, and use of adjunct airways. Because face-mask ventilation is generally the first approach if an unexpected airway or respiratory event occurs, having the appropriately sized mask is important preoperatively. The mask should cover from the bridge of the nose to the cleft of the chin, and not cover the eyes. If the mask is too small or too large, proper ventilation will be ineffective. The proper size of oral and nasopharyngeal airways should

also be chosen preoperatively. The oral airway should be measured from the commissure to the angle of the mandible, and the nasopharyngeal airway from the nostril to the angle of the mandible. Again, improper size will contribute to airway obstruction rather than facilitate opening the airway. It is generally thought that because of the stiff and narrow epiglottis and the narrow mandibular space, a straight laryngoscope blade is the best choice for pediatric patients. A #2 straight blade is appropriate for ages 2 to 10 years. After 10 years of age a curved blade, a #3, can be substituted for intubation if desired. Tracheal tube sizes can be found on the Broselow tape or can be determined by the formula 4 + age/4. Traditionally, uncuffed tubes were used in children younger than 8 years because early endotracheal tubes were not designed for children and it was thought that an increased chance of injury might result with the funnel-shaped pediatric larynx. This long-held belief is being reconsidered, and several studies have shown no difference in postextubation stridor, reintubation, or need for tracheotomy in cuffed and uncuffed tubes in the pediatric patient.[35–38] The advantages of the cuffed tubes in the operating room (OR) setting is that there seems to be fewer repeat laryngoscopies because of "leak" of an uncuffed tube, lower fresh gas flow rates, reduced anesthetic pollution of the OR, and more accurate end-tidal CO_2 readings. The advantage for the OMS of a cuffed tube for a pediatric patient in the emergency setting is that higher peak pressures may be able to be delivered with a more accurate fit of the endotracheal tube. If a cuffed tube is selected for a pediatric patient, a half-size smaller than given by the formula (4 + age/4) is used.

If face-mask ventilation is not effective with oral or nasal airways, an LMA or other supraglottic device can be considered for rescue if the obstruction is supraglottic. The LMAs Classic, Proseal, and Unique are available. The LMA would not be appropriate in the case of anaphylaxis, vomiting and aspiration, foreign body in the airway, or severe bronchospasm, as it does not protect against aspiration, airway pressures cannot be managed above 20 cm of water (except for the LMA Proseal), and it cannot protect the patient in the case of laryngeal edema. Sizes of LMAs for pediatric and adult patients are shown in **Table 10**.[30]

The Broselow tape has been discussed earlier, and is an invaluable resource for equipment and drug dosages used in pediatric resuscitation. It was designed to be used for a supine patient rather than a patient in a dental chair. For all patients undergoing anesthesia, but especially pediatric patients, obtaining an accurate weight and height are important preoperatively. The other convenient manner by which to calculate pediatric dosages is to download applications for smart phones. Upon input of the pediatric weight, the application provides dosages for emergency medications.

Fluid replacement should be performed with normal saline or lactated Ringer solution. Solutions containing D5W should be avoided, as the free water leaves the intravascular space rapidly. Fluid replacement should follow the "4:2:1" rule, as shown in **Box 4**. In general, procedures in the office are short (<1 hour) and are associated with minimal blood loss, so calculation of additional fluid requirements is not necessary. Intravenous access can be difficult in a child, particularly during resuscitation, and this author feels that is important to have an intraosseous kit available to reestablish IV access if it is lost. Kits are available as manual insertion or powered motor insertion devices. The intraosseous kit can be placed in many locations, but generally for young children the proximal tibia 2 fingerbreadths

---

Box 4
Fluid management

Fluid Maintenance

4 mL/kg/h for the first 10 kg

2 mL/kg/h for the second 10 kg

1 mL/kg/h for each additional kg

Fluid deficit is calculated based on amount of time in nothing by mouth status (NPO). The maintenance rate is calculated and multiplied by the time NPO. Half is given back in the first hour, then the remainder is given back over the next several hours. For most office-based procedures the patient is discharged home before this second time frame. (For most office-based procedures, surgical blood loss and insensible losses are not important, and there is generally no urinary loss to calculate for replacement.)

---

below and medial to the tibial tuberosity is the location of choice. For older children, the distal tibia 2 fingerbreadths above the medial malleolus may be a good alternative, owing to increased cortical thickness at the proximal site. All medications that can be given intravenously can be given intraosseously at the same dose, and are followed by a saline flush. A popular kit is the EZ-IO[tm] by Vidacare (Shavano Park, TX), which has a powered drill with 3 available 15-gauge needle lengths: 15 mm (3–39 kg), 25 mm (>40 kg), and 45 mm (for patients with excessive tissue thickness).

Cardiac arrest in the pediatric population is almost always secondary to respiratory arrest. Defibrillation may need to be performed, and is part of the pediatric cardiac arrest algorithm. Pediatric pads or paddles are manufacturer specific, but generally the largest pads that can fit on the chest wall without touching are acceptable. Dose attenuators for defibrillation energy are generally required for pediatric patients younger than 8 years or weighing less than 25 kg.[6] The exact dose for pediatric defibrillation is not known, but 2 to 4 J/kg is thought to be the correct initial starting energy level. Recent changes in pediatric resuscitation emphasize good-quality cardiopulmonary resuscitation (CPR), to "push hard and push fast" and compress the chest about half the depth of the rib cage, and to minimize interruptions in compressions. An important difference in bradycardia management in the pediatric patient in comparison with the adult is that CPR is initiated when the pulse rate is less than 60 beats/min, and epinephrine is given before atropine as the initial pharmacologic management.

Table 10
Weight of patients and inflation volumes of laryngeal mask airways

1	<5 kg	4 mL
1.5	5–10 kg	7 mL
2	10–20 kg	10 mL
2.5	20–30 kg	14 mL
3	30 kg to small adult	20 mL
4	Adult 50–70 kg	30 mL
5	Large adult 70–100 kg	40 mL
6	Adult >100 kg	50 mL

Monitoring for pediatric patients is the same as for older patients and should include pulse oximetry, end-tidal CO_2 (an AAOMS requirement starting in January 2014), pulse rate, blood pressure, temperature, electrocardiogram, and usually a precordial stethoscope as well. For very young children the self-adhesive disposable pulse oximeter probe generally works better than the standard finger probe, but for the age ranges seen in OMS offices the standard probe generally works well.

Management of the pediatric patient in the OMS office can be rewarding and challenging. Full use of knowledge, training, experience, and judgment, as well as an understanding of the physiologic and pharmacologic differences in pediatric age groups, will allow the OMS to provide safe and effective care in the office and determine which cohort of pediatric patients are best managed in the ASC or hospital setting.

REFERENCES

1. Office anesthesia evaluation manual. 8th edition. AAOMS Publications; 2012.
2. Kain ZL. Preoperative psychological preparation of the child for surgery: an update. Anesthesiol Clin North America 2005;23(4):591–614, vii.
3. Hannullah RS. Selection of patients for paediatric ambulatory surgery. Can J Anaesth 1991;38:887–90.
4. Hannullah RS. Who benefits when parents are present in during anaesthesia induction in their children? Can J Anaesth 1994;41:271–5.
5. Hannullah RS. Paediatric ambulatory anaesthesia: role of parents. J Clin Anesth 1995;7:597–9.
6. Chamedies L, Samson R, Schexnayder S, et al, editors. Pediatric advanced life support provider manual. American Heart Association; 2011.
7. Broselow pediatric emergency tape. Lincolnshire (IL): Armstrong Medical Industries; 2007. Vital Signs, Inc.
8. Stoelting RK, Dierdorf SF. Anesthesia and co-existing disease. 4th edition. Philadelphia: Churchill Livingstone; 2002. p. 282–4, 687–90.
9. Miloro M, et al. Peterson's principles of oral and maxillofacial surgery. 2nd edition. Hamilton (London): BC Decker; 2004. p. 103–5.
10. Dembo J. Pediatric anesthesia. Oral Maxillofac Surg Clin North Am 1992;4(4):837–8.
11. Fonseca R, Barber D, Matheson J. Oral and maxillofacial surgery. 2nd edition. St Louis (MO): Saunders; 2009. p. 93–6.
12. Karlis V, Appelblatt R, Bourell L, et al. Pediatric outpatient anesthesia and sedation. Selected Readings in Oral and Maxillofacial Surger 2010; 18(2):1–4.
13. Burgoyne LL, Anghelescu DL. Intervention steps in treating laryngospasm in pediatric patients. Paediatr Anaesth 2008;18:297–302.
14. Weiss M, Engelheat T. Cannot ventilate—paralyze! Paediatr Anaesth 2012;22(12):1147–9.
15. Michota F, Frost S. Procedure related risk, anesthesia related risk, provider related risk, perioperative risk. Med Clin North Am 2002;86(4):731–48.
16. Cote C, Notterman DA, Karl HW, et al. Adverse sedation events in pediatrics: a critical incident analysis of contributing factors. Pediatrics 2000;105: 805–14.
17. Cote C, Karl HW, Notterman DA, et al. Adverse sedation events in pediatrics: analysis of medications used for sedation. Pediatrics 2000;106: 603–44.
18. Callahan KA, Panter TM, Hall TM, et al. Peak flow monitoring in pediatric asthma management. J Pediatr Nurs 2010;25:12.
19. Sauder RA, Lenox WC, Tobias JD, et al. Methylprednisolone increases sensitivity to beta-adrenergic agonists within 48 hours in Basenji greyhound. Anesthesiology 1993;79(6):1278–83.
20. Tait AR, Malviya S, Voepel-Lewis T, et al. Risk factors for perioperative adverse respiratory events in children with upper respiratory tract infections. Anesthesiology 2001;95:299–306.
21. Cohen MM, Cameron CB. Should you cancel the operation when a child has an upper respiratory infection? Anesth Analg 1991;72:282–8.
22. Rolf N, Cote CJ. Frequency and severity of desaturation events during general anesthesia in children with and without upper respiratory tract infections. J Clin Anesth 1992;4:200–3.
23. Maxwell LG, Yaster M. Perioperative management issues in pediatric patients. Anesthesiol Clin North America 2000;18(3):601–32.
24. Greeley WJ. Pediatric cardiovascular anesthesia. Anesth Analg 1998;(Suppl):45–56.
25. Hedley A, Ogden C, Johnson C, et al. Prevalence of overweight and obesity among US children, adolescents and adults. 1999-2002. JAMA 2004; 23:291.
26. Available at: www.cdc.gov/healthyweight/assessing/bmi/children_bmi/about_childrens_bmi.html.
27. Cohn S, Smetana G, Weed H. Perioperative medicine. New York: McGraw-Hill; 2006. p. 210.
28. Rhodes E, Ferrari L, Wolfsdorf J. Perioperative management of the pediatric patient with diabetes mellitus. Anesth Analg 2005;101:986–99.
29. Available at: http://dailymed.nlm.nih.gov/dailymed/archives/fdaDrugInfo.cfm?archiveid=4936.
30. Muraro A, Roberts G, Clark A, et al, EAACI Task Force on Anaphylaxis in Children. The management of anaphylaxis in childhood: position paper of the European academy of allergology and clinical immunology. Allergy 2007;62:857–71.
31. Quarnstom F, Donalson M. Triazolam use in the dental setting: a report of 270 uses over 15 years. Gen Dent 2004;52:496–501.

32. Friedberg B, Sigl J. Clonidine premedication decreases propofol consumption during BIS monitored propofol-ketamine technique for office-based surgery. Dermatol Surg 2000;26(9):848–52.

33. Bergandahl HT, Lonnqvist PA, Esksborg S. Clonidine in paediatric anaesthesia: review of the literature and comparison with benzodiazepines for premedication. Acta Anaesthesiol Scand 2006;50:135–43.

34. Hall D, Rezvan E, Tatakis D. Oral clonidine pretreatment prior to venous cannulation. Anesth Prog 2006; 53(2):34–42.

35. Newith C, Rachman B, Patel N, et al. The use of cuffed vs uncuffed endotracheal tubes in pediatric intensive care. J Pediatr 2004;144(3):333–7.

36. Khine H, Corddry DH, Kettrick RG, et al. Comparison of cuffed versus uncuffed endotracheal tubes in young children during general anesthesia. Anesthesiology 1997;86(3):627–31.

37. Cox RG. Should cuffed endotracheal tubes be used routinely in children? Can J Anaesth 2005;52:669–74.

38. Available at: http://lmana.com/files/prosealquick-reference-card.pdf.

Respiratory Anesthetic Emergencies in Oral and Maxillofacial Surgery

Daniel J. Gesek Jr, DMD

KEYWORDS

- Anesthesia • Airway emergencies • Laryngospasm • Bronchospasm • Airway obstruction

KEY POINTS

- Respiratory anesthetic emergencies are the most common complications encountered during anesthesia administration.
- Asthma is the most common chronic inflammatory respiratory disease and affects 6% of the US population.
- Laryngospasm is a protective mechanism preventing irritants from entering the lower airway.
- The most common airway anesthesia emergencies include laryngospasm, bronchospasm, airway obstruction, and emesis and aspiration.

INTRODUCTION

Respiratory anesthetic emergencies are the most common complications encountered during the administration of anesthesia in both the adult and pediatric populations.[1–26] Regardless of the depth of anesthesia, a thorough review of the patients' health history, including the past medical history, medication list, prior anesthesia history, and complex physical examination, is critical in the promotion of safety in the oral and maxillofacial surgery office. The effective management of respiratory anesthetic emergencies includes both strong didactic and clinical skills.

There are multiple disease states that affect the pulmonary system. These states include asthma, chronic obstructive pulmonary disease (COPD), and respiratory infections. Patients with these types of respiratory diseases present many challenges during the perioperative period in the office-based setting. It is with a thorough knowledge, excellent training, and clinical skills that the oral and maxillofacial surgeon is uniquely qualified to perform both surgical and anesthetic procedures in the outpatient setting.

RESPIRATORY PHYSIOLOGY

The primary function of the lungs is to oxygenate the blood perfusing through the pulmonary vasculature and remove the byproduct of metabolism carbon dioxide. This gas exchange occurs between the alveoli of the lungs and the blood in the pulmonary capillary system. Oxygen diffuses through the capillary walls into the plasma and binds to hemoglobin molecules. To establish gas exchange in the pulmonary system, there must be ventilation of the alveoli, diffusion through the capillary membranes, and circulation or perfusion of the pulmonary capillary bed.

A very important aspect of the use of oxygen during anesthesia is preoxygenation. Preoxygenating patients with 100% oxygen before the induction of anesthesia will maintain higher levels of tissue oxygenation during periods of apnea. The use of preoxygenation will greatly aid the

There are no conflicts of interest and no financial disclosures.
Private Practice, 2047 Park Street, Jacksonville, FL 32204, USA
E-mail address: dsgesek@comcast.net

Oral Maxillofacial Surg Clin N Am 25 (2013) 479–486
http://dx.doi.org/10.1016/j.coms.2013.04.004

surgeon during anesthetic induction, when there may be periods of apnea, ventilatory difficulty, and airway control issues.

The respiratory system, as noted earlier, functions by delivering oxygen to the arterial blood supply, which is then delivered to the body's tissues. The oxygen found in the arterial blood is 98% bound to hemoglobin molecules located in the red blood cells. The remaining 2% is diffused in the plasma. This ratio produces a pressure called the *arterial oxygen tension* (Pao$_2$). This pressure gradient is how the unbound oxygen enters the plasma and is delivered to the tissues of the body. There is a commonly known relationship between the hemoglobin saturated with oxygen (Sao$_2$) and the pressure gradient by dissolved oxygen (Pao$_2$). This relationship is classically illustrated by the oxygen-hemoglobin dissociation curve (**Fig. 1**). It is this curve that we use to assess a patient's oxygenation status.

COMMON RESPIRATORY DISEASES

There are many diseases of the respiratory tract that can alter the physiology of gas exchange and, thus, the administration of an anesthetic. A thorough history and physical examination are critical in the decision-making process of an anesthesia plan and before the induction of that anesthetic. A few of the major disease processes that affect the respiratory system include asthma, COPD, and upper respiratory infections (URI). URIs can adversely affect the airway. For example, in children a URI can cause hyperreactivity of the airway for up to 6 weeks after the infection. For this reason, the recommendation for postponing any anesthetic for 2 weeks after any clinical signs

or symptoms is commonplace and recommended by the American Society of Anesthesiologist (ASA).

Chronic pulmonary diseases are characterized as obstructive or restrictive. Obstructive airway disease is the most frequent cause of pulmonary dysfunction. Two of the most common obstructive airway diseases are asthma and COPD. Changes in airway resistance will lead to ventilation-perfusion mismatches. These mismatches result in arterial hypoxemia while on room air. Carbon dioxide is chronically retained, leading to respiratory acidosis. All obstructed airway diseases will manifest dyspnea, coughing, wheezing, and sputum production.

Restrictive pulmonary diseases have decreased lung compliance resulting in decreased lung volumes. This decrease translates to a decreased in vital capacity or forced expiratory volume in the first second of expiration (FEV$_1$), which is the classic sign of restrictive diseases. The main complaints of patients with restrictive diseases include dyspnea and rapid, shallow breathing. Acute episodes of restrictive pulmonary diseases are caused by leakage of intravascular fluid into the interstitium of the lungs and alveoli manifesting as pulmonary edema. Acute diseases include adult respiratory distress syndrome, aspiration pneumonia, and pulmonary edema. Chronic restrictive diseases are caused by pulmonary fibrosis. Sarcoidosis is the main chronic restrictive disease. Other causes include the interference of lung expansion, which includes pulmonary effusions, obesity, pregnancy, and ascites.

Asthma

Asthma is the most common chronic inflammatory respiratory disease, and it affects upwards of 6%

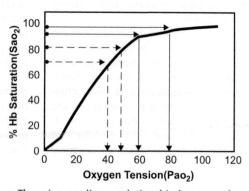

Extrapolations	
Hb Saturation (Sao$_2$)	Arterial Tension (Pao$_2$)
95	80
90	60
80	50
70	40

Fig. 1. The oxygen-hemoglobin dissociation curve. There is a nonlinear relationship between the percentage of total Sao$_2$ and Pao$_2$, as demonstrated by the oxygen-hemoglobin dissociation curve. Hemoglobin saturations of 95% and more sustain Pao$_2$ at or more than 80 mm Hg, preventing hypoxemia. At 90% saturation, the curve becomes steep; within a relatively narrow period, the percent hemoglobin saturation and Pao$_2$ decline dramatically. Hb, hemoglobin. (*Data from* Guyton AC. Textbook of medical physiology. 8th edition. Fort Worth (TX): Harcourt College Publishers; 1991. p. 436.)

of the US population. Asthma is defined by the presence of chronic inflammation of the respiratory tract submucosal tissue, hyperreactivity to various stimuli, and reversible expiratory airflow obstruction. The irritability of the airway will manifest as wheezing and coughing. An acute asthma attack can result in bronchospasm.

Asthma is further defined as either intrinsic (nonspecific factors) or extrinsic (allergen mediated). Intrinsic causes include infectious, exercise-induced, or emotional changes. A thorough history can help differentiate between intrinsic and extrinsic.

Frequently asked questions include the following:

1. What causes your asthma attacks?
2. When where you first diagnosed?
3. Have you ever been to the emergency department or hospitalized?
4. When was your last attack?
5. What medications do you currently use?
6. Have there been any recent changes in your medications?
7. When was the last time you used your rescue medications?
8. How frequently do you use your inhaler?

The clinical manifestations of asthma are secondary to the edema, mucous production, and constriction of the smooth muscle of the airway. This effect is a reactionary effect from the release of histamine from mast cell degranulation (immunoglobulin E mediated) and cytokines from leukocytes.

The bronchoconstriction is mainly countered by beta (B) agonists, such as albuterol, which stabilize the mast cells and prevents their degranulation. Albuterol is the most common B agonist rescue inhaler used today. There are many other medications used in the treatment of asthma (chronic and acute flare-ups). Other medications used to treat acute asthma attacks include epinephrine in doses of 0.2–0.5 mL of 1:1000 aqueous solution for adults and .01 mg/kg to a maximum dose of 0.5 mg for children. Other medications used perioperatively include corticosteroids, metered dose inhalers, and nebulizer therapy.

A thorough history is important when treating patients with asthma. Other useful tests/studies to consider are pulmonary function tests, chest radiographs, and preoperative medical consultations. Caution should be used when sedating patients with asthma. The control of the asthmatic airway is critical. Consideration should be given to pretreating patients with asthma with B agonist inhalers and corticosteroids. Patients should be instructed to bring their rescue inhaler to their surgical appointment regardless of whether the oral

and maxillofacial surgeon has emergency rescue inhalers.

Some medications should be administered with caution in patients with asthma. One such class in particular is the narcotics. Narcotics can cause respiratory depression, rigid chest, and mast cell degranulation, which can manifest as a bronchospasm; emergency measures must be initiated immediately on recognition of these unfolding events.

COPD

COPD is a disease process that includes airflow obstruction caused by either chronic bronchitis or emphysema. There are 2 major types of COPD: chronic bronchitis and emphysema.

Chronic bronchitis
Chronic bronchitis (blue bloaters) is the chronic secretion of mucous into the bronchi causing increased airflow resistance. These patients develop arterial hypoxemia, hypercarbia, and cor pulmonale. Patients with chronic bronchitis have a chronic productive cough that is present for at least 2 consecutive years.

Emphysema
Emphysema (pink puffers) is the abnormal persistent enlargement of the airway distal to the terminal bronchioles along with the destruction of the walls without fibrosis. This condition is characterized by the loss of elasticity causing collapse of the airway during exhalation, which will lead to increased airway resistance. Clinically, patients with emphysema will have dyspnea, cough, sputum production, and decreased exercise tolerance.

Although both asthma and COPD exhibit similar clinical findings, the signs and symptoms are reversible for asthma and irreversible for COPD. COPD typically consists of chronic bronchitis, emphysema, and peripheral airway disease. Patients will exhibit hypercarbia, hypoxemia, and heart failure (cor pulmonale). Clinically these patients can tolerate elevated levels of carbon dioxide and decreased oxygen levels, which are the driving force of respiration. It has been shown that patients can tolerate oxygen concentrations of 40% or less without decreasing the respiratory drive. To maintain adequate oxygen levels under sedation, the use of a nasal cannula or nasal hood at 1 to 4 L/min oxygen can be safely used without affecting hypoxic drive.

COMMON RESPIRATORY EMERGENCIES IN ADULTS
Laryngospasm

A laryngospasm is a spasm of the intrinsic muscles of the larynx causing closure of the airway at the level of the vocal cords. It is a protective reflex mechanism that prevents irritants, such as blood, saliva, or irrigation, as well as solid materials from entering the lower airway. A laryngospasm is classified as complete or incomplete (partial). The classic sign is a high-pitched stridor or crowing for a partial laryngospasm and silence for a complete obstruction. Patients with a laryngospasm can also exhibit paradoxic chest wall and abdominal movements and oxygen desaturation.

The cause of a laryngospasm includes local irritants and the depth of anesthesia. In consciously sedated patients, these irritants will cause the spasm of the intrinsic muscles of the larynx, but the swallowing mechanism will clear the airway. In deeply sedated patients, these mechanisms can be absent causing the laryngospasm because of the inability of the musculature to function properly and clear the airway.

Preventing a laryngospasm should include proper airway maintenance. The surgeon routinely uses a throat pack or partition to keep foreign material out of the airway. Proper suctioning techniques aid in airway control. Head positioning (sniffers position) will position the airway in a straight-line physiologic position. Finally, the depth of anesthesia can sensitize the airway causing irritability. This situation is most commonly seen when the sedation is inadequate.

If a laryngospasm is suspected, the surgery shall be stopped and the surgical site packed off. The proper head position will assist in airway control. The airway should be suctioned to clear any foreign bodies, including blood, saliva, and irrigation. Also, 100% oxygen should be administered via a full face mask. By depressing the chest, the surgeon may elicit a huff of air indicating a patent airway.

With a continuing laryngospasm, the next step is to attempt ventilation of patients with a full face mask and 100% oxygen. If patients cannot be ventilated, a small dose of succinylcholine 0.15 to 0.30 mg/kg intravenously (IV) in adults is used to break the spasm and initiate ventilation. This dose will work for smaller individuals or a partial spasm. In larger individuals or a complete spasm, 0.3 to 0.6 mg/kg IV should be considered. If successful, the airway is maintained along with proper ventilatory support until the return of spontaneous respiration. If the spasm continues, an intubating dose of succinylcholine 1 mg/kg should be administered along with endotracheal intubation.

In the office setting, emergency services (911) should be called early in any anesthesia emergency. If there is a suspected familial history of malignant hyperthermia, the drug rocuronium can be used at a dose of 0.6 to 1.2 mg/kg IV. Succinylcholine acts as a triggering agent for MH. The onset of rocuronium is 1 to 2 minutes, and the duration of action is anywhere from 20 to 60 minutes. Therefore, with the use of rocuronium, prolonged ventilator support will be necessary. The reversal agent for rocuronium is Sugammadex. This drug is likely to receive approval by the Food and Drug Administration in 2013.

Bronchospasm

A bronchospasm is a reflex bronchiolar constriction that can be centrally mediated or a local response to airway irritation. This constriction can be elicited by stimuli, such as secretions, blood, or foreign bodies. The clinical manifestations include expiratory wheezing and increased airway resistance. Increased airway resistance can make ventilation difficult in deeply anesthetized patients. In consciously sedated patients, tachypnea and dyspnea are commonly seen.

In the oral and maxillofacial surgery office, most patients are anesthetized without the use of a secure airway like an endotracheal tube or laryngeal mask airway (LMA). Further, these patients are spontaneously breathing with supplemental oxygen. If a bronchospasm is suspected, nonsedated or minimally sedated patients may be able to inhale a B agonist inhaler, such as albuterol (4–8 puffs). In moderately to deeply sedated patients, 100% oxygen with a full face mask should be immediately initiated. If patients can be ventilated, nebulized albuterol (6–10 puffs) can be administered.

After the use of a B agonist, if the bronchospasm is still present, subcutaneous epinephrine in doses of 0.3 to 0.5 mg of 1:1000 is used. IV epinephrine should be used carefully in patients exhibiting hypertension because of the potential cardiac side effects. Boluses of 10 to 20 µg of a 1:10 000 solution of epinephrine is titrated to effect. If after all the prior medications are administered and there is still difficulty ventilating patients, intubation should be considered. The airway of choice in this situation is the endotracheal tube. Other reasons for a secure airway in this anesthetic emergency include continuing hypoxemia, muscle weakness, and worsening obtundation.

Once patients are intubated, a B agonist, such as Albuterol, can be given through the endotracheal tube. Albuterol is the most common B agonist used today for the treatment of a bronchospasm in doses of 6 to 10 puffs. Other treatments include deepening the level of anesthesia, especially if using bronchodilating inhalation agents. Further treatments include continued hydration and humidification of the airway during the use of inhaled gases.

Airway Obstruction

Airway obstruction is one of the more common anesthetic emergencies. The obstruction of the airway is usually located in the upper airway (supraglottic region) and is caused by the loss of pharyngeal muscle tone. With the loss of muscle tone, the tongue is displaced posteriorly and occludes the airway. The deeper the plane of anesthesia, the more common the possibility of developing an obstructed airway. Other causes of airway obstruction include foreign bodies, such as teeth, aspirate, prosthetic devices, or surgical instruments.

The clinical signs of obstruction include paradoxic breathing with sterna retraction and abdominal muscle activity. These abnormal movements manifest as a rocking motion. A partial obstruction may also exhibit stridor.

The initial treatment of an airway obstruction includes simple airway opening techniques, including the head tilt–chin lift maneuver. Following the chin lift, the jaw thrust can be used. Grabbing the tongue with gauze, a tissue forceps, or suture and pulling it forward also can be used to open the oropharyngeal airway. If the airway obstruction is not cleared with these positional changes, the next recommended treatment in both conscious and unconscious patients is to deliver chest or abdominal thrusts to increase airway pressure. Producing increased airway pressures produced by the chest or abdominal thrust can force the foreign body into the pharynx. In obese patients or pregnant woman, the chest thrust over the sternum is used instead of the abdominal thrust over the sternum. Complications of the thrust maneuvers include rib fracture and laceration of abdominal or thoracic viscera. The abdominal thrust can be effective in both conscious and unconscious patients.

Blind finger sweeps are no longer used in unconscious patients per the American Heart Association. Another technique that works well is to visualize the airway while performing a laryngoscopy and retrieving any foreign matter with the Magill forceps. If these maneuvers are unsuccessful, attempts to give positive pressure ventilation with a full face mask is initiated. Blind finger sweeps in children are not indicated because it can push the object further down the airway.

Adjunctive airway equipment to be considered includes oral and nasal airways, LMA sized to fit, and endotracheal tube intubation. If the simpler techniques are not effective, more invasive airway management is necessary. There are multiple noninvasive options; but if these are ineffective, then surgical airways are required. These surgical airway options include transtracheal catheterization, cricothyrotomy, and tracheostomy.

Emesis and Aspiration

There are many causes of nausea and vomiting, including anxiety, narcotics, pain, and anesthesia. Gastric emptying times can also be increased by any of these. Emesis of gastric contents in anesthetized patients can lead to aspiration. Aspiration can exhibit as hypoxemia, tachycardia, tachypnea, bronchospasm, hypotension, and atelectasis. The volume and the pH of the aspirate dictate the severity of the injury. There are medical conditions that can increase the likelihood of aspiration. These conditions include obesity, hiatal hernia, pregnancy, gastroesophageal reflux disease, and obstruction of the gastrointestinal tract.

The prevention of aspiration during anesthesia includes following the ASA's fasting guidelines. Most oral and maxillofacial surgeons recommend fasting for 8 hours before the administration of an office-based anesthetic, but the ASA's recommendations are the following:

ASA's fasting guidelines	
Ingested Materials	**Minimum Fasting Periods**
Clear liquid	2 h
Breast milk	4 h
Infant formula	6 h
Nonhuman milk	6 h
Light meal	6 h
Fatty meal	8 h

The clinical signs of aspiration, including rales, dyspnea, tachycardia, bronchospasm, and partial airway obstruction, will occur with a liquid aspirate. A solid aspirate can cause partial or complete airway obstruction.

When vomiting or regurgitation occurs in anesthetized patients with an unsecured airway, patients should be placed in the Trendelenburg position with the head down. Patients should also be rolled to the right side using gravity and natural anatomy to minimize aspiration damage to the left lung. The oropharynx should be suctioned free of debris, and 100% oxygen via a full face mask should be started. The oropharynx should be cleaned of any solid particulate matter with the finger-sweep technique, forceps, or large-bore suction. Liquid materials are removed with aggressive suctioning techniques.

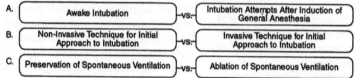

DIFFICULT AIRWAY ALGORITHM

1. Assess the likelihood and clinical impact of basic management problems:
   A. Difficult Ventilation
   B. Difficult Intubation
   C. Difficulty with Patient Cooperation or Consent
   D. Difficult Tracheostomy

2. Actively pursue opportunities to deliver supplemental oxygen throughout the process of difficult airway management

3. Consider the relative merits and feasibility of basic management choices:

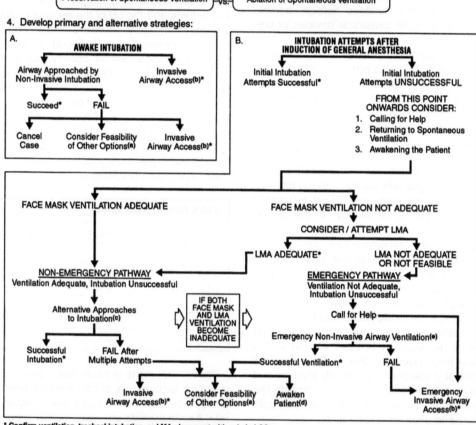

4. Develop primary and alternative strategies:

* Confirm ventilation, tracheal intubation, or LMA placement with exhaled CO_2

a. Other options include (but are not limited to): surgery utilizing face mask or LMA anesthesia, local anesthesia infiltration or regional nerve blockade. Pursuit of these options usually implies that mask ventilation will not be problematic. Therefore, these options may be of limited value if this step in the algorithm has been reached via the Emergency Pathway.

b. Invasive airway access includes surgical or percutaneous tracheostomy or cricothyrotomy.

c. Alternative non-invasive approaches to difficult intubation include (but are not limited to): use of different laryngoscope blades, LMA as an intubation conduit (with or without fiberoptic guidance), fiberoptic intubation, intubating stylet or tube changer, light wand, retrograde intubation, and blind oral or nasal intubation.

d. Consider re-preparation of the patient for awake intubation or canceling surgery.

e. Options for emergency non-invasive airway ventilation include (but are not limited to): rigid bronchoscope, esophageal-tracheal combitube ventilation, or transtracheal jet ventilation.

Fig. 2. Difficult airway algorithm. (*From* American Society of Anesthesiologists Task Force on Management of the Difficult Airway. Practice guidelines for management of the difficult airway: an updated report by the American Society of Anesthesiologists Task Force on Management of the Difficult Airway. Anesthesiology 2003;98(5):1269–77; with permission.)

If patients show signs of respiratory compromise, the airway should be intubated. During the intubation, any solid material should be removed with the aid of Magill forceps and large-bore suction. The patient should be ventilated with 100% oxygen. Care should be taken to watch for signs and symptoms of bronchospasm and treat as necessary.

If the particles are large enough, a bronchoscopy may be necessary to remove the foreign material from the lungs. Antibiotics are only recommended if the aspirate is highly contaminated with bacteria. Steroids are shown not to be useful for treating aspiration. Bronchial lavage has a minimal effect because of the rapidity with which the mucosal surfaces of the lung are damaged because of the low pH aspirate. Hospitalization and the need for aggressive ventilatory support may be required depending on the severity of the symptoms.

Emergency Protocols

Laryngospasm

- Administer 100% oxygen via nasal or full face mask
- Pack surgical site to control bleeding
- Suction oral cavity, oropharynx, and hypopharynx with tonsil suction tip
- Pull tongue and/or mandible forward
- Depress patient's chest and listen for rush of air
- Break spasm with positive pressure ventilation with 100% oxygen and full face mask
- Administer IV dose succinylcholine (partial spasm 10–20 mg IV, complete spasm 20–40 mg, or rocuronium 0.6–1.2 mg/kg IV may require prolonged ventilatory support)
- Administer intubating dose of succinylcholine and intubate airway (alternately, use rocuronium)

Bronchospasm

- Administer 4 to 8 puffs of B agonist via inhaler or nebulizer (2–4 puffs for pediatric patients)
- 100% oxygen via full face mask
- If sedated, use albuterol nebulizer via face mask
- 0.3 to 0.5 mg epinephrine (1:1000 solution) subcutaneous
- Consider reversal of sedative medications
- Consider intubation to secure airway

Emesis and aspiration

- Trendelenburg position with head down at least 15° and rolled to right
- Clear airway of vomitus with suction and Magill forceps
- If no change, intubate airway, 100% oxygen

Difficult airway

- Chin lift/jaw thrust
- Pull tongue forward, reposition airway
- Full face mask, 100% oxygen, positive pressure ventilation
- Consider oral and nasal airways, LMA
- Consider intubation
- Consider cricothyrotomy needle versus surgical
- Consider tracheostomy
- See **Fig. 2**, the difficult airway algorithm

REFERENCES

1. Committee on Anesthesia of American Association of Oral and Maxillofacial Surgerons, Schwartz P, Gesek DJ, Kaplan C. Office anesthesia evaluation manual. 8th edition. Chicago: AAOMS Publications; 2012.
2. Stoelting RK, Dierdorf SF. Anesthesia and coexisting disease. 4th edition. Philadelphia: Churchill Livingstone; 2002. p. 105–29.
3. OMS reference guide, American Association of Oral and Maxillofacial Surgeons Resident Organization 2010.
4. Levine WC, Allain RM, Alston TA, et al. Clinical anesthesia procedures of the Massachusetts General Hospital. 8th edition. Philadelphia: Lippincott, Williams, and Wilkins; 2010. p. 498–503.
5. Stoelting RK, Miller RD. Basics of anesthesia. 4th edition. Philadelphia: Churchill Livingstone; 2000. p. 271–81.
6. Becker DE, Haas DA. Recognition and management of complications during moderate and deep sedation. Part 1: respiratory considerations. Anesth Prog 2011;58:82–92.
7. Becker DE. Preoperative medical evaluation: part 2: pulmonary, endocrine, renal, and miscellaneous considerations. Anesth Prog 2009;56:135–45.
8. Bruells CS, Rossaint R. Physiology of gas exchange during anaesthesia. Eur J Anaesthesiol 2011;28(8): 570–9.
9. Orfanos JG, Quereshy FA. Causes of difficult airway. Atlas Oral Maxillofac Surg Clin North Am 2010;18:1–9.
10. AAOMS Parameters of Care 2012.
11. Strauss RA, Noordhoek R. Management of the difficult airway. Atlas Oral Maxillofac Surg Clin North Am 2010;18:11–28.
12. Kluger MT, Visvanathan T, Myburgh JA, et al. Crisis Management during anaesthesia: regurgitation,

vomiting, and aspiration. Qual Saf Health Care 2005; 14:e4, 1–5.

13. Isaacs RS, Sykes JM. Anatomy and physiology of the upper airway. Anesthesiol Clin North America 2002;20:733–45.

14. Apfelbaum JL, Connis RJ, Nickinovich DG, et al. Practice advisory for preanesthesia evaluation. Anesthesiology 2012;116:522–38.

15. Boynes SG, Lewis CL, Moore PA, et al. Complications associated with anesthesia administered for dental treatment. Gen Dent 2010;58:e20–5.

16. Watson CB. Respiratory complications associated with anesthesia. Anesthesiol Clin North America 2002;20:275–99.

17. Qaseem A, Wilt TJ, Weinberger SE, et al. Diagnosis and management of stable chronic obstructive pulmonary disease: a clinical practice guideline update for the American College of Physicians, American College of Chest Physicians, American Thoracic Society, and European Respiratory Society. Ann Intern Med 2011;155:179–91.

18. Stephens MB, Yew KS. Diagnosis of chronic obstructive pulmonary disease. Am Fam Physician 2008;78(1):87–92.

19. Evensen AE. Management of COPD exacerbations. Am Fam Physician 2010;81(5):607–13, 616.

20. Pollart SM, Elward KS. Overview of changes to asthma guidelines: diagnosis and screening. Am Fam Physician 2009;78(9):761–7.

21. Elward KS, Pollart SM. Medical therapy for asthma: updates from the NAEPP guidelines. Am Fam Physician 2010;82(10):1242–51.

22. Yamakage M, Iwasaki S, Namiki A. Guideline-oriented perioperative management of patients with bronchial asthma and chronic obstructive pulmonary disease. J Anesth 2008;22:412–28.

23. Tait AR, Malviya S. Anesthesia for the child with an upper respiratory tract infection: still a dilemma? Anesth Analg 2005;100:59–65.

24. Infosino A. Pediatric upper airway and congenital anomalies. Anesthesiol Clin North America 2002; 20:747–66.

25. Doyle DJ, Arellano R. Upper airway diseases and airway management: a synopsis. Anesthesiol Clin North America 2002;20:767–87.

26. Miller RD, Eriksson L, Fleisher LA, et al. Miller's anesthesia. 7th edition. Philadelphia: 2010. p. 361–92, 1067–150, 2419–60.

Cardiovascular Anesthetic Complications and Treatment in Oral Surgery

Edward C. Adlesic, DMD

KEYWORDS

- Perioperative hypertension • Antihypertensive agents • Cardiovascular anesthetic complications
- Oral surgery

KEY POINTS

- Perioperative hypertension is a common problem.
- If hypertension is left untreated in patients at risk, infarctions and stroke are possible.
- There are limited choices of antihypertensive agents for the office.
- Aggressive antihypertensive therapy is not indicated because most of the episodes seen in the office are hypertensive urgencies and not emergencies.
- Hypotension is usually managed by decreasing the depth of anesthesia, intravenous fluids, and then vasopressors, typically ephedrine or phenylephrine.
- Consider treatment of hypotension whenever the mean arterial pressure decreases less than 60 mm Hg, especially for patients in a beach chair–head elevated position to reduce the risk of hypoperfusion of the brain causing possible infarction or cognitive defects.

HYPERTENSION

Hypertension (HTN) is a common disease with a worldwide incidence of 1 billion individuals. It is found in all societies except primitive, isolated countries; it accounts for about 6% of all deaths. The World Health Organization predicts that one-third of the world's population will have HTN by the 2025.[1]

In the United States, there are approximately 72 million patients with HTN. The incidence increases with age: 30% of people older than 20 years and 60% to 70% of people older than 70 years. Patients who are normotensive by 55 years of age still have a 90% chance of developing HTN.[2]

Adult men have a higher incidence than women, but the reverse is seen in the senior population. The incidence in blacks is twice that of Caucasians, and their morbidity and mortality from coronary artery disease (CAD), stroke (cerebrovascular accidents [CVA]), left ventricular hypertrophy (LVH), myocardial infarction (MI), and renal failure is more pronounced.

HTN is a major risk factor for the development of cardiovascular, cerebrovascular, and renal diseases. Appropriate antihypertensive therapy reduces these risks, but only 29% of patients with HTN seek care; of those patients, only 49% have the appropriate therapy and control of the disease. If patients are well controlled, stroke reduction is 35% to 40%, MIs are reduced by 20% to 25%, and heart failure (HF) reduction is greater than 50%.[3]

The Seventh Report of the Joint National Committee on Prevention, Detection, Evaluation, and Treatment of High Blood Pressure (JNC 7) established categories for HTN and outlined the steps for management. The 3 categories are illustrated in **Table 1**.

4780 Liberty Avenue, Pittsburgh, PA 15224, USA
E-mail address: edward_adlesic@msn.com

Oral Maxillofacial Surg Clin N Am 25 (2013) 487–506
http://dx.doi.org/10.1016/j.coms.2013.04.002
1042-3699/13/$ – see front matter © 2013 Elsevier Inc. All rights reserved.

Table 1
The Seventh Report of the Joint National Committee on Prevention, Detection, Evaluation, and Treatment of High Blood Pressure Classification (adults aged 18 years or older)

Blood Pressure	Systolic Blood Pressure (mm Hg)	Diastolic Blood Pressure (mm Hg)
Normal	<120	<80
Prehypertension	120–139	80–89
Stage I HTN	140–159	90–99
Stage II HTN	≥160	≥100

Data from Holm SW, Cunningham LL, Bensadoun E, et al. Hypertension: classification, pathophysiology, and management during outpatient sedation and local anesthesia. J Oral Maxillofac Surg 2006;64:111–21.

A new category was created called prehypertension. Prehypertension is defined as a systolic blood pressure (SBP) of 130 to 139 mm Hg and a diastolic BP (DBP) of 80 to 90 mm Hg. Patients in this category are *twice as likely* to have HTN than patients with lower BPs.

Historically, antihypertensive therapy targeted DBP control, but current data show elevations in SBP as a greater risk for cardiovascular disease (CVD), especially in patients older than 50 years. For patients between the ages of 40 and 70 years, each incremental increase of 20 mm Hg in SBP and/or 10 mm Hg increase in DBP, doubles their risk for CVD. This effect occurs over a pressure range of 115/75 to 185/115 mm Hg.

The management of HTN requires a multimodal approach. Medications are almost always the primary step, but other treatments are initiated simultaneously with these drugs. Lifestyle changes are indicated. Diets are necessary to induce weight loss in overweight and obese patients; this includes a low-fat, sodium-restricted diet for chronic BP control. Patients also need to increase their aerobic physical activity and reduce their alcohol intake to a daily maximum of 3 oz of 80-proof spirits, 24 oz of beer, or 10 oz of wine.

BP can be controlled by antihypertensive medications, but most patients will require *2 or more agents*. Typically, the thiazide diuretics are the first-line agents used in HTN, and they are augmented as needed by beta-blockers (BB), calcium channel blockers (CCB), angiotensin-converting enzyme inhibitors (ACEI), and angiotensin receptor blockers (ARB). Some practitioners will skip the diuretic and immediately go to the other agents. The metabolic syndrome is an example whereby many patients are not on diuretics, and the first-line drug used is an ACEI agent. The goal is to reduce BP to less than 140/90 in most patients, but an additional reduction to less than 130/80 is the goal for patients with diabetes or renal disease. In most patients, once the SBP goal is achieved, the DBP will be controlled (**Fig. 1**).[4]

In special circumstances, as illustrated later, certain agents are more effective than others in controlling HTN. Existing comorbidities make one drug better than another (**Table 2**).

TYPES OF HTN

Essential HTN (also know as primary or idiopathic HTN) is of an unknown cause, but there is a familial incidence. It accounts for 80% to 90% of all HTN. Patients typically have an increased sympathetic discharge with an increased beta-receptor activity. The incidence increases with age; it frequently has associated comorbidities, like diabetes, obesity, and obstructive sleep apnea.[5]

Secondary HTN accounts for the remaining 5% to 20% of cases, with renal disease being the primary cause. The causes of secondary HTN are listed in **Box 1**.[6]

PATHOLOGIC EFFECTS OF HTN

HTN is a major risk factor for developing CVD, which is the leading cause of death in patients with HTN. In trying to pump blood against elevated

Fig. 1. Initial drug therapy for HTN. (*Data from* Chobanian AV, Barkis G, Black HR, et al. JNC-7 report: detection, evaluation, and treatment of high blood pressure. JAMA 2003;289(19):2560–72.)

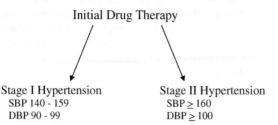

Initial Drug Therapy

Stage I Hypertension
SBP 140 - 159
DBP 90 - 99

1st Drug = Thiazide Diuretic
or skip diuretic and start
one of the following agents
ACEI, ARB, BB, CCB

Stage II Hypertension
SBP ≥ 160
DBP ≥ 100

2 Drug Combination: Thiazide Diuretic +
ACEI, or ARB, or BB, or CCB

Table 2
HTN management special circumstances: agents to consider

Medication	HF	Post MI	Diabetes	Chronic Kidney Disease
Diuretic	Yes	No	Yes	No
BB	Yes	Yes	Yes	No
ACEI	Yes	Yes	Yes	Yes
ARB	Yes	No	Yes	Yes
CCB	No	No	Yes	No

Data from National Heart, Lung, and Blood Institute; National Institutes of Health. Seventh Report of the Joint National Committee on Prevention, Detection, Evaluation, and Treatment of High Blood Pressure (JNC 7). NIH Publication No. 04-5230. Available at: www.nhlbi.nih.gov/guidelines/hypertension. Accessed November 10, 2012.

BPs (afterload), structural and functional defects develop in the heart. LVH, a thickening of the heart wall muscle mass, develops resulting in a less compliant heart that is unable to effectively withstand the increases in left ventricular end diastolic pressures and volumes (LVEDP and LVEDV). The end result is myocardial ischemia, injury, infarction, dysrhythmias, and HF.

Cardiovascular effects from HTN are far more common than the cerebrovascular effects, but the central nervous system (CNS) complications from hypertension can be just as significant. HTN increases a patients' risk for cerebral ischemic infarcts and hemorrhagic stroke. This risk is amplified in patients older than 65 years. These patients are also at an increased risk for cognitive dysfunction and dementia.

Box 1
Causes of secondary HTN

Renal disease

Pheochromocytoma

Oral contraceptives

Obesity and obstructive sleep apnea

Primary aldosteronism

Hyperthyroid

Hypothyroid

Cushing syndrome

Postoperative hypertension

Drugs of abuse

    Cocaine, amphetamines, and alcohol

Hyperparathyroid

In severe HTN, the autoregulation of cerebral blood flow fails and ischemia, edema, or encephalopathy can develop. In normotensive patients, blood flow is maintained over a mean arterial pressure (MAP) of 50 to 150 mm Hg; but in severe HTN, there is vasodilation and hyperperfusion of cerebral tissues that can cause death within hours if not managed properly.

Renal disease is the most common cause of secondary HTN. Patients with chronic renal failure have an 80% incidence of HTN.[7]

METABOLIC SYNDROME

The metabolic syndrome is a combination of HTN, insulin resistance, and dyslipidemia. In the United States, 44% of the population who are older than 50 years have metabolic syndrome. The incidence increases with age, resulting in rates of 34% in men and 35% in women. These patients are at increased risk for CAD, stroke, and diabetes.

The primary approach to treatment is weight loss. A low-carbohydrate diet will lead to rapid weight loss, but a diet of fruits, vegetables, whole grains, lean poultry, and fish is the preferred long-term diet. Diet control needs to be followed by an increase in physical activity and reduced alcohol intake just like in any patient with HTN. BP control is usually accomplished by the use of angiotensin agents, either ACEI or ARB, which have been found to not only decrease BP but to also decrease the onset of type 2 diabetes (**Table 3**).[5]

PHYSIOLOGIC EFFECTS OF HTN

With new-onset HTN, there is an increased sympathoadrenal activity that results in changes in cardiac output (CO), heart rate, systemic vascular resistance (SVR), and circulating blood flow.

Table 3
Risk factors for metabolic syndrome

	Men	Women
BP	≥130/85	≥130/85
Abdominal waist size	>102 cm	>88 cm
Fasting glucose	>100 mg/dL	>100 mg/dL
Triglycerides	>150 mg/dL	>150 mg/dL
HDL cholesterol	<40 mg/dL	<50 mg/dL

Abbreviation: HDL, high-density lipoprotein.

Data from National Heart, Lung, and Blood Institute; National Institutes of Health. Seventh Report of the Joint National Committee on Prevention, Detection, Evaluation, and Treatment of High Blood Pressure (JNC 7). NIH Publication No. 04-5230. Available at: www.nhlbi.nih.gov/guidelines/hypertension. Accessed November 10, 2012.

Vasoconstriction of the arterial vessels causes an increase in SVR, so there is an increase in the afterload that the heart pumps against. The vasoconstriction also reduces the pooling of blood in the venous vessels, so there is an increase in blood return to the heart and, therefore, an increased preload; this results in an increase in the heart rate and the CO.

The resultant increase in BP (HTN) and heart rate (tachycardia) is not without adverse side effects. There are imbalances between oxygen supply and demand. The increased myocardial oxygen consumption can lead to ischemia, injury, and infarction. Tachycardia and HTN are the two most important determinants of imbalances in oxygen supply and demand. These effects are tolerated in young adults, but they are significant in the middle-aged and senior populations.

Coronary blood flow is dependent on diastolic filling time and pressure. If there is a decrease in filling time caused by tachycardia or an increase in LVEDP and LVEDV caused by HTN, coronary blood flow and volume will be decreased and ischemia will result. The resultant ischemia causes a decrease in CO over time, and this ultimately leads to signs of congestion and HF (**Table 4**).[8]

ANESTHESIA AND HTN

Patients with HTN can develop exaggerated hypotension and HTN perioperatively. With chronic HTN, there is a relative decrease in intravascular volume; if the anesthetic agents cause vasodilation, the decreased intravascular volume cannot fill those dilated vessels. The result is a decrease in venous return to the heart, a decrease in CO, and an exaggerated hypotensive event.

Chronic HTN also causes vascular smooth muscle hypertrophy. Surgical stimulation can activate the sympathetic nervous system; this results in vasoconstriction of the hypertrophic muscle in those vessels, and you see an exaggerated hypertensive event. This reaction is not uncommon during intubation or the maintenance phase of anesthesia if patients are not in a deep enough stage of anesthesia.[6]

Table 4
Heart rate and cycle time

Heart Rate (beats per min)	Diastolic Time	Systolic Time
60	66% of cycle	33% of cycle
90	50% of cycle	50% of cycle
120	Diastolic < systolic	Systolic > diastolic

PERIOPERATIVE HTN

Perioperative HTN does increase the risk of ischemia, infarction, HF, CVA, and renal disease. The incidence of complications is 30% in patients with untreated HTN, 36% in poorly controlled patients, and 16% in well-controlled patients. The overall incidence of perioperative HTN is 25%.[9]

Patients with pre-HTN or stage 1 HTN (SBP 120–159 mm Hg or DBP 80–99 mm Hg) do not have an increased risk for cardiovascular complications. The parenteral use of antihypertensive agents is unnecessary preoperatively, and there is no apparent benefit in delaying the surgery. During surgery, if an acute exacerbation occurs, medications are indicated to control BP, and patients' antihypertensive medications should be maintained during the perioperative period.

Patients with a DBP less than 110 mm Hg behave very similar to normotensive patients. BPs that are less than *180/110 without evidence of target organ disease* are not independent risks for perioperative cardiovascular complications. Therefore, it is unnecessary to reduce these pressures to normal before surgery. In fact, aggressive lowering of BP (too fast, too low) may increase the risk of ischemic injury to the heart, brain, and kidneys.

Surgery must be deferred regardless of BP in the presence of ischemia, HF, renal failure, or CNS dysfunction. Patients at high risk (previous stroke or active CAD) should have surgery postponed when the *SBP is more than 180 mm Hg or the DBP is more than 110 mm Hg.* These patients need optimization of BP before surgery to reduce risks.

Surgery in patients with poorly controlled HTN has increased complications. The decision to proceed with surgery is based on the surgical risk (low vs high), comorbidities, and patients' presentation. Patients with no evidence of target organ disease despite BPs of 180/110 or more may still be candidates for elective surgery. There is no data to support delaying surgery solely based on the BP reading. If you decide to proceed, those patients will need parenteral perioperative antihypertensive medications. BB like metoprolol or labetalol are typical agents that are used along with a benzodiazepine to reduce anxiety. The target BP decrease should be no greater than 20% of the baseline. These cases are not office-based cases. They should be done in a hospital-based ambulatory center or an in-patient facility.

Pulse pressure (PP) is the difference between the SBP and the DBP. Patients with PPs greater than 80 mm Hg have a greater risk for perioperative stroke, death, and renal dysfunction. Increased PPs in ambulatory patients is a better indicator of cardiovascular and cerebrovascular risk than SBP or DBP readings.

Studies have shown that death rates in the middle-aged and senior populations are highest in patients with HTN with an *SBP more than 160 and a DBP less than 70, which result in PPs more than 90 mm Hg*. The morbidity and mortality rates increase as PPs increase more so than increases in SBP at fixed PPs. This increase is caused by decreased coronary perfusion and increased myocardial oxygen consumption in pumping blood against the increased afterload.[10]

OFFICE SURGERY AND HTN

Patients with an SBP of 180 mm Hg or more and/or a DBP of 110 mm Hg or more may be at low risk in the absence of target organ damage, but they still have risks. It would be wise to defer elective office surgery and anesthesia until the BP can be optimized. Anecdotally, surgeons try test doses of sedation to see if the BPs can be lowered; if so, they assume that patients have white coat syndrome, and this is why the pressure is elevated. Anxiety may be a contributing factor, but these patients can still develop HTN/hypotension episodes under anesthesia. A more conservative approach would be to discuss these patients with the physician to see if additional antihypertensive agents are indicated and then proceed with surgery.

The JNC-7 report classifies a SBP of more than 180 mm Hg and a DBP of more than 110 mm Hg as a hypertensive crisis. This crisis can be further classified as an emergency or an urgency, and the treatments differ for both.

Hypertensive emergencies result in target organ damage. It was first described in 1914 as severe HTN with signs of vascular injury to the heart, brain, kidney, and eyes. In 1939, the term *malignant hypertension* was used to describe the event. Before the use of antihypertensive agents, 7% of patients with HTN suffered an emergency, and there was a 79% 1-year mortality rate.

In the United States, men have twice the incidence as women. The elderly and black populations have a higher incidence than middle-aged white men. Sympathetic stimulation with the release of vasoconstrictors increases the SVR and subsequently damage the endothelial lining of vessels. Ischemia develops over time, and the renin angiotensin system is activated to cause additional vasoconstriction. The overall result is end organ hypoperfusion, ischemia, and dysfunction.[11]

The most common clinical signs are dyspnea, chest pain, headache, altered mental status, and focal neurologic deficits. Patients who present with severe HTN should be examined to rule out target organ injury.[8]

BRAIN

As BP increases, intracranial pressure and cerebral blood flow increase. This increase disrupts the blood-brain barrier and causes fluid leakage and cerebral edema. As this process progresses, hypertensive encephalopathy develops; although it is uncommon, it is a true emergency. Clinical signs include severe, generalized headache; confusion; somnolence; projectile vomiting; visual disturbances (blurred vision to blindness); and transient focal neurologic deficits.[12]

Retinal examination shows arteriolar spasm, exudates, hemorrhage, cotton wool spots, and papilledema. This progressive deterioration may take 12 to 24 hours before all the signs are evident. Treatment is to reduce the MAP 10% to 15%, with a maximum reduction of 20% in the first hour. Further reduction in pressure to 160/100 is done over the next 2 to 6 hours. If the reduction is too rapid, cerebral perfusion decreases and cerebral ischemia and infarcts can develop (**Table 5**).[13]

Hypertensive urgencies are elevations in BP of more than 180/120, but there is no target organ disease. These patients are usually given oral antihypertensive agents to reduce BP over several hours or days. In the perioperative setting, this is usually not possible because the patients are under anesthesia. The potential problem with not treating these patients is that the urgency may be a transitioning period, which can lead to a true emergency. In this setting, parenteral agents are used, but aggressive therapy is to be avoided. Avoid lowering too fast and too low to prevent hypoperfusion and prolonged postoperative hypotension.[14]

HTN during elective office anesthesia is usually a hypertensive urgency, not an emergency. There is no target organ failure. Patients who present to the office with well-controlled HTN *have less than a*

Table 5 Target organ disease	
	Cerebral Infarction
Brain	Intracranial hemorrhage Hypertensive encephalopathy Subarachnoid hemorrhage
Heart	Ischemia, injury, infarction Dysrhythmias Pulmonary edema HF
Kidney	Renal ischemic injury Renal failure

10% risk of developing SBP of more than 160 mm Hg intraoperatively. Data support low complication rates perioperatively as long as the preoperative BP is less than 180/110.[2]

Intraoperative HTN

Fluctuations in BP are very common during anesthesia induction and intubation. These fluctuations happen with both normotensive patients and patients with HTN. Patients with HTN will exhibit the most dramatic changes in pressure.

In normotensive patients, general anesthesia induction can increase BP by 20 to 30 mm Hg and elevate the heart rate by 15 to 20 beats per minute. In patients with HTN, there can be increases in BP up to 90 mm Hg and increases in heart rate up to 40 beats per minute.[15]

Intraoperatively, the BP usually decreases from direct vasodilation of vessels by the anesthetic agents and inhibition of the sympathetic nervous system. In normotensive patients, BP will decrease up to 30 mm Hg; in the patients with HTN, this decrease can exceed 60 mm Hg. This hypotension can result in hypoperfusion with ischemia, dysrhythmias, HF, and renal failure. Goldman[16] found that intraoperative hypotension (BP <50% of baseline or a 33% decrease for 10 or more minutes) will increase these risks. Beyer and colleagues[17] found that HTN will increase the risk of intraoperative dysrhythmias and hemodynamic changes by 40%. During surgery, fluctuations in MAP more than 20% will increase postoperative cardiovascular complications.

The management of intraoperative HTN is complicated by patients' comorbidities, volume status, anesthetic depth, and choice of anesthetic agents (**Box 2**).

ACUTE POSTOPERATIVE HTN

It is not uncommon to see postoperative HTN. There is no universally accepted definition for acute postoperative HTN (APH). Some practitioners define APH as an SBP of more than 20% of the baseline preoperative pressure or an increase in DBP of more than 110 mm Hg. Others use an SBP of more than 160 mm Hg, a DBP of more than 90 mm Hg, or an MAP that exceeds 110 mm Hg. Regardless of the definition, APH can increase the risk of cardiovascular and cerebrovascular complications (**Box 3**).

The onset is usually within 10 to 15 minutes after surgery, but it can take up to 2 hours to develop. The duration is less than 6 hours, and the incidence is 4% to 35%. The major component of APH is activation of the sympathetic nervous system as demonstrated by the increased plasma concentration of circulating catecholamines. The renin angiotensin system is a minor component in APH (**Box 4**).[18]

One specific cause of APH is the clonidine withdrawal syndrome. Although rare, it can happen because patients are NPO for anesthesia and they do not take the oral clonidine, and there is no parenteral substitute in the United States. The reaction develops 18 to 24 hours after the drug is stopped. Patients have increased sympathetic stimulation with rebound HTN.

If oral clonidine is stopped for surgery, a transdermal clonidine patch is available for use until patients can take oral medications. Patients who also use nonselective BB are at an increased risk because the beta-2 sites (vasodilation) are blocked, and the alpha vasoconstrictor sites are now unopposed, which leads to significant HTN. Dexmedetomidine may have some use in these cases because of its alpha-2 agonist activity (vasodilation).

MEDICATIONS FOR PERIOPERATIVE HTN

Perioperative HTN management should include the use of sedation, either moderate or deep, to reduce the anxiety component of HTN. Pain management using profound local anesthesia and perioperative opioids is appropriate as is optimal oxygenation

---

Box 2
Causes of intraoperative HTN

Intubation and airway manipulation

Light anesthesia and pain

Exogenous epinephrine

Hypoxia and hypercarbia

Hypovolemia

Hypothermia

Volume overload and/or bladder distention

Holding perioperative antihypertensive medications

Box 3
Acute postoperative HTN complications

Myocardial ischemia and infarction

Cerebral ischemia and infarction

Dysrhythmias

Congestive HF

Pulmonary edema

Intracranial bleeding

Incisional bleeding

| Box 4 |
Causes of APH
Pain and anxiety
Hypoxia and hypercarbia
Hypothermia
Volume overload and/or bladder distention
Emergence delirium
Endotracheal tube irritation
Rebound HTN from withholding antihypertensives

and ventilation. Antihypertensive medications are usually maintained perioperatively, but patients may still require intraoperative medications to control the BP.

The ideal antihypertensive agent should have a rapid onset and short duration of action to avoid prolonged recovery times. Bolus agents are preferable to infusion agents in the office because they can be given fast and they do not require additional equipment to administer the drug. These agents should also have minimal side effects that will not disrupt cardiac conduction or reduce myocardial contractility. Agents that vasodilate the arteriolar resistance vessels are good because they decrease afterload and myocardial oxygen consumption, and any agent that has limited reflex tachycardia is good because it too will limit oxygen consumption.[19]

BB

BB have a long history in the management of HTN. They have been found to decrease post-MI mortality. Perioperatively, they reduce ischemia and attenuate fluctuations in intraoperative BP. Patients at risk for cardiovascular complications have less perioperative events while maintaining the beta agent. There are fewer episodes of ischemia, infarction, dysrhythmias, HF, or death. However, these agents are not without risk. Deveraux[20] found that although the risk of perioperative MI is reduced, the risk for stroke actually increased.

Should BB Be Maintained Perioperatively?

Major cardiovascular complications, such as infarctions or unstable angina, only occur in 1% of elective inpatient surgery; but that risk can increase to 5% in patients who have underlying CVD.[21]

In high-risk patients undergoing high-risk surgery, there is a benefit to perioperative BB therapy. Withdrawal of the BB is associated with an increased mortality at 30 days and 1 year.[22]

For office and ambulatory surgery, if patients are not taking a BB and there is no indication for long-term beta blockade, there is no indication to support the initiation of BB therapy.[23]

BB reduce BP by decreasing the heart rate and myocardial contractility. The result is a decrease in CO and BP. Most patients using BB are on selective BB to limit side effects. However, at high doses, even the selective beta-1 agents lose selectivity and have crossover effects that inhibit beta-2 vasodilation. BB are not used in acute HF because they reduce heart rate and contractility in a failing heart. These agents are also restricted in patients with atrioventricular (AV) heart block.

SHOULD BB BE USED IN PATIENTS WITH OBSTRUCTIVE AIRWAY DISEASE?

There are 3 types of beta-receptors. Beta-1 receptors are typically found in the heart and when activated cause an increase in heart rate and force of myocardial contraction. These receptors also compose up to 30% of the beta-receptors in the alveolar walls of the lung. Beta-2 receptors cause bronchial and vascular smooth muscle to dilate. These receptors are also found in the heart and account for about 20% to 25% of those beta-receptors. The role of beta-3 receptors is still to be determined.

Nonselective BB like propranolol act on beta-1 and beta-2 receptors. Patients with asthma or chronic obstructive pulmonary disease (COPD) that are exposed to these drugs orally can see a 66-fold increase in airway hyperresponsiveness and a 6-fold increase to intravenous (IV) drug exposure as compared with the response in nonasthmatic patients. Therefore, nonselective BB should not be used in these patients because of a potentially life-threatening bronchospastic response.[24]

Studies have shown that cardioselective BB do not cause significant changes in patients' forced expiratory volume in 1 second or affect the response of rescue beta-2 agents. Patients with COPD typically have more significant airway disease than most patients with asthma, and they are also more prone to have a coexisting CVD. If these patients require antihypertensive therapy and would benefit from the use of a cardioselective BB, they should not be withheld.

Because of its short duration and demonstrated lack of airway dysfunction in patients with asthma, IV esmolol may be useful in perioperative HTN. Labetalol may also have a role because of its alpha-1 blockade. Alpha-1 antagonists are weak bronchodilators, and they also have antihistamine and antiserotonin activity.

However, some investigators caution against using these agents in patients with airway hyper-responsiveness. Certainly, they would be contraindicated in patients with acute bronchospasm, but elective anesthesia would also be contraindicated in these patients. It remains up to the practitioner to assess risk versus benefit in this group of patients with perioperative HTN.[25,26]

ESMOLOL

Esmolol is an ultrashort-acting beta-1 selective blocker. The elimination half-life is about 8 minutes because of hydrolysis of its ester linkage by red blood cell esterases. This metabolism is independent of renal or liver function. The onset of action is 60 seconds after the IV bolus dose, and the duration is about 10 to 20 minutes after the infusion is stopped.[18]

Esmolol competitively blocks the beta-1 receptor; but at high doses, there is also beta-2 blocking. This crossover can precipitate bronchospasm in patients with reactive airway disease, asthma, or COPD. There is less risk of bronchospasm with esmolol versus labetalol because of esmolol's short duration of action. Esmolol has no direct vasodilation effects. The reduction in BP is by decreasing heart rate and myocardial contractility. Clinical effects are a reduction in heart rate, CO, SBP, and DBP.[10]

Esmolol is an excellent agent for perioperative HTN, especially when tachycardia is present. This BB reduces BP, but it reduces heart rate to a greater degree than BP. It should not be used in patients who present with bradycardia, acute HF, or AV heart block (second or third degree).[27]

In most cases, an IV bolus is given over 30 seconds to 1 minute, and this is followed by an infusion because of the short duration of the agent. An alternative approach presented in an American Dental Society Anesthesiology (ADSA) I general anesthesia review program is to give an IV bolus of 5 to 10 mg (0.5 mg/kg). As with other techniques, this dose would be given over 30 seconds, and you will see a decrease in heart rate of 1 beat per minute for every 1 mg of drug given. The maximum dose of esmolol by any schedule is 300 mcg/kg/min (**Tables 6** and **7**).

LABETALOL

Labetalol is a nonselective BB and a selective alpha-1 blocker. Beta blockade is 5 to 10 times greater than the alpha blockade, but the beta-1 and beta-2 sites are blocked to the same degree. The ratio of alpha to beta blockade is 1:7. **Unlike other BB, labetalol maintains CO, and the heart**

Table 6
Esmolol dosing schedules

Bolus Dose Schedule	Infusion Dosage Schedule
80 mg over 30 s	150 mics/kg/min
500 mics/kg over 1 min	25–200 mics/kg/min
500 mics/kg over 1 min	25–50 mics/kg/min then increase the dosage by 25 mics/kg/min q 10–15 min

rate is either maintained or slightly reduced. SVR is decreased, but cerebral, coronary, and renal blood flow is maintained.[18]

The onset of action is 2 to 5 minutes, with a peak effect within 5 to 15 minutes. The duration of action is 2 to 4 hours. Metabolism occurs in the liver. Labetalol, like esmolol, is an effective medication for **perioperative HTN with tachycardia.** It should not be used in bradycardia, HF, or AV heart block. Its use in airway disease is controversial. Certainly it would not be used in acute bronchospasm.

As stated previously, with most of these antihypertensive agents, it is better to go low, go slow in an office setting because we can precipitate other complications that can be worse. Although the initial bolus dose of labetalol is 20 mg IV, a conservative approach would be to give 5 to 10 mg IV with incremental dosing in 5 to 10 minutes at 20 mg or more. The use of 1 to 2 mg/kg as an initial dose should be avoided because significant hypotension can occur. The maximum daily dose of labetalol is 300 mg in 24 hours (**Table 8**).[10,28]

Table 7
AAOMS office anesthesia manual for esmolol

Bolus Dose	Infusion Dose
80 mg (1 mg/kg) over 30 s	150 mics/kg/min to a maximum of 300/mics/kg/min
500 mics/kg over 1 min	50 mics/kg/min for 4 min, reevaluate, and if needed, try the bottom dose schedule
500 mics/kg over 1 min	100 mics/kg/min up to maximum of 300 mics/kg/min

Abbreviation: AAOMS, American Association of Oral and Maxillofacial Surgeons.
Data from Office Anesthesia Evaluation Manual. 8th edition. Rosemont (IL): American Association of Oral & Maxillofacial Surgeons; 2012.

Table 8
Labetalol dosing

Initial Bolus	Repeat Bolus in 10 min
5–10 mg IV	20 mg IV
20 mg IV	20–80 mg IV
5–20 mg IV over 2 min	2 mg/min up to 300 mg maximum dose
Infusion of 0.5–2.0 mg/min	Increase by 0.5 mg/min q 15 min up to maximum of 6 mg/min

Data from Office Anesthesia Evaluation Manual. 8th edition. Rosemont (IL): American Association of Oral & Maxillofacial Surgeons; 2012; and Hays A, Wilkerson T. Management of hypertensive emergencies. AACN Adv Crit Care 2010;21(1):5–14.

METOPROLOL

Metoprolol is a beta-1 selective blocker. Like the other BB, it reduces BP and CO by decreasing the heart rate and myocardial contractility. A secondary effect on BP is its suppression of the sympathetic nervous system to pain and anxiety. Patients who use metoprolol for maintenance therapy for HTN have decreased renin release and decreased levels of angiotensin II.

IV metoprolol is used to control the ventricular response in atrial fibrillation and paroxysmal supraventricular tachycardia (PSVT). It is not a first-line drug for perioperative HTN; as a solo agent, it is not always effective. If a vasodilating antihypertensive agent is used to reduce BP, a reflex tachycardia will occur. If metoprolol is added to the treatment, it will prevent the reflex tachycardia.

The initial dose is 1 to 2 mg IV. The onset of action is 2 to 3 minutes, with a peak effect within 20 minutes. The duration of action is 4 hours. Additional doses of metoprolol of 1.25 to 5.0 mg can be given every 6 hours.[15]

Other BB that can be used for perioperative HTN include the following: Propranolol is a nonselective BB that is rarely used for perioperative HTN because there are better cardioselective BB. Atenolol, a cardioselective BB, has a slow onset, so it is not a first-line agent. Nebivolol is a third-generation BB that also has vasodilating properties. Both arteries and veins are dilated through the L-arginine-nitric acid pathway. It is a BB plus a vasodilator, which makes it a promising agent for the future.

CCB

There are 6 types of CCB. The L-type agents act on vascular and myocardial functions. This drug class inhibits the influx of extracellular calcium (Ca) ions through the Ca channels. This inhibition causes vascular smooth muscle to vasodilate, and it inhibits myocardial contractions and cardiac conduction pathway transmissions.

There are 3 classes of L-type CCB

Phenylalkylamines: verapamil
Dihydropyridines: nifedipine, amlodipine, nicardipine (Cardene), and clevidipine (Cleviprex)
Benzothiapines: diltiazem

The dihydropyridines are used as vasodilators, whereas the phenylalkylamines and the benzothiapines are antidysrhythmics.

DIHYDROPYRIDINES

These drugs include nifedipine, nicardipine, and clevidipine. They are selective for vascular smooth muscle with cerebral vessels having the highest affinity followed in descending order by coronary, muscle, and renal vessels. There is little to no activity on cardiac muscle contractility or sinoatrial node transmission. The net effect of these agents is vasodilation, which acts to reduce BP.

Nicardipine is a second-generation dihydropyridine. In cerebral vessels, it dilates small resistance arterioles to relieve cerebral ischemia without changing intracranial pressure or intracranial volume. Nicardipine reduces SVR by vasodilation and reduces coronary ischemia by increasing coronary blood flow. There will be an increase in the heart rate and CO, whereas the afterload is decreased. Side effects are headache, hypotension, and nausea and vomiting.[11]

Nicardipine is usually given as an infusion, and the dose is independent of weight. Nicardipine comes in premixed bags for IV infusion use.

Nicardipine: Use 20 mg in 200 mL fluid, 40 mg in 200 mL fluid, or 2.5 mg/mL in a 10-mL vial.

Dosing instructions

The initial dosage is 5 mg/h as an IV infusion. This dosage is increased by 2.5 mg/h every 5 minutes for a rapid reduction of BP. For a gradual reduction of BP, the dosage can be increased by 2.5 mg/h every 15 minutes. This dosing is done until the BP is controlled or a maximum dosage of 30 mg/h.

When the target pressure is achieved, the dosage is reduced by 3 mg/h. This dosage is single use only; discard any unused portion. Do not mix or run the drug in the same line as other medications.

Nicardipine is an excellent drug for perioperative HTN. The onset of action is 5 to 15 minutes, with a duration of 4 to 6 hours. At present because of its cost and the need for infusion administration, this agent has limited usefulness in the office. However, bolus nicardipine has been used to control BP during cardiac surgery and to limit the cardiovascular response in rapid sequence intubations.

An IV bolus of 0.5 to 1.0 mg decreased the SBP by 32 to 36 mm Hg. It also decreased the MAP by 21 to 24 mm Hg, with a maximum response in about 60 seconds in both instances. IV doses of 20 mics/kg have been used for intubations with an onset of action in 2.5 ± 0.6 minutes and a duration of 24 ± 5 minutes.[29,30]

Diltiazem and Verapamil

These CCB can reduce BP, but the side effects outweigh the benefits. IV diltiazem will lower BP within 5 minutes, but heart blocks and dysrhythmias are also seen. Verapamil side effects seen when used to manage HTN include electrocardiogram (ECG) PR interval prolongation, along with second- and third-degree AV heart block. These agents are used to treat PSVT and to control the ventricular rates in atrial fibrillation and atrial flutter.[31,32]

Clevidipine

Clevidipine is an ultrashort-acting third-generation dihydropyridine CCB. The onset of action is within 2 to 4 minutes from the start of the infusion, and there is a return to baseline pressures within 10 to 15 minutes after stopping the infusion. The short duration is caused by redistribution effects similar to what is seen with propofol. The rapid metabolism is from tissue and red blood cell esterase hydrolysis.

This agent reduces SVR by arterial smooth muscle vasodilation, so there is a decrease in the afterload. There is no effect on venous capacitance vessels, so the preload of the heart is maintained. CO increases, as does coronary blood flow; but unlike other vasodilators, there is no reflex tachycardia seen with clevidipine. Clinically, there is a reduction in SBP, DBP, and MAP.[33]

Dosing schedule for clevidipine

The initial dosage is 1 to 2 mg/h. This dosage may be doubled at 90-second intervals until you approach the target BP reduction. As the pressure approaches the target pressure, the dosage is increased by less than double at an interval of every 5 to 10 minutes.
Most patients reach the target reduction at rates of 4 to 6 mg/h in less than 30 minutes.
The maximum dosage is 32 mg/h.
Use clevidipine 0.5 mg/mL in 50-mL or 100-mL vials.

Clevidipine is a lipid emulsion, so as with propofol, there is a concern in patients with soy and egg allergy. The unused portion of the drug must be discarded after 4 hours to avoid contamination. Side effects include onset of atrial fibrillation, headache, flushing, fever, and nausea and vomiting. The advantages of clevipidine are its ultrashort half-life, along with ease of titration, predictable response, and lack of toxicity and drug interactions.[34]

HYDRALAZINE

Hydralazine is a direct arteriolar vasodilator with little to no effect on venous capacitance vessels. The drug causes reflex sympathetic activity with an increase in circulating catecholamines. This vasodilation and sympathetic discharge causes an increase in CO, myocardial contractility, and reflex tachycardia.

The tachycardia will increase the myocardial oxygen demand and myocardial oxygen consumption, so hydralazine should be avoided in patients at risk for myocardia ischemia. Cerebral vessels also vasodilate and that will allow an increase in intracranial pressure. The clinical relevance of this effect is debatable; but to be safe, hydralazine is contraindicated in closed head injury.

The onset of activity is 5 to 15 minutes, but the onset may be followed by an unpredictable and severe decrease in BP that can last for up to 12 hours. The circulating blood half-life is 3 hours, but the drug's clinical half-life is up to 10 hours. The duration of action is between 2 to 10 hours, depending on the ability of the liver to metabolize the drug. The maximum decrease in BP in most cases is 10 to 80 minutes after bolus injection. Clinically, there is a decrease in SBP, DBP, and MAP.[11,35]

There are multiple dosing guidelines found in the literature. The reason is that the response is unpredictable and the risk of prolonged hypotension is real. In using this drug, a conservative approach is necessary; and we need to remember that although the perioperative BP readings may be high (SBP ≥180 mm Hg), most of these cases, at least initially, are urgencies and not emergencies. We have the time to slowly decrease the BP.

One approach to consider

The initial dose of hydralazine is 2.5 to 5.0 mg IV over 2 minutes. Wait for 10 to 15 minutes, then give a repeat of the initial dose or increase that dose. The maximum dose in the office should be 20 to 25 mg (Table 9).[36]

Hydralazine has been used as an office treatment of perioperative HTN for many years. It is

Table 9
Hydralazine dosing

Initial Dose Bolus	Repeat Dose Bolus
10–20 mg IV	None given
10–50 mg IM dose not IV	None given
5–10 mg IV over 2 min	5–20 mg IV q 6 h
10–20 mg IV	Repeat q 4–6 h
2.5–5.0 mg IV	None given
3–20 mg IV	Repeat q 20–60 min
AAOMS manual, eighth edition 5 mg IV	Titrate up to 25 mg

Abbreviations: AAOMS, American Association of Oral and Maxillofacial Surgeons; IM, intramuscularly.

no longer a first-line agent because there are other options with less risk of hypotension and tachycardia-induced ischemia. This availability of other options is certainly true in a hospital setting. But in the office, these newer agents are not readily available; they are expensive, and they require infusion technology. When left with hydralazine as a treatment option, we need to assess the risk of such treatment in our consultation visit. In doing so, the potential harm to patients may lead us to doing this case in a facility that has more medication options. It is up to each practitioner to make that judgment.

NITROGLYCERIN

Nitroglycerin (NTG) is primarily an antianginal agent because it dilates coronary arteries, relieves coronary vessel spasms, and increases blood flow to ischemic myocardial tissues. At low doses, it is a potent venodilator decreasing the preload and the LVEDP and LVEDV. The result is a decrease in myocardial oxygen demand and a relief of ischemia and pain. The decrease in BP is secondary to reductions in the preload and CO. These effects are seen regardless of the route of administration (sublingual, patch, or IV).

At higher doses of NTG, arterial vessels dilate, which then decreases the afterload of the heart. This decrease makes it easier to pump blood to the aorta with less myocardial oxygen consumption. **The IV dosage of NTG is 5 to 10 mics/min** or 0.075 to 0.15 mics/kg/min. This dosage can be **increased by 5 to 10 mcg/min every 3 to 5 minutes.**

The onset of action is within 2 to 5 minutes, with a duration of 10 to 20 minutes after the infusion is stopped. Side effects are headache, reflex tachycardia, and, on rare occasions, methemoglobinemia.[18]

APH can lead to hypovolemia. If NTG is administered in the presence of hypovolemia, an exaggerated hypotensive episode will follow. NTG is not a first-line agent for APH because of this possibility along with the reflex tachycardia that most always occurs at doses of NTG that can decrease BP. NTG is an adjunct therapy to other antihypertensive medications in patients that present with acute ischemia, infarction, or pulmonary edema, which are situations when you need a decrease in preload, afterload, and myocardial oxygen consumption.[1]

Before NTG is used, patients should be asked about erectile dysfunction medications, the phosphodiesterase-5-inhibitors. Patients need a 48-hour washout period for these agents, otherwise NTG can cause severe hypotension that may be unresponsive to most vasopressors.

Is There a Role for Sublingual NTG in Office Perioperative HTN?

Most practitioners have limited choices for managing HTN in the office. Typical IV agents are labetalol, esmolol, and possibly hydralazine. A beta agent is not a good choice for a hypertensive event in patients with acute, severe bronchoconstriction. Patients with acute angina who are hypertensive do not need an agent like hydralazine whereby the tachycardia will make the ischemia worse, so what is left?

In this circumstance, the use of low-dose sublingual NTG can help. It certainly is indicated in patients who are anginal; in patients with asthma, if you do not have hydralazine, the NTG can be helpful. Where is the peer-reviewed literature to back this up? At present, it is lacking, but there are practitioners who use it.

A recommendation found in a 2005 ADSA General Anesthesia Review course outlines the use of sublingual NTG for HTN. Using 0.4-mg sublingual tablets, 1 to 2 tablets are placed under the tongue. The onset of action is within 15 to 20 minutes, with a duration of 5 to 7 minutes, and the onset may be faster. It may be more useful to use ACLS dosing guidelines of every 5 minutes. Anecdotally, emergency medical services (EMS) providers that treat far more cardiac complications than OMFS, use sublingual NTG for HTN on route to the hospital. Anesthesiologists have used NTG spray for short-term hypertensive reactions from exogenous epinephrine; in the cardiac catheterization laboratory, cardiologists have used the spray during their procedures. Because of a lack of published data, a recommendation cannot be made; but practitioners do use off-label treatments. It is up to the surgeon to make that call.

CLONIDINE

Clonidine is a centrally acting alpha-2 adrenergic receptor agonist that prevents the release of norepinephrine from the sympathetic nervous system and acts on CNS I-1 receptors to cause centrally mediated vasodilation and hypotension. Clinically, there is a reduction in peripheral vascular resistance, heart rate, and BP.[18]

As an anesthetic agent, it reduces the MAC (minimum alveolar concentration) of volatile gases and opioid requirements for pain. It also reduces the sympathetic response to intubation. In the United States, it is only available in oral and transdermal patches, but other countries have an IV formulation.[15]

There is a lack of published data to support the routine use of clonidine for acute postoperative HTN, most likely because of the lack of an IV route of administration. However, there are data for the perioperative effects of clonidine. Oral or transdermal clonidine the night before surgery decreases the MAP for up to 24 to 48 hours and reduces the levels of circulating catecholamines.[37]

Wallace[38] studied preoperative clonidine in patients at risk for CAD who required noncardiac surgery. They used a 0.2-mg oral dose plus an applied transdermal patch the night before surgery; they also gave patients a 0.2-mg oral dose 1 hour before surgery. Patients continued to receive 0.2 mg oral clonidine postoperatively for 4 days, and the patch was removed at that time. The results showed less episodes of perioperative HTN and ischemia. The patients did have more episodes of tachycardia than patients on BB, but the ischemia improvement was similar to the BB.

Side effects are headache, nausea and vomiting, and hypotension that responds to IV fluids. These reactions occur within 30 minutes to 1 hour after taking the drug, but they can last up to 10 hours.[3]

There is a role for clonidine in office anesthesia. Friedberg uses an office plastic surgery technique where clonidine is given preoperatively taking the place of midazolam, and this is followed by an intravenous anesthetic consisting of ketamine and propofol.

Another indication for clonidine would be patients with HTN who present in the office for a minor oral surgical procedure under local anesthesia but have a BP more than 180/100. When you ask patients about antihypertensive medication compliance, they tell you, "I take my meds daily, my BP is high just because I am here." The primary care physician (PCP) tells you, "The BP is controlled and this is just white coat syndrome, so just take out the teeth."

Clonidine is useful here. It can be given 0.1 to 0.2 mg orally as a solo agent or it can be combined with an anxiolytic. Clonidine will decrease BP, and it also has a sedative effect. The patch is not useful because it takes too long for an effect.

PHENTOLAMINE

Phentolamine is a pure alpha-adrenergic antagonist. The primary indication for this agent is a catecholamine-induced hypertensive emergency like a pheochromocytoma or an monoamine oxidase inhibitor hypertensive crisis. It is not a first-line drug for perioperative HTN.

The dosage in perioperative HTN is 1 mg every 5 to 10 minutes, with a range of 1 to 5 mg. The onset of action is within 1 to 2 minutes, with a duration of 3 to 15 minutes. Side effects include flushing and headache. This agent is often difficult to obtain because it is rarely indicated, so its usefulness as compared with other agents is minimal.[19,39]

NITROPRUSSIDE

No discussion of the management of acute HTN is complete without nitroprusside. It was the gold standard of care for hypertensive emergencies. The drug is both a venous and arterial vasodilator that reduces preload, afterload, and peripheral venous resistance. IV infusion has a near-immediate response, with a range of 1 to 2 minutes; once the infusion is stopped, the duration of action is about 2 minutes.

The side effects are problematic. Cerebral blood flow is diminished, whereas the intracranial pressure is increased. In the heart, coronary steal (a process whereby blood flow is diverted away from ischemic areas) happens frequently. Renal function and blood flow are also decreased.[39]

Cyanide and thiocyanate toxicity are side effects from prolonged infusions of nitroprusside. Nitroprusside metabolism releases cyanide, which is then detoxified by circulating thiosulfate molecules. The amount of cyanide depends on the amount of available thiosulfate in the circulation.

Infusions of nitroprusside exceeding 4 to 5 mics/kg/min for as little as 2 to 3 hours cause cyanide toxicity. Signs include headache, anxiety, confusion, lethargy, and coma. Cardiovascular signs are ischemia, dysrhythmias, AV heart block, and cardiovascular collapse. Patients may also report nausea and vomiting, abdominal pain, and increased salivary flow.[1]

To prevent cyanide toxicity, thiosulfate is added to the infusion at a ratio of 10:1. It will not decrease the antihypertensive effect of nitroprusside. The byproduct of cyanide metabolism by thiosulfate is thiocyanate, which is 100 times less toxic than cyanide.[2]

> **The dosage for nitroprusside is 0.25 to 0.5 mics/kg/min increased by 0.5 mics/kg/min every 5 to 10 minutes. Do not exceed a total dosage of 5 mics/kg/min.**

Nitroprusside is no longer a first-line agent for hypertensive urgencies and emergencies. Its renal, cerebral, and cardiac side effects are significant. In addition, it is mandatory to use arterial line catheters to monitor BPs with this agent. There is no reason to consider the use of this drug in an office.[11]

RENIN ANGIOTENSIN SYSTEM

This system regulates BP and intravascular volume. Antihypertensive drugs in the category are ACEI and ARB. ACEI block the conversion of angiotensin I to angiotensin II, a vasoconstrictor. ARB block the effect of circulating angiotensin II.

Intraoperative HTN can be treated with enalaprilat, an ACEI. It will reduce MAP, SBP, DBP, and the preload. The vasodilation decreases the afterload, but there is no reflex tachycardia. Enalaprilat maintains cerebral blood flow with no change in intracranial pressure.

The dose is 0.015 mg/kg or 0.625 to 1.25 mg IV over 5 minutes, and it can be repeated in 20 to 30 minutes if the first dose was ineffective. Additional doses can be given every 6 hours. The onset of action is within 15 minutes; it peaks in 1 hour, and the duration of action is more than 4 hours. This drug would not be a first-line agent for perioperative HTN.[10,18]

OFFICE AND AMBULATORY ANESTHESIA AND ANTIHYPERTENSIVE AGENTS
Do We Hold These Agents or Maintain Them During Surgery?

BB should be maintained perioperatively, and this was discussed earlier in the article.

CCB may not be cardioprotective during surgery, but there is no evidence to suggest any detrimental effects, so they too are maintained perioperatively.

ACEI and ARB
These drugs are frequently used to manage HTN, HF, and chronic renal failure. Pharmacologically they should be cardioprotective during surgery, but they are the most likely antihypertensive agents to cause significant intraoperative hypotension. This hypotension is less responsive to IV fluid challenges and vasopressors like ephedrine, phenylephrine, and epinephrine. At present, there is controversy as to holding these drugs preoperatively or maintaining them perioperatively.[23]

During the first 30 minutes of anesthesia, there is greater volatility in BP. This volatility is related to possible decreased intravascular volume from being NPO or chronic HTN. Anxiety also has a role, and the pharmacology of the anesthetic induction drugs has a major role. After the first 30 minutes, BP changes tend to be less volatile and more stable.

ACEI and ARB have a typical half-life of about 10 hours. Comfere and colleagues[40] examined the incidence of hypotension during the first 30 minutes of anesthesia in patients who stopped their medications in **less than 10 hours and 10 hours or more preoperatively.** The incidence of moderate hypotension (SBP ≤85 mm Hg) was 60.4% in the less-than-10-hour group and 46.3% in the 10-hour-or-more group. There was no difference between groups in the incidence of severe hypotension (SBP ≤65 mm Hg), and there was no difference in the response to vasopressor treatment.

The presence of other antihypertensive drugs did not affect the incidence of hypotension. They concluded that ACEI and ARB drugs are significant risk factors for moderate hypotension during the first 30 minutes of general anesthesia. Because this hypotension did not result in significant adverse effects, there is no support for stopping these drugs preoperatively in all patients. However, a practitioner should consider holding these drugs for patients that cannot tolerate acute hypotensive episodes.[40]

ARB induce more profound and more frequent episodes of intraoperative hypotension than do ACEI. When diuretics are combined with ARB drugs, the hypotension is more exaggerated. Brabant[41] reported that perioperative hypotension occurred in 100% of patients who maintained their ARB the morning of surgery. Bertrand and colleagues[42] found that intraoperative hypotension was greater and required more vasopressor treatment when the ARB was taken the morning of surgery.

WHAT SHOULD WE DO?

If ACEI and ARB drugs are not stopped, the risk of hypotension is significant; but it still can occur if the drugs are stopped 24 hours before surgery. Although omitting 1 dose does not seem to cause adverse effects, most of the hypotensive episodes will respond to IV fluids and the usual vasopressors found in the office. For office anesthesia, the risk is minimal if ACEI and ARB drugs are maintained. However, consideration should be given to holding the morning dose of the diuretic because it exacerbates the level of hypotension with ACEI and ARB. We can further decrease the risk of hypotension by infusing at least 500 ml of lactated ringers (LR) or normal saline (NSS) for our office anesthetics. The first treatment of hypotension is a fluid challenge, so butterfly IV anesthesia without IV fluids needs to be abandoned.[23]

GENERAL MANAGEMENT OF PERIOPERATIVE HTN

HTN with Bradycardia

Where do we start the treatment, the bradycardia or the HTN? If you initiate treatment aimed at the bradycardia, you can make the situation worse. There is already an increased afterload consuming myocardial oxygen, so if you speed up the rate, you increase myocardial oxygen demands and decrease coronary oxygen supply. In this case, the use of the anticholinergic drug atropine should be avoided.

How do we treat the HTN? BB are not a good choice because they work by decreasing the heart rate, and patients are already bradycardic. There are many other drugs that can be used, but the question is what do we have in the office? The most likely agents would be hydralazine or NTG tablets.

HTN with Tachycardia

Patients who have CVD do not tolerate prolonged tachycardia or HTN. These two factors significantly increase the heart's need for coronary blood flow to prevent ischemia. In this case, you need to assess the level of anesthesia. Are patients too light? Do patients need an increase dose of opioids for pain, or do they need additional local anesthesia?

The antihypertensive management in this case would be a BB. The BB will decrease the heart rate and lower the BP. Esmolol or labetalol would be excellent agents to use in this case.

PCP AND EMERGENCY DEPARTMENT REFERRALS

In the office, patients with stage 1 HTN (SBP 140–159 mm Hg, DBP 90–99 mm Hg) with no symptoms pose little risk for treatment in the office. They need to be referred to their PCP for a nonurgent appointment. What is your protocol for patients with HTN who arrive in the office for treatment but their BP is more than180/120? By JNC guidelines, this is a hypertensive crisis, and treatment depends on differentiating an emergency versus an urgency. Our primary obligation to these patients is to inform them of the pressure

reading and explain why this should not be ignored. A referral is made that day to their PCP or to the emergency department. They will make the diagnosis of emergency or urgency and proceed from there.

A brief history and physical examination is necessary in these cases. Are antihypertensive medications being prescribed for patients and, in fact, are they taking them as directed? Do they have a past history of MI, HF, stroke? Do they use any recreational drugs?

At present are they experiencing chest pain, dyspnea, severe headache, confusion, visual disturbances, or nausea and vomiting. Call the PCP with the findings; if they are unavailable, tell patients you think it is in their best interest to go to the emergency department. Expect patients to be resistant, but tell them there is a possibility of complications, including *heart attack* if this is not addressed. It is up to patients to take responsibility, but no oral surgery care will be done until this is addressed.

The emergency department or the PCP is necessary to rule out target organ disease. Fundoscopic examination will rule out hemorrhage, exudates, and papilledema. A 12-lead ECG and troponin levels are indicated for cardiac at-risk patients, and a neurologic evaluation should also be done.

If there is no evidence of end organ damage, this is a hypertensive urgency. In newly diagnosed patients, the emergency department may refer to the PCP for an urgent (1–5 days) follow-up. Some patients may be given an antihypertensive medication in the emergency department and kept for a few hours for observation.

In rare cases, patients may be admitted, especially if they have no PCP of record and will not be able to find a physician in the next few days. BP therapy is started; patients are admitted; social work arranges for follow-up.

In cases of a hypertensive emergency, patients are admitted for antihypertensive therapy. The MAP will be reduced 20% to 25% over the first hour, and then target BP is achieved over the next 6 hours.[43]

Anecdotally, some of us have had the experience of sending a patient to the emergency department for severe BP and received a call questioning our reasoning for this nonurgent referral. It is not our responsibility to make the diagnosis of a hypertensive urgency versus and emergency; we need a **physician to rule out the possibility of a hypertensive emergency**.

COSTS OF ANTIHYPERTENSIVE AGENTS

The past few years have seen critical shortages of medications along with costs that have increased dramatically. Availability of drugs used on a daily basis is unpredictable and frustrating. The following chart lists agents discussed in this article along with estimated pricing, which varies frequently (**Table 10**). Also, tables of stage I and II hypertension drug therapy are presented (**Tables 11** and **12**).

PERIOPERATIVE HYPOTENSION

Syncope is the most common medical emergency in the dental office. Hypotension develops as a result of peripheral venous pooling of blood. This condition causes a decrease in the preload, so BP decreases and cerebral blood flow is decreased to the point of a loss of consciousness. During the third trimester of pregnancy, patients in the supine position will experience the supine hypotensive syndrome from compression of the inferior vena cava. The treatment is to turn patients onto their left side to reestablish vena cava blood flow. Patients can also experience hypotensive episodes if they stand up too quickly from the dental chair. This postural hypotension frequently occurs in the senior population, but medications with this side effect can make patients in any age group more susceptible.

Patients are NPO before anesthesia, so they do have an intravascular volume deficit; but this minor decrease in volume by itself is unlikely to cause hypotension. Patients arriving in the office for anesthesia usually do not have preoperative hypotension and tachycardia. Their anxiety is more likely to present as minor elevations in BP as compared with their consultation BP along with tachycardia. However, the combination of volume status from being NPO and anesthetic induction medications can cause a hypotensive episode. Propofol and/or volatile anesthetic gases are known to decrease BP.

During the maintenance phase of anesthesia, medications can continue to affect BP. Propofol, when used as a solo general anesthetic agent, will decrease BP. The amounts of propofol needed to maintain that general anesthetic state can decrease MAP to a point of hypoperfusion that will require small doses of vasopressors.

Allergic reactions during anesthesia are another source of hypotension, so the anesthesia team needs to monitor patients for signs of rash, hives, or angioedema during the case. Other causes of hypotension include hypoxia and hypercarbia; but with the use of the precordial stethoscope, pulse oximetry, and capnography, early detection and intervention can eliminate these as causes of hypotension.

Rare but possible causes of hypotension are pneumothorax and pulmonary embolism. Medication errors are another possibility.[44]

Initial Management of Hypotension

The first step would be to place patients in a supine position and possibly elevate the legs. The next step is to evaluate patients for the cause of the event.

Oxygenation and ventilation need to be assessed. Surgeons will need to auscultate all of the lung fields and then check the equipment. Is the oxygen delivery system working and is it connected to the patients? Are the monitor alarms disabled? Is the pulse oximeter probe connected? Is the capnograph connected?

Table 10
Estimated costs of antihypertensive agents

Drug	Size	Average Cost ($)	Availability Usual Supply Houses
Labetalol	5 mg/mL 20 mL	5.00–6.00	Yes
Esmolol	10 mg/mL 10 mL	22.00–26.00	Yes
Metoprolol	5 mg/5 mL	7.00–20.00	Yes
Hydralazine	20 mg/mL	18.00–20.00	Yes
NTG	5 mg/mL 10 mL	8.00–9.00	Yes
Diltiazem	5 mg/mL 5 mL	3.50–4.00	Yes
Verapamil	2.5 mg/mL 2 mL	5.00–10.00	Yes
Enalaprilat	1.25 mg/mL 2 mL	9.00–10.00	Yes
Phentolamine	5 mg/2 mL	95.00–112.00	Yes
Clevidipine	0.5 mg/mL	>>100.00	No
Nicardipine	25 mg/mL	>>100.00	No

Costs accessed on the Internet on 11/29/2012 from multiple sites and then averaged. Prices and availability vary weekly.

Table 11		
Stage I HTN drug therapy		
BP	**Primary Drug**	**Alternative Drugs**
SBP 140–159	Thiazide	ACEI
DBP 90–99	diuretic	
		BB
		ARB
		CCB

Data from National Heart, Lung, and Blood Institute; National Institutes of Health. Seventh Report of the Joint National Committee on Prevention, Detection, Evaluation, and Treatment of High Blood Pressure (JNC 7). NIH Publication No. 04-5230. Available at: www.nhlbi.nih.gov/guidelines/hypertension. Accessed November 10, 2012.

Medications: What was the **last syringe used? Was it the right drug? What was the dose?** Is the infusion pump working, and is it set at the proper infusion rate?

TREATMENT OF PERIOPERATIVE HYPOTENSION

Before vasopressors are given, the depth of anesthesia should be reduced and a bolus of IV fluid should be tried. The dose can be up to 10 mL/kg, and a typical starting dose in adults is 250 mL of LR or NSS. These doses can be repeated as needed.

If an allergic reaction is suspected, then epinephrine should be the agent of choice. An intramuscular adult dose is 0.3 mg of 1:1000. In the event of a severe reaction, an IV dose of 10 to 20 μg of 1:10 000 can be used but expect to see cardiac side effects. If this is the start of an anaphylactic reaction, the side effects from the IV epinephrine are far less a problem than the cardiac arrest that will follow if we do not use the epinephrine. If an allergic reaction is not suspected, epinephrine

Table 12	
Stage II HTN drug therapy	
SBP ≥160	**Thiazide Diuretic Plus**
DBP ≥100	**One of the Following**
	ACEI
	BB
	ARB
	CCB

Data from National Heart, Lung, and Blood Institute; National Institutes of Health. Seventh Report of the Joint National Committee on Prevention, Detection, Evaluation, and Treatment of High Blood Pressure (JNC 7). NIH Publication No. 04-5230. Available at: www.nhlbi.nih.gov/guidelines/hypertension. Accessed November 10, 2012.

will not be the drug of choice for the perioperative hypotension.

Patients that present with hypotension and bradycardia (heart rate <60 beats per minute) are sometimes treated with an anticholinergic agent like atropine. The dosage is 0.5 mg IV every 3 to 5 minutes up to a maximum dose of 3.0 mg. It may be difficult to get vials of 0.5 mg or 1.0 mg unless you order a prefilled syringe. Most of the time, atropine comes in 0.4 mg/mL, so this dose can be used. The reasoning behind this technique is that if you increase the heart rate, cardiac output will increase and BP increases will follow. A better alternative would be to use ephedrine or phenylephrine.

Ephedrine is an alpha and beta agonist that increases heart rate, SBP, and DBP. It affects venous constriction more than arterial constriction, and this results in an increase in preload and CO to increase BP. There is a minor increase in afterload but far less than the preload, so it is easier for the heart to eject blood; so there is less myocardial oxygen consumption than with epinephrine. Side effects that may be beneficial are bronchodilation and a minor antiemetic effect.

The dosage in adults is **5 mg IV bolus every 5 to 10 minutes as needed**. The onset of action is within 10 minutes, with a peak effect in 20 minutes. The duration of action is 4 hours. The drug comes in a **50-mg/1 mL vial, so it is diluted in 9 mL of fluid making the dose 5 mg/mL.** In patients with CVD, ephedrine should be limited to cases of hypotension without tachycardia.

Phenylephrine is an alpha agonist that causes vasoconstriction. It too has more of an effect on venous vessels than arterial, so the preload is increased, which increases CO and BP. This drug causes a reflex bradycardia, so it is an excellent choice in patients with hypotension plus tachycardia.

Phenylephrine 1% usually comes in a 10-mg/1 mL vial. This drug requires a double dilution technique to get to the 100-μg/mL dose. The phenylephrine is diluted into 9 mL of fluid, and then 1 mL from that syringe is diluted into another 9 mL of fluid. This now gives you a concentration of 100 μg/mL.

The dose is 100 μg in adults. The onset of action is within 2 to 3 minutes, with a duration of 15 minutes. Repeat dosing in every 5-minute intervals.

How Do You Manage a Case of Refractory Perioperative Hypotension?

Most patients respond to vasopressors like ephedrine or phenylephrine along with IV fluids. If that is ineffective, epinephrine mini-boluses of 10 μg IV can be started, and the dose can be increased up to 20 mics as needed. An infusion of 2 to 10 mics/min can be titrated to an effect. Diluting 1 mg of epinephrine in 500 mL of D5 W yields a 2 µg/mL concentration. The use of epinephrine for hypotension is a treatment of last resort because of potential side effects. If patients require this type of support, EMS should be called for immediate transfer to a hospital.

Patients taking ACEIs or ARBs are well known to have more episodes of perioperative hypotension, and they are also less likely to respond to the vasopressors discussed earlier, including epinephrine. Vasopressin, a peptide hormone secreted by the hypothalamus, can stimulate **V_1** receptors found in vascular smooth muscle; this results in vasoconstriction.

Vasopressin can be given as an **IV bolus starting at 0.4 U every 10 minutes; if that is ineffective, it can be increased to 2 U every 10 minutes, or an infusion of 0.04 U can be started and increased as needed.** Vasopressin has a half-life of only 6 minutes and has a side effect of decreasing renal perfusion, so urine output must be monitored. The cost of vasopressin is approximately $5.00 for a dose of 20 U/1 mL.[45]

CONTROLLED HYPOTENSIVE ANESTHESIA

Controlled hypotensive anesthesia has been used for more than 50 years. The benefits are a reduction in blood loss with less need for blood transfusions, a clear view of the operating field, and a reduction in surgical time. Multiple agents have been used in this technique: volatile anesthetic gases, sodium nitroprusside, IV NTG, and nicardipine.[46]

It is defined as a reduction in SBP to 80 to 90 mm Hg or a reduction in MAP to 50 to 65 mm Hg. In normotensive healthy patients, reductions in MAP to 55 to 65 mm Hg did not result in target organ damage from hypoperfusion. A growing concern in all of anesthesia is postoperative cognitive dysfunction. Choi and colleagues[47] studied the effects of NTG and nicardipine hypotensive anesthesia on cerebral oxygen saturation, and they found that at MAP of 60 to 65 mm Hg, the saturation was unaffected and cerebral cognitive function was not impaired.

The vasodilating agents used in these techniques can cause a reflex tachycardia. It will not occur in all cases, but the incidence has been reported to be about 70%. The concern is the increased myocardial oxygen consumption from the tachycardia. BB have been used both preoperatively and intraoperatively to reduce tachycardia. Preoperative propranolol, 10 mg orally, and

esmolol 0.5 mg/kg IV for intraoperative heart rates of more than 95 beats per minute have been found to be safe and effective.[48,49]

Controlled hypotension requires indwelling arterial line catheters to monitor BP along with urine output measurements to decrease the risk of hypoperfusion. In the future, the use of cerebral oximetry may become a standard of care to decrease the risk of postoperative cognitive dysfunction.

CONTROVERSIES IN PERIOPERATIVE HTN AND HYPOTENSION

In an operating room, most of our surgery is done in the supine position on an operating room table. However, in the office, our patients are in a dental chair and the surgeon is usually standing. This means that patients are in a head-up position of 30° or more. **Does this place patients at an increased risk of cerebral hypoperfusion?**

Cerebral autoregulation is the body's ability to maintain cerebral blood flow over a range of BP. For normotensive patients, this range is reported to be a MAP of 50 to 150 mm Hg. With chronic HTN, there is a shift to the right, so an MAP of 50 mm Hg will now result in hypoperfusion of the brain, placing patients at risk for injury, ischemic infarcts, or postoperative cognitive dysfunction. Immink and colleagues[50] reported the range of cerebral autoregulation to be 60 to 150 mm Hg, and a range of 115 to 170 mm Hg in patients with HTN. The upper limits cannot be tested in humans, so these values come from studies in baboons.

In normotensive patients despite cerebral autoregulation, the baseline cerebral blood flow in the supine position can decrease by 14% to 21% when patients stand up. Any elevations in head position **more than 20° from the horizontal position** will cause a decrease in cerebral blood flow. In awake patients, these effects are compensated by increases in the SVR to maintain flow; but during anesthesia, the vasodilating anesthetic agents block this sympathetic response.[51]

Cerebral perfusion pressures even in awake patients **will decrease by 15% when they sit down**, so it is safe to assume that during anesthesia, those pressures will decrease to a greater degree from the anesthetic agents.[52]

Since 2007, the Anesthesia Patient Safety Foundation has been investigating the effects of patient positioning and controlled hypotensive anesthesia on cerebral blood flow. Some of their preliminary findings are quite revealing.

During surgery in a supine position, the BP measured at the arm is equal to the BP in the brain. However, in a head-up position, the cerebral BP is less than the arm reading. This difference is 1 mm

Hg for each vertical measurement of 1.25 cm as measured from the arm to the external auditory meatus of the ear (level of the base of the brain).[52]

Drummond,[53] in a review of the literature, now recommends a lower limit of 70 mm Hg for autoregulation in the supine position for normotensive patients. One of his reasons is that 45% of patients have an incomplete Circle of Willis, which decreases autoregulation function. The workshop findings also recommended that surgery done in a beach chair position (head elevated 30°–90° from horizontal) should have BP adjusted for hydrostatic gradients from the arm to the ear and that controlled hypotensive anesthesia should be avoided in this position. Reductions in baseline pressures **should not exceed 30% in the sitting position**.[53]

Sanders and colleagues,[54] in an editorial, recommended that in patients with HTN and those with vascular disease hypoperfusion and hyperperfusion must be avoided. Their goal is to avoid HTN (SBP >160 mm Hg) and to keep hypotension to no greater than a 20% decrease in baseline pressure.

To no one's surprise, there are also studies that say this risk of stroke and cognitive dysfunction is being overstated because the incidence of perioperative stroke in noncardiac and non-neurosurgery is low (0.1%), and most of the reported strokes are thromboembolic in nature. Data also show that during sleep, BP decreases about 30% from baseline, so intraoperative pressure decreases of 30% are acceptable, but you must keep in mind that this is in the supine position. The American College of Surgeons National Surgical Quality Improvement Program's report in 2011 failed to establish perioperative hypotension as a risk factor for stroke in noncardiac and non-neurologic surgery.[55,56] The debate will continue, and we need to remain in the loop for further information.

SUMMARY

Perioperative HTN does increase the risk of ischemia, infarction, HF, and stroke. For office-based anesthesia/surgery, it would be best to defer patients with an *SBP* of *180* mm Hg or more and a *DBP* of *110* mm Hg or more until their BP can be optimized. The antihypertensive agents that are typically found in offices will allow us to treat most of the hypertensive episodes that we will encounter, but we also have to realize that there are other agents that may be better in some instances but are, as yet, impractical for office use. The agents that we should consider stocking are esmolol, labetalol, NTG (spray or tablets), and maybe hydralazine.

Patients on maintenance antihypertensive agents should have those agents maintained during surgery, and this includes BB, CBC, and, in most cases, the angiotensin blockers ACEI and ARB. However, if patients are on a diuretic in addition to the angiotensin agents, that diuretic may be held preoperatively to reduce the incidence of hypotension.

Hypotension is usually managed by decreasing the depth of anesthesia, administering IV LR or NSS, and then adding vasopressors. Most offices have phenylephrine and ephedrine for these episodes, along with the ability to administer mini-bolus epinephrine. There may be an indication for vasopressin, and that decision should be up to the individual practitioner.

A conservative approach for perioperative hypotension prevention and management would be to replace NPO fluid deficits with IV fluids preoperatively and intraoperatively. Vasopressors should be used when MAP decreases to less than 60 mm Hg in normotensive, healthy adolescents or adults. Most patients will tolerate baseline BP decreases of 30% without the risk of target organ damage, especially cerebral ischemia or postoperative cognitive deficits. However, there is an increasing concern, especially in the elderly, about postoperative cognitive deficits from the agents that are being used and the level of hypotension intraoperatively. We need to keep abreast of current literature regarding these issues.

REFERENCES

1. Marik PE, Varon J. Perioperative hypertension: a review of current and emerging therapeutic agents. J Clin Anesth 2009;21:220–9.
2. Varon J, Marik PE. Perioperative hypertension management. Vasc Health Risk Manag 2008;4(3):615–27.
3. Holm SW, Cunningham LL, Bensadoun E, et al. Hypertension: classification, pathophysiology, and management during outpatient sedation and local anesthesia. J Oral Maxillofac Surg 2006;64:111–21.
4. Chobanian AV, Barkis G, Black HR, et al. JNC-7 report: detection, evaluation, and treatment of high blood pressure. JAMA 2003;289(19):2560–72.
5. Chobanian AV, Barkis G, Black HR, et al. JNC-7 report. Available at: http://www.nhlbi.nih.gov/guidelines/hypertension. Accessed November 10, 2012.
6. Kaplan N. Overview of hypertension in adults. In: UptoDate; 2012. Available at: http://www.uptodate.com. Accessed November 10, 2012.
7. Kotchen T. Hypertensive vascular disease. In: Fauci A, Kasper D, Longo D, et al, editors. Harrisons principles of internal medicine. 17th edition. New York: McGraw Hill Medical; 2008. p. 1549–62.

8. Gaudio AR, Chelazzi C, Villa G, et al. Acute severe hypertension: therapeutic options. Curr Drug Targets 2009;10:788–9.

9. Weksler N, Klein M, Szendro G. The dilemma of immediate preoperative hypertension. J Clin Anesth 2003;15:179–83.

10. Fontes M, Varon J. Perioperative hypertensive crisis. Int Anesthesiol Clin 2012;2:40–58.

11. Marik P, Rivera R. Hypertensive emergencies: an update. Curr Opin Crit Care 2011;17:569–80.

12. Mansoor GA, Frishman WH. Comprehensive management of hypertensive emergencies and urgencies. Heart Dis 2002;4:358–71.

13. Desai RG, Muntazar M, Goldberg ME. Strategies for managing perioperative hypertension. Curr Hypertens Rep 2009;11:173–7.

14. Aggarwal M, Khan I. Hypertensive crisis: emergencies and urgencies. Cardiol Clin 2006;24:135–46.

15. Ahujka K, Charap M. Management of perioperative hypertensive urgencies with parenteral medications. J Hosp Med 2012;5:e11–6.

16. Goldman L. Mutifactorial index of cardiac risk in noncardiac surgery: ten year status report. J Cardiothoracic Anesth 1987;1:237–44.

17. Beyer K, Taffe P, Halfon P, et al. Hypertension and intraoperative incidents. Anaesthesia 2009;64:494–502.

18. Haas C, LeBlanc J. Acute postoperative hypertension: a review of therapeutic options. Am J Health Syst Pharm 2004;61:1661–75.

19. Feneck R. Drugs for perioperative control of hypertension. Drugs 2007;7(14):2023–44.

20. Deveraux PJ. Effects of extended release metoprolol in patients for non-cardiac surgery. Lancet 2008;37:1839–47.

21. Harte B. Perioperative beta blockers in non cardiac surgery. Cleve Clin J Med 2008;75(7):513–9.

22. Wallace A. Perioperative beta blockade and postoperative mortality. Anesthesiology 2012;113(4):794–805.

23. Smith I, Jackson I. Beta blockers, calcium channel blockers, angiotensin receptor blockers. Curr Opin Anaesthesiol 2010;23:687–90.

24. Cazzola M, Noschese P, D'Amato G. Pharmacologic treatment of uncomplicated arterial hypertension in patients with airway dysfunction. Chest 2002;121:230–41.

25. Albouaini K, Andron M, Alahmar A, et al. Beta blockers in patients with COPD. Int J Chron Obstruct Pulmon Dis 2007;2(4):535–40.

26. Sheppard D. Effects of esmolol on airway in patients with asthma. J Clin Pharmacol 1986;26:169–74.

27. Kovac AL. Comparison of nicardipine versus esmolol in hemodynamic response to emergence and intubation. J Cardiothorac Vasc Anesth 2007;21:45–50.

28. Hays A, Wilkerson T. Management of hypertensive emergencies. AACN Adv Crit Care 2010;21(1):5–14.

29. Moon Y, Lee S, Lee J. Optimal dose of esmolol and nicardipine for cardiovascular stability during rapid sequence induction. J Clin Anesth 2012;24:8–13.

30. Cheung A, Guvak D, Weiss S, et al. Nicardipine intravenous bolus dose for acutely increasing blood pressure during general anesthesia. Anesth Analg 1999;89:1116–23.

31. Reams GD. Efficacy, ECG, and renal effects of intravenous diltiazem. Am J Cardiol 1987;60(17):781–841.

32. Chun G. Rapid acting parenteral antihypertensive agents. J Clin Pharmacol 1990;30(3):195–209.

33. Ndefo UA, Erowele GI, Ebiasah R, et al. Clevidipine: a new intravenous option for the management of acute hypertension. Am J Health Syst Pharm 2010;67:351–60.

34. Kenyon K. Clevidipine: an ultra short calcium channel antagonist for acute hypertension. Ann Pharmacother 2009;43:1258–65.

35. Rhoney D, Peacock F. Intravenous therapy for hypertensive emergencies, part I. Am J Health Syst Pharm 2009;66:1343–52.

36. Shepherd AM. Differential hemodynamic and sympathoadrenal effects of nitroprusside and hydralazine. J Cardiovasc Pharmacol 1986;8:527–33.

37. Dorman T. Effects of clonidine: a prolonged postoperative sympathetic response. Crit Care Med 1997;25:1147–52.

38. Wallace A. Effect of clonidine on cardiovascular morbidity and mortality for non cardiac surgery. Anesthesiology 2004;101:284–93.

39. Ram C, Silverstein T. Treatment of hypertensive urgencies and emergencies. Curr Hypertens Rep 2009;11:307–14.

40. Comfere T, Sprung J, Kumar M, et al. Angiotensin system inhibitors in general surgery population. Anesth Analg 2005;100:636–44.

41. Brabant SM. Hemodynamic effects of anesthesia induction in angiotensin II receptor antagonists. Anesth Analg 1999;88:1388–92.

42. Bertrand M, Godet G, Meersscharet K, et al. Should angiotensin II antagonists be discontinued before surgery. Anesth Analg 2001;92:26–30.

43. Baumann B, Cline D, Pimenta E. Treatment of hypertension in the emergency room. J Am Soc Hypertens 2011;5(5):366–77.

44. Morris RW, Watterson LM, Westhorpe RN, et al. Crisis management during anesthesia: hypotension. Qual Saf Health Care 2005;14:e11–8.

45. Wheeler A, Turchiano J, Tobias J. A case of refractory intraoperative hypotension treated with vasopressin infusion. J Clin Anesth 2008;20:139–42.

46. Petrozza P. Induced hypotension. Int Anesthesiol Clin 1990;28(4):223–9.

47. Choi S, Lee S, Jung Y, et al. Nitroglycerin and nicardipine induced hypotension does not affect cerebral oxygen saturation and cognitive function. J Oral Maxillofac Surg 2008;66:2104–9.

48. Apipan B, Rummusak D. Efficacy and safety of oral propranolol premedication to reduce reflex tachycardia. J Oral Maxillofac Surgery 2010;68:120–4.

49. Hanamoto H, Sugimura M, Boku A, et al. Small bolus esmolol prevents reflex tachycardia. J Oral Maxillofac Surg 2012;70:1045–51.

50. Immink RV, van den Born BJ, van Montfrans GA, et al. Impaired cerebral autoregulation in patients with malignant hypertension. Circulation 2004; 110:2241–5.

51. Moraine JJ, Berre J, Melot C. Is cerebral perfusion pressure a major determinant of cerebral blood flow during head elevation. J Neurosurg 2000;92: 606–14.

52. Cullen DJ, Kirby RR. Beach chair position may decrease cerebral perfusion: catastrophic outcomes have occurred. APSF Newsletter 2007; 22(2):25–7.

53. Lee L, Caplan R. APSF workshop cerebral perfusion experts head up cases. APSF Newsletter 2009–2010;24(4):45–8.

54. Sanders RD, Degas V, Young WL. Cerebral perfusion under pressure: is the autoregulation plateau a level playing field for all. Anaesthesia 2011;64: 968–71.

55. Lam AM, Baldwin G. Blood pressure and adverse perioperative neurologic outcomes: an uncomfortable position. Anesth Analg 2012;114:1156–9.

56. Mashour GA, Shanks AM, Kheterpal S. Perioperative stroke and associated mortality after noncardiac, nonneurologic surgery. Anesthesiology 2011; 114:1289–96.

Anesthetic Emergencies in Oral Surgery
Malignant Hyperthermia, Endocrinopathy, and Neurologic Events

Andrew Herlich, DMD, MD

KEYWORDS

- Anesthesia emergencies • Treatment • Malignant hyperthermia • Endocrinopathies
- Neurologic events

KEY POINTS

- Serious anesthesia emergencies are infrequent but do occur in the office-based practice.
- Preparedness for the emergencies is important, including practicing emergency drills.
- The overarching theme for caring for these emergencies is the urgent transfer of most of the patients to the emergency room of an acute care facility for definitive treatment and successful outcomes.

Significant anesthetic emergencies in oral and maxillofacial surgery office are rare events. The safety record of anesthesia in the office environment is excellent with reasonable data.[1,2] However, emergencies still occur and preparedness is the key to ameliorating the impact of these events. This article addresses several of these emergencies that have a great impact despite their infrequent occurrence. The oral and maxillofacial surgeon should always consider the emergency transfer of patients who have had a significant emergent event to the nearest emergency room of an acute care facility for definitive care.

MALIGNANT HYPERTHERMIA

Malignant hyperthermia (MH) occurs in the office environment and some fatalities have occurred despite proper care and preparation. The Malignant Hyperthermia Association of the United States (MHAUS)[3] has several resources to support clinicians whose patients may have malignant hyperthermia. MHAUS has a 24-hours-per-day, 7-days-per-week phone support answered by volunteer anesthesiologists with extensive knowledge of MH. The phone service is called the MH Hotline and the phone number is 1-800-644-9737 (1-800-MH-Hyper). The service is free of charge, and the help is invaluable. The volunteer anesthesiologists give whatever advice is needed during an ongoing crisis or are available prospectively for advice for cases with potential problems. Valuable information for patients and clinicians alike are available on the MHAUS Web site at www.MHAUS.org.

MH is autosomal dominant inheritable disease with variable penetrance. Its frequency in the United States is approximately 1000 cases per year. Survival has increased dramatically since early use of intravenous dantrolene therapy more than 33 years ago.[4] Before the use of dantrolene therapy, the mortality of MH was approximately 90%.

Disclosures: None.
Department of Anesthesiology, University of Pittsburgh School of Medicine, 1400 Locust Street, Suite 2192, Pittsburgh, PA 15219, USA
E-mail addresses: herlicha@upmc.edu; anherlich@comcast.net

Oral Maxillofacial Surg Clin N Am 25 (2013) 507–514
http://dx.doi.org/10.1016/j.coms.2013.03.005

Once MH is suspected, any triggering agents must be ceased. If an anesthesia machine with volatile anesthetics has been used, converting to bag-valve endotracheal tube ventilation is appropriate. A newer approach to the management of the volatile agents incorporates the use of charcoal filters on both the expiratory and inspiratory limbs of the anesthesia circuit. These filters absorb the volatile agents from the anesthesia machine to levels of less than 5 parts per million (ppm) in less than 2 minutes and effectively maintain those levels for more than 1 hour. Depending on the severity of the event, the carbon filters may need to be changed. It is not always possible to have a clean anesthesia machine in the office-based environment; the charcoal filters are effective and a reasonable substitue in an MH crisis. They are also easily replaced.[5]

Signs of MH include unexplained tachycardia, rapid increase in end-tidal carbon dioxide levels, tachypnea, hyperthermia, masseter muscle spasm, and generalized muscle rigidity. In the office-based environment, an early call (911) for transfer of the patient to an acute care facility capable of treating MH is mandatory.[6] A call to the Malignant Hyperthermia Hotline should also be included in the early processes if there are personnel to so assist. Steps to reduce the severity of the reaction include the rapid administration of dantrolene 2.5 mg/kg as the anchor of treatment. This initial treatment should be followed by additional doses of 1 mg/kg as clinical signs and symptoms continue. In addition, administration of intravenous normal saline, active cooling of body surface areas, and control of dysrhythmias with appropriate therapies is crucial. The most common cause of rhythm disturbances during an MH crisis is related to hyperkalemia. Treatment of hyperkalemia requires glucose and insulin administered intravenously, vigorous diuresis with fluids and furosemide, as well as intravenous calcium chloride (via central intravenous access) or calcium gluconate in peripheral intravenous access. The glucose and insulin combination and calcium force the excess potassium intracellularly, whereas furosemide provides kaliuresis, which is the renal excretion of potassium. Attention to this detail is imperative: hyperkalemia and coagulopathy are likely the two greatest causes of death from MH. Coagulopathy is a late occurrence; it is usually the result of severe hyperthermia in excess of 41°C.[7]

In principle, MH does not preclude surgery and anesthesia on an ambulatory basis in the hospital or ambulatory surgical center. With common sense, it should not preclude surgery in the office-based environment. Although other publications issue a precautionary note regarding MH-susceptible patients being too risky for the office-based environment, routine dental procedures occur daily in MH-susceptible patients without triggering an MH crisis. In the absence of nontriggering anesthetics, prepared practitioners should not fear that MH-susceptible patients are at any greater risk than non–MH-susceptible patients, with the exception of patients with exertional heat–related illness and central core myopathy.[8,9]

In addition, there is controversy within the oral and maxillofacial surgical community about how much dantrolene should be available in the office environment. The American Association of Oral and Maxillofacial Surgeons Office Evaluation Manual, eighth edition, 2012, suggests that dantrolene be readily available at any time if triggering agents are present in the office. The greatest controversy is centered on the issue of having only succinylcholine available as a potential triggering agent without volatile anesthetic agents. A recent publication recommended that dantrolene still be available in the office because there have been instances of succinylcholine alone triggering MH. They also suggested that more epidemiologic data be available in the future to either refute or support the need for dantrolene under these circumstances.[10] There have been adverse reactions to the administration of intravenous dantrolene. The common complications include muscle weakness, gastrointestinal upset, and phlebitis. Serious complications associated with the administration of dantrolene were most likely caused by medical comorbidities rather than the drug itself.[11] However, the complications of the administration are outweighed by the risks of not administering the drug. Many lives have been saved because of the appropriate administration of dantrolene.

A suggested list of rescue medications and equipment is provided in the MH medication and equipment list (**Box 1**).

ENDOCRINOPATHIES

There are several endocrinopathies that could require emergent treatment in the oral and maxillofacial surgeon's office. Although there have been other books and reviews discussing endocrinopathies in the dental office, most of these are rarely if ever seen by the oral and maxillofacial surgeon. On a survey of large anesthesia and surgery departments at an academic medical center, the number of attending physicians who had seen or treated many of these acute endocrinopathies was very small. In a sampling of more than 300 faculty physicians with greater than 15 years of

Box 1
MH medication and equipment list
(www.MHAUS.org)

Drugs

36 vials of dantrolene (powder); 20 mg/vial reconstituted with 36 vials of sterile water, 60 mL each

Sodium bicarbonate 8.4% (50 mEq) × 5 ampules dextrose 50 g × 2 insulin 100 units regular (drug refrigerator)

Furosemide/Lasix 40-mg vials × 4

Calcium gluconate 1000 mg × 4

Calcium chloride 1000 mg × 2

Lidocaine 100 mg/5 mL × 10 or 100 mg/10 mL × 10 or amiodarone 300 mg ampules × 3

Equipment

Large intravenous catheters (sizes 18, 16, 14)

60-mL syringes × 5 for reconstitution/delivery of dantrolene

Minimum of 3 L of cold normal saline for patient cooling (500-mL or 1000-mL bags are appropriate)

A supply of ice with large and small plastic bags for patient cooling (substitute ice packs for wounds)

Helpful stationary supplies for event: MHAUS event logs, MHAUS wall poster for treatment, MHAUS/The Society for Ambulatory Anesthesia transfer guidelines

postresidency practice, none had ever seen thyroid storm, myxedema coma, adrenal collapse, or acute parathyroid dysfunction (Herlich A, unpublished data, 2012).

GLYCEMIA CONTROL

Treating diabetics on an ambulatory basis has become the norm rather than the exception. The goal should be to maintain the euglycemic state and rapidly return the patient to an environment in which they can manage their food intake and glucose control.[12] To prevent postoperative nausea and vomiting (PONV), it is a common practice to administer dexamethasone intravenously as part of multimodal therapy. Two articles in the anesthesia literature have implied that this practice should be examined in patients with glucose control problems. In nondiabetic patients undergoing craniotomy, a single dose of perioperative dexamethasone significantly increased the blood glucose levels and peak 9 hours after surgery.[13] Another study examined the use of dexamethasone for postoperative PONV in morbidly obese patients undergoing gastroplasty. These investigators also found significant postoperative blood glucose levels in patients who received dexamethasone compared with the control group in patients with impaired glucose tolerance.[14] A recent article in the clinical nutrition literature investigated outcomes of both hypoglycemia and hyperglycemia in the diabetic patient who is critically ill. The article emphasized that hyperglycemia in the critically ill diabetic patient had a stronger association with mortality than in the nondiabetic patient. Hypoglycemia was associated with increased mortality in both the nondiabetic and diabetic patient. In addition, glycemic variability had a stronger association with mortality in nondiabetic critically ill patients than in critically ill diabetic patients.[15] One review suggested that diabetic ketoacidosis (DKA) and hyperglycemic hyperosmolar nonketotic (HHNK) state are increasing in frequency as well as increasing mortalities with the extremes of age.[16] Acute status changes in the diabetic patient should therefore prompt transfer to an acute care environment as quickly as possible for accurate and expeditious treatment.

The diabetic patient may present to the office with clinically significant hypoglycemia. Symptoms include confusion, dizziness, diaphoresis, tachycardia, hunger, tremulousness, and possibly seizure activity. Simple treatment can vary from supplementing the patient with any oral glucose-containing solutions to providing dextrose in the patient's intravenous fluids. Intravenous dextrose is available in ampules of 50 mL at 25% and should be administered in increments of 1 to 2 mL/kg until symptoms are corrected or reasonable blood glucose is achieved by a point-of-care testing device for blood glucose. Any patient who has an abnormal level of consciousness should not be encouraged to correct their hypoglycemia via the oral route because aspiration may be a risk. If intravenous access is not possible or has infiltrated, intramuscular glucagon is an appropriated alternative.

The severe hyperglycemic state may present as DKA or as a nonketotic hyperglycemic patient. In both circumstances, the patient requires rapid transfer to a hospital setting wherein appropriate fluid and medication correction are indicated. Nevertheless, immediate emergent treatment requires appropriate recognition. Patients are usually tachypneic, tachycardic, have abdominal pain, temperature alteration, and ketones on their breath if they present with DKA. The office-based management requires immediate administration of intravenous normal saline and regular insulin

100 units per vial to run at 0.1 units/kg/h. Frequent blood glucose assays are mandatory because these patients' blood glucose levels may decrease precipitously. By the time the patient reaches the acute care/hospital setting, serum potassium, phosphate, significant acidosis, and correction of electrolytes, including sodium, are required. The use of sodium bicarbonate is strongly discouraged unless the patient's arterial blood gas pH is less than 7.0.

The initial management approaches are the same for both DKA and HHNK state.[17] The average patient who presents with DKA has 5 to 10 L (100 mL/kg) free water deficit. The correction for this free water deficit takes many hours and should not be administered rapidly. Dextrose 5% with 0.45 normal saline is the preferred fluid with concomitant insulin infusion. Total body potassium deficit may be large and this should not be corrected rapidly either. Rapid potassium correction is likely to create life-threatening arrhythmias and too rapid a correction of free water creates the risk of central pontine myelinolysis, which may also have a high mortality. In contrast, the patient with hyperglycemic, hyperosmolar syndrome may have twice the free water deficit of the patient with DKA. The onset of HHNK state is usually a more prolonged and insidious process. In pediatric cases of HHNK, many of these patients are obese. The ability to diagnose dehydration in this population becomes more difficult.[18] In the case of pediatric HHNK, insulin boluses are discouraged. Insulin infusions are less precipitous with respect to glucose reduction. Despite its name, HHNK only presents with coma 30% of the time. Another proportion of patients presents with focal neurologic injury or seizures. Supportive care including fluid replacement and blood pressure support are the most important issues for these patients in an office-based environment.[17] As previously emphasized, the remainder of the complex treatment of these patients must be performed in a hospital environment because blood sugar, fluid, and electrolyte status can be closely observed and rapidly treated as changes occur in the patient.[19] Target blood sugar should be approximately 150 mg/dL and a blood glucose level of less than 100 mg/dL is associated with poor neurologic outcomes. These data are extrapolated from the current critical care literature.[20]

PHEOCHROMOCYTOMA

The perioperative initial finding of an unsuspected pheochromocytoma is a challenge in the office-based environment. The oral and maxillofacial surgeon may encounter this neoplasm but is rarely the first clinician to see this patient. Unexpected tachycardia, hypertension, diaphoresis, fever, and orthostatic hypotension may be the first clues to this problem.[21,22] The differential diagnosis of pheochromocytoma includes thyroid storm, MH, neuroleptic malignant syndrome, serotonin syndrome, or cocaine intoxication. Most pheochromocytomas are norepinephrine-secreting masses. The patient may be asymptomatic in the upright position, such as walking, whereas the seated patient may become symptomatic leaning forward or when intravenous anesthetic agents are administered. Induction of anesthesia may initiate a hyperdynamic episode of a pheochromocytoma that had not been diagnosed before the anesthetic. Unknown pheochromocytomas that are encountered intraoperatively for the first time may have mortalities as high as 50% from myocardial infarctions or strokes.[23] The hallmark of treating these patients involves alpha-blockade and beta-blockade because a large catecholamine surge may overcome only alpha-blockade or beta-blockade alone. Labetalol is the most appropriate intravenous agent in the oral and maxillofacial surgeon's office. However, caution is needed because labetalol has been associated with precipitating congestive heart failure.[24] Using pure beta-blockade without alpha-blockade may also result in congestive heart failure. For rhythm disturbances combined with hypertensive crises, magnesium sulfate has been successfully used for years. A loading dose of 1 to 2 g over 20 minutes followed by 1 to 2 g/h is a satisfactory dosing regimen. In 1985, the first report of its use in patients with pheochromocytomas was reported.[25] It has subsequently been used successfully in the intraoperative management of patients with pheochromocytomas and with minimal complications.[24] Drugs that should not be used in patients with pheochromocytomas include meperidine, droperidol, ketamine, and ephedrine. Morphine, as histamine releaser, has also been associated with triggering a hemodynamic crisis.[26] A case report also indicated that metoclopramide (Reglan) has also been implicated in unmasking a previously unknown pheochromocytoma.[27] Indirect-acting agents that include ephedrine are likely to initiate a hypertensive and tachycardic response. If a bolus vasopressor is needed, phenylephrine 50 to 100 µg per bolus are less likely to precipitate problems.

ADRENAL INSUFFICIENCY

Clinically significant adrenal insufficiency occurring in the oral and maxillofacial surgeon's office is a rare event unless the patient has been taking high-dose steroids. Lability of blood pressure, especially unexplained mild to moderate hypotension, may be the key to the diagnosis. There is not widespread literature to support the concept that this event is common or serious.[28] Most patients with a history of adrenal insufficiency are known before induction of anesthesia or sedation. Nevertheless, there are appropriate treatments for these patients if an episode is encountered. Because glucocorticoids assist catecholamines to increase vascular tone,[26] the immediate administration of glucocorticoids such as hydrocortisone 100 mg helps to reverse the hypotensive episodes. However, preoperative administration of glucocorticoids to prevent adrenal insufficiency varies among investigators, degree of surgical invasiveness, and duration and location of the procedure.[29] Etomidate should not be used in patients with adrenal insufficiency because it inhibits steroid synthesis, which in turn may cause acute adrenal insufficiency.[30]

HYPERTHYROIDISM

Thyroid storm, the most severe form of hyperthyroidism, is very uncommon in the United States in the era of modern medicine. Its onset may occur at any time from the perioperative period to 48 hours after surgery.[26] Symptomatic patients are usually well recognized before surgery and anesthesia. Elective surgery is postponed until they are functionally euthyroid. The differential diagnosis is similar to pheochromocytoma, MH, or cocaine toxicity. These patients present with tachycardia, labile blood pressure, and hyperthermia. Unlike neuroleptic malignant syndrome, these patients are not stuporous but may be delirious. If a patient presents with atrial fibrillation and fever, thyroid storm may be the cause.[31]

Because the mortality of thyroid storm varies from 10% to 75%, emergent treatment is required and should take place in a critical care environment as soon as possible.[26] Treatment includes hydrocortisone 100 mg to reduce the peripheral conversion of thyroxine (T4) to triiodothyronine (T3), sodium iodide, 500 mg to 1 g intravenously to promote the Wolff-Chaikoff (negative feedback for thyroid hormone synthesis) effect, propylthiouracil orally, and, most importantly, beta-blocker therapy, which reduces the peripheral conversion of T4 to T3. Emergent transfer of the patient from the office-based environment is mandatory. The patients require critical care observation for optimal and rapid recovery.

HYPOTHYROIDISM

Hypothyroidism usually has an insidious onset and does not require treatment on an emergent basis in the oral and maxillofacial surgeon's office. The administration of anesthesia in the patient with overt hypothyroidism (severe) may initiate hypothyroid coma. Unusual sensitivity to sedatives suggests hypothyroidism in unsuspected patients. Elective procedures must be postponed until the patient is optimized. Careful titration of levothyroxine is mandatory and should take place over several days in patients with suspected coronary artery disease. Rapid administration of levothyroxine and the administration of large doses may result in an acute myocardial infarction.[32] Patients with severe hypothyroidism are likely to require stress doses of hydrocortisone because patients with overt hypothyroidism are likely to manifest adrenocortical insufficiency. Complete reversal of all symptoms of hypothyroidism including muscular weakness may take many months. The patient is biochemically euthyroid by thyroid-stimulating hormone, T3, and T4 assays.[32]

NEUROLOGIC EMERGENCIES
Syncope

Establishing the cause of syncope is important and has a so-called 6P outline: preprodomal activity, prodromal activity such as visual symptoms and nausea, predisposing factors, precipitating causes, passerby or witness verification, and the postictal phases including frank seizure activity. Prodromal symptoms classically include nausea, weakness, diaphoresis, and loss of visual clarity.[33]

Pediatric syncope is usually accompanied by much concern from family members and clinicians. Despite the concern, a review in the pediatric cardiology literature indicates that less than 10% of patients evaluated had significant disorder.[34,35] Causes of pediatric syncope are either cardiac or noncardiac. In the pediatric population, neutrally mediated syncope (noncardiac) is more likely than cardiac.[36] The most common cause of syncope is vasodepressor (vasovagal) syncope. However, an in-depth history is the key to uncovering the cause. Treatment is supportive; use of the recumbent position is usually sufficient along with encouragement and appropriate education. If there is persistent bradycardia, intravenous administration of atropine 12 μg/kg (0.4 mg equivalent in the adult) helps to ameliorate the symptoms. Recurrent syncope should prompt a referral to a cardiologist. In the office-based environment, prolonged recovery or uncovering an arrhythmia should prompt the oral and maxillofacial surgeon to transfer the patient to the emergency room of the hospital for further definitive assessment and treatment. Cardiac causes of syncope are associated with 85% of sudden deaths in children and adolescents, and 17% of young athletes who have sudden death have a history of syncope.[35] Frequent common causes of syncope include psychological causes, which are seen in adolescents and not in children younger than 10 years of age. A cause of syncope in adolescent girls that should be considered before treatment by the oral and maxillofacial surgeon is pregnancy and pregnancy-related issues such as an ectopic pregnancy. Calling the emergency medical system (911) and establishing intravenous access with a non–dextrose-containing intravenous solution is imperative before transfer to an acute care facility. An ectopic pregnancy requires emergent transfer to a hospital and surgery to remove the ectopic fetus and correct additional bleeding sources.

Adult syncope tends to a more cardiac cause and is more common than pediatric syncope. However, in all age groups, vasovagal causes are still the most common cause of syncope.[37] Cardiac causes of syncope include many rhythm disturbances, most notably prolonged QT syndrome, Wolff-Parkinson-White syndrome, and the Brugada syndrome. The Brugada syndrome is notable for familial sudden death in young adults, caused by a right bundle branch block, and ST elevation in the right precordial leads (V1–V3), and it is unrelated to any structural, electrolyte, or ischemic disturbances.[38] Treatment of syncope in the adult is similar to that of pediatric syncope. Administer oxygen, establish intravenous access, and improve circulation by changing the patient's position by placing the patient in the recumbent or upright position, depending on the position in which the patient was in at the time of the prodrome or syncope. Some elderly patients may require intravenous fluids to improve their recovery profile from syncope because dehydration in the elderly patient is a common finding.

Seizures

Oral and maxillofacial surgeons are faced with several encounters in their practice lifetimes with patients who have seizures in their offices. A history of seizures is helpful, but other possibilities include head trauma, headaches, nuchal rigidity, febrile illness, and current anticoagulant therapy.[39] Most of these patients have readily identifiable causes of seizures that are likely self-limiting. Systemic reaction to local anesthesia from an inadvertent injection into a vein or artery has a rapid onset of seizure activity. Two-thirds of all systemic reactions were seizure activity according to one prominent report.[40] The use of bupivacaine

and etidocaine are specifically notable for problems.[41] Children are particularly vulnerable to local anesthesia–induced seizure activity in the presence of sedation.[42] If an oral and maxillofacial surgeon's practice uses a eutectic mixture of local anesthesia before placing intravenous access, care must taken to prevent a toxic reaction. The mixture (eutectic mixture of local anesthetics) should not be placed on denuded or injured skin. It should also be used with great care in the young pediatric patient population.[43] Treatment consists of airway management with the administration of oxygen; supportive care; and either a benzodiazepine, such as midazolam in small incremental doses, methohexital; or propofol in small doses if needed because of sustained activity. All sustained new-onset seizures require immediate assessment in the emergency department of an acute care facility.

Perioperative Stroke

Perioperative stroke varies in occurrence from 0.05% to 7% of patients. Many strokes occur in the postoperative period, including after discharge from the postanesthetic care unit.[44] As a result, patients who may have had a perioperative stroke in the oral and maxillofacial surgeon's office may not be known to the practice unless high-risk patients are followed by postoperative phone calls. Patients who are predisposed to perioperative stroke are those with advanced age, previous stroke, atrial fibrillation, vascular disease, and metabolic disease. Additional factors include female gender, diabetes, chronic obstructive pulmonary disease, smoking, chronic heart failure, and low ejection fraction.[45] Prevention of perioperative stroke requires optimization of risk factors, including use of antiplatelet therapy.[46,47] If a stroke evolves during procedures in the office, straightforward treatment is necessary. Classic findings of an acute stroke include acute facial asymmetry, slurring of the speech, limb function asymmetry, and patients stating that they are experiencing the worse headache of their lives. Effective treatment must include the termination of the surgical procedure as soon as it is safe to do so. If there is concern about the airway, the airway needs to be protected from possible aspiration of gastric contents by intubation of the trachea. Blood pressure that is abnormally increased should be carefully and gently lowered to less than 180 mg Hg systolic and 110 mm Hg diastolic. Drugs such as labetalol 5 to 10 mg every 10 to 15 minutes are helpful in controlling the patient's blood pressure. Esmolol in 10-mg to 20-mg increments helps to lower the patient's heart rate if it is unacceptably high (greater than 100 beats per minute.) Dramatic lowering of blood pressure may worsen the effects of the stroke in the watershed region. Most importantly, when calling 911, it is imperative for the caller in the oral and maxillofacial surgeon's office to indicate that there is a stroke in evolution. If the region where the oral and maxillofacial surgeon practices is sufficiently large, there may be a specific stroke center for patient transfer. Transferring the patient to a non–stroke center inevitably results in delay and aggressive inpatient stroke care. Early acute stroke care involves computed tomography scans; thrombolysis of clot, if appropriate; and possibly interventional radiologic procedures to remove the clot. On rare occasions, emergent craniotomy to evacuate a large extravascular clot may be indicated.

COAGULATION EMERGENCIES

Most procedures in the oral and maxillofacial surgeon's office are related to dentoalveolar surgery. Several investigators have suggested that it is safe to proceed with such surgery in patients who are taking anticoagulants.[48] Topical hemostatic agents such as oxycellulose, compression suture closure, and gauze compression are the bulwarks of treating hemorrhage during oral and maxillofacial surgery.[49] If unpredictable hemorrhage occurs during dentoalveolar surgery, the same principles apply for emergent treatment: compression of the wound by suture, topical hemostatic agents, and gauze compression. If a coagulopathy is suspected, then transfer of the patient to the emergency department of an acute care facility for component specific treatment of the coagulopathy. The emergency department has the advantage that specific tests are available for diagnosing the problem and treating appropriately.

REFERENCES

1. Perrott DH, Yuen JP, Andresen RV, et al. Office-based ambulatory anesthesia: outcomes of clinical practice of oral and maxillofacial surgeons. J Oral Maxillofac Surg 2003;61:983–95.
2. Perrott DH. Anesthesia outside the operating room in the office-based setting. Curr Opin Anaesthesiol 2008;21:480–5.
3. Available at: www.MHAUS.org. Accessed December 20, 2012.
4. Friesen CM, Brodsky JB, Dillingham MF. Successful use of dantrolene sodium in human malignant hyperthermia syndrome: a case report. Can Anaesth Soc J 1979;26:319–21.
5. Birgenheirer N, Stoker R, Westenkow D, et al. Activated charcoal effectively removes inhaled

anesthetics from modern anesthesia machines. Anesth Analg 2011;112:363–70.
6. Larach MG, Hirshey SJ, Belani KG, et al. Creation of a guide for the transfer of care of the malignant hyperthermia patient from ambulatory surgery centers to receiving hospital facilities. Anesth Analg 2012;114:94–100.
7. Bouchama A, Knochel JP. Heat stroke. N Engl J Med 2002;346:1978–88.
8. Capacchione JF, Muldoon SM. The relationship between exertional heat illness, exertional rhabdomyolysis, and malignant hyperthermia. Anesth Analg 2009;109:1065–9.
9. Klingler W, Rueffert H, Lehmann-Horn F, et al. Core myopathies and risk of malignant hyperthermia. Anesth Analg 2009;109:1167–73.
10. Dexter F, Epstein RH, Wachtel RE, et al. Estimate of the relative risk of succinylcholine for triggering malignant hyperthermia. Anesth Analg 2013;116:118–22.
11. Brandom BW, Larach MG, Chen MS, et al. Complications associated with the administration of dantrolene 1987 to 2006: a report from the North American Malignant Hyperthermia Registry of the Malignant Hyperthermia Association of the United States. Anesth Analg 2011;112:1115–23.
12. Joshi GP, Chung F, Vann MA, et al. Society for Ambulatory Anesthesia consensus statement on perioperative blood glucose management in diabetic patients undergoing ambulatory surgery. Anesth Analg 2010;111:378–87.
13. Lukins MB, Manninen PH. Hyperglycemia in patients administered dexamethasone for craniotomy. Anesth Analg 2005;100:1129–33.
14. Nazar CE, Lacassie HJ, López RA, et al. Dexamethasone for postoperative nausea and vomiting prophylaxis: effect on glycaemia in obese patients with impaired glucose tolerance. Eur J Anaesthesiol 2009;26:318–21.
15. Krinsley JS, Meyfroidt G, van den Berghe G, et al. The impact of premorbid diabetic status on the relationship between the three domains of glycemic control and mortality in critically ill patients. Curr Opin Clin Nutr Metab Care 2012;15:151–60.
16. Kitabachi AE, Umpierrez GE, Miles JM, et al. Hyperglycemic crises in adult patients with diabetes. Diabetes Care 2009;32:1335–43.
17. Kitabchi AE, Nyenwe EA. Hyperglycemic crises in diabetes mellitus: diabetic ketoacidosis and hyperglycemic hyperosmolar state. Endocrinol Metab Clin North Am 2006;33:725–51.
18. Zeitler P, Haqq A, Rosenbloom A, et al. Hyperglycemic hyperosmolar syndrome in children: pathophysiological considerations and suggested guidelines for treatment. J Pediatr 2011;158:9–14, 14.e1–2.
19. Weber JM. Diabetic ketoacidosis. In: Schaider JJ, Barkin RM, Hayden SR, et al, editors. Rosen & Barkin's 5-minute Emergency Medicine Consult.

4th edition. Philadelphia: Wolters Kluwer/Lippincott Williams & Wilkins; 2011. p. 308–9.

20. Jacobi J, Bircher N, Krinsley J, et al. Guidelines for the use of an insulin infusion for the management of hyperglycemia in critically ill patients. Crit Care Med 2012;40:3251–76.

21. Lord MS, Augoustides JG. Perioperative management of pheochromocytoma: focus on magnesium, clevidipine, and vasopressin. J Cardiothorac Vasc Anesth 2012;26:526–31.

22. Kumar V, Spivey J, Arthur M, et al. Pheochromocytoma detected during anesthesia induction. J Cardiothorac Vasc Anesth 2011;25:e43–4. Available at: http://www.jcvaonline.com/article/S1053-0770(11)00439-3/fulltext. Accessed January 02, 2013.

23. Hong JC. Pheochromocytoma. In: Singh-Radcliff N, editor. The 5-minute anesthesia consult. Philadelphia: Wolters Kluwer/Lippincott Williams & Wilkins; 2013. p. 656–7.

24. James MF, Cronjé L. Pheochromocytoma crisis: the use of magnesium sulfate. Anesth Analg 2004;99: 680–6.

25. James MF. The use of magnesium sulfate in the anesthetic management of pheochromocytoma. Anesthesiology 1985;62:188–90.

26. Kohl BA, Schwartz S. How to manage perioperative endocrine insufficiency. Anesthesiol Clin 2010;28: 139–55.

27. Sheinberg R, Gao WD, Wand G, et al. A perfect storm: fatality resulting from metoclopramide unmasking a pheochromocytoma and its management. J Cardiothorac Vasc Anesth 2012;26:161–5.

28. Gibson N, Ferguson JW. Steroid cover for dental patients on long-term steroid medications: proposed clinical guidelines based upon a critical review of the literature. Br Dent J 2004;197:681–5.

29. Jung C, Inder WJ. Management of adrenal insufficiency during the stress of medical illness and surgery. Med J Aust 2008;188:409–13.

30. Lundy JB, Slane ML, Frizzi JD. Acute adrenal insufficiency after a single dose of etomidate. J Intensive Care Med 2007;22:111–7.

31. Ghobral MW, Ruby EB. Coma and thyroid storm in apathetic thyrotoxicosis. South Med J 2002;95: 552–4.

32. Murkin JM. Anesthesia and hypothyroidism: a review of thyroxine physiology, pharmacology, and anesthetic implications. Anesth Analg 1982;61:371–83.

33. Mossier J, Keim SA. Syncope. In: Schaider JJ, Barkin RM, Hayden SR, et al, editors. Rosen and Barkin's 5 minute emergency medicine consult. 4th edition. Philadelphia: Wolters, Kluwer/Lippincott, Williams & Wilkins; 2011. p. 1088–9.

34. Johnsrude CL. Current approach to pediatric syncope. Pediatr Cardiol 2000;21:522–31.

35. Fischer JW, Cho CS. Pediatric syncope: cases from the emergency department. Emerg Med Clin North Am 2010;28:501–16.

36. Del Rosso A, Alboni P, Brignole M, et al. Relation of clinical presentations of syncope to the age of patients. Am J Cardiol 2005;96:1431–5.

37. Marrison VK, Fletcher A, Parry SW. The older patient with syncope: practicalities and controversies. Int J Cardiol 2012;155:9–13.

38. Wilde AA, Antzelevitch C, Borggrefe M, et al. Proposed diagnostic criteria for the Brugada syndrome: consensus report. Circulation 2002;106:2514–9.

39. Gupta A, Smith-Coggins R. Seizures, adult. In: Schaider JJ, Barkin RM, Hayden SR, et al, editors. Rosen and Barkin's 5-minute emergency consult. 4th edition. Philadelphia: Wolters Kluwer/Lippincott Williams & Wilkins; 2011. p. 1004–5.

40. Di Gregorio G, Neal JA, Rosenquist RW, et al. Clinical presentation of local anesthetic systemic toxicity: a review of published cases, 1979 to 2009. Reg Anesth Pain Med 2010;35:181–7.

41. Bacsik CJ, Swift JQ, Hargreaves KM. Toxic systemic reactions of bupivacaine and etidocaine. Oral Surg Oral Med Oral Pathol Oral Radiol Endod 1995;79: 18–23.

42. Moore PA. Adverse drug interactions in dental practice: interactions associated with local anesthetics, sedatives and anxiolytics. J Am Dent Assoc 1999; 130:541–54.

43. Rincon E, Baker RL, Iglesias AJ, et al. CNS toxicity after topical application of EMLA cream on a toddler with molluscum contagiosum. Pediatr Emerg Care 2000;16:252–4.

44. Ng JL, Chan MT, Gelb AW. Perioperative stroke in noncardiac, nonneurosurgical surgery. Anesthesiology 2011;115:879–90.

45. Selim M. Perioperative stroke. N Engl J Med 2007; 356:706–13.

46. Szeder V, Torbey MT. Prevention and treatment of perioperative stroke. Neurologist 2008;14:30–6.

47. Au V, Smith-Coggins R. Cerebral vascular accident. In: Schaider JJ, Barkin RM, Hayden SR, et al, editors. Rosen and Barkin's 5 minute emergency consult. 4th edition. Philadelphia: Wolters Kluwer/Lippincott Williams & Wilkins; 2011.

48. Beirne OR. Evidence to continue oral anticoagulant therapy for ambulatory oral surgery. J Oral Maxillofac Surg 2005;63:540–5.

49. Karsh ED, Erdogan O, Esen E, et al. Comparison of the effects of warfarin and heparin on bleeding caused by dental extraction: a clinical study. J Oral Maxillofac Surg 2011;69:2500–7.

Managing the Untoward Anesthetic Event in an Oral and Maxillofacial Surgery Practice

Steven I. Kaltman, DMD, MD*, Michael Ragan, DMD, JD, LLM,
Osbel Borges, DMD

KEYWORDS

- Anesthesia certification • Untoward anesthesia event • Emergency medicine protocol
- Professional liability • Apology • Second victim

KEY POINTS

- There has been a significant increase in the number of outpatient surgical procedures and administration of sedation/anesthesia in the United States, resulting in a greater risk of an untoward anesthesia event.
- An untoward anesthesia event must be reported to the practitioner's professional liability insurance carrier and State Board of Dentistry/Regulatory agencies as soon as possible after such events.
- Compliance with training programs and familiarity with established emergency protocols are essential for all oral and maxillofacial surgery (OMS) staff involved with patient care.
- Disclosure of information associated with an untoward anesthetic outcome, as well as the apology that is often appropriated after such an event, should be discussed with the OMS's counsel.
- A cataclysmic patient injury or death can lead to significant emotional distress for the oral maxillofacial practitioner and their team, which can potentially lead to significant and permanent psychological limitations.

Dentistry through the legacy of Horace Wells, DDS and William T.G. Morton, DDS has a rich history in the administration of anesthesia to alleviate pain and anxiety. For oral and maxillofacial surgeons, the administration of sedation and general anesthesia in the office setting has been a hallmark of the specialty for many decades. The safe and efficient use of outpatient surgical anesthesia modalities is a significant part of the training and expertise of the oral and maxillofacial surgeon.[1–7]

The most recent anesthesia morbidity and mortality data reported by the Oral and Maxillofacial Surgeons National Insurance Company (OMSNIC) from 2000 to 2011 show that the average oral and maxillofacial surgeon performs 669 office anesthetic procedures per year, of which 71% are general anesthetics and 29% are sedation anesthetics, for a total of 33,191,562 cases over the 11-year period. Ninety-one in-office cases of death and brain damage were reported, along with 33 cases of hospital death and brain damage for a total of 124 cases and an average in-office mortality rate of 1 per 364,742. According to this report, the average oral and maxillofacial surgeon will perform 20,070 in-office anesthetics over a 30 year period. Considering a mortality rate of 1/364,742, these data suggest that 1 in 18 oral

Department of Oral and Maxillofacial Surgery, College of Dental Medicine, Nova Southeastern University, 3200 South University Drive, Fort Lauderdale, FL 33328, USA
* Corresponding author.
E-mail address: skaltman@nova.edu

Oral Maxillofacial Surg Clin N Am 25 (2013) 515–527
http://dx.doi.org/10.1016/j.coms.2013.03.006
1042-3699/13/$ – see front matter © 2013 Elsevier Inc. All rights reserved.

and maxillofacial surgeons will experience an in-office death over their career, and as this report accounts for 49,581 oral and maxillofacial surgeon years, it can be extrapolated that 1 in 545 oral and maxillofacial surgeons will experience an office anesthetic death per year.[8]

The experience of the oral and maxillofacial surgery (OMS) practice and the administration of sedation/anesthesia during ambulatory surgery reflect an excellent safety record. Over the life of an OMS practice, there is a small but definable chance that an untoward anesthesia event (UAE) will occur, placing all oral and maxillofacial surgeons performing outpatient anesthesia at risk of experiencing a UAE resulting in cataclysmic injury to the patient or death. Although adverse outcomes are rare, they can have considerable traumatic psychological and professional consequences for the surgeon involved. Although oral and maxillofacial surgeons are highly trained in the management of the airway and managing complications and emergencies associated with the administration of anesthesia, this training does not prepare them to handle the aftermath of an untoward outcome or adverse event. Unfortunately, when bad outcomes do occur there are 2 sets of victims. The first set of victims and the most affected is the patient and the families. The doctor is the second victim suffering from the same bad outcome, having to deal with devastation, pain, frustration, overwhelming stress and anxiety negatively affecting their health and interpersonal relationships.[9] Bad outcomes do occur to good doctors who are good practitioners and when things go wrong it may or may not be to the result of negligence. It is not uncommon for the doctor to experience a long and extremely stressful legal process involving complex inter-actions with attorneys, courtrooms, and juries. Ironically, as surgeons, we have well-established guidelines and procedural algorithms for our surgical and anesthesia practice but no such guidelines to follow to help us deal with crisis management if we encounter a bad outcome. There is little written in the literature to guide us through the misfortune of an adverse outcome. The goal of this article is to develop guidelines to educate the doctor, the second victim, on how to manage a bad outcome and how to navigate through a difficult and arduous process.

CERTIFICATION FOR ADMINISTRATION OF SEDATION/ANESTHESIA

Within the United States, the practice of OMS is regulated by each state's Dental Practice Act, which sets out the requirements for certification for the administration of the various levels of sedation and anesthesia. The certification process involves an application and the provision of credentials and/or additional training to be confirmed by the appropriate certification. It is not expected that an oral maxillofacial surgeon will require a significant amount of additional education or training based on the amount of anesthesia training provided within OMS residency programs in North America. It is important that the oral maxillofacial surgeon is cognizant of the training requirements for the OMS team.

It is imperative that each practitioner in the OMS is current with their Advanced Cardiac Life Support (ACLS) certification and that the requisite emergency monitoring and resuscitation equipment, pharmaceutical agents, current permits, and so forth are maintained.

In addition, many states require inspection of the ambulatory facility in which the sedation/anesthesia is to be administered. The regulatory inspection of the facilities may be performed on an annual basis or by unannounced inspections. The OMS practitioner must be aware of the requirements for the display of appropriate state Department of Health and Board of Dentistry certification documents.

MEDICAL EMERGENCY RESPONSE OFFICE PROTOCOL

Each OMS office must maintain a medical emergency response office protocol document (the Protocol) outlining, with specificity, the procedures for responding to the occurrence of an UAE or other medical emergency. This Protocol must include documentation of regular medical emergency response office education and training including practice sessions and unannounced emergency response drills. The documentation must include the date, time and names of the OMS team participants present for the emergency training, and the documentation of attendance must be dated and signed by all participants.

The Protocol must contain certification that each member of the OMS team has received requisite training in medical emergency response, ACLS certification, has maintained said training and is up to date with all required credentials. Copies of the certification for continuing education programs necessary for maintaining the office certification for sedation/anesthesia administration should be maintained as part of the Protocol document.

The Protocol document must contain the specific delegation of medical emergency response duties and responsibilities for each member of the OMS team. Each member of the OMS team must be aware of, trained, and examined in their specific duties in the event of a medical emergency. The following are essential components of this protocol outlining specific team member responsibility:

- The Protocol must include specific designation of the team members who are to assist the oral maxillofacial surgeon with the direct ventilation/resuscitation efforts on the patient.
- The Protocol must specify which members of the OMS team are responsible for documentation of the patient's vital signs, including O_2 saturation, heart rate, blood pressure, respiration, skin tone, pallor, and any other signs of distress. It is imperative to designate 1 or more members of the OMS team specifically to document, in hand written notes or on the electronic health care record, the patient's vital signs, the type, time, and duration of all manner of ventilation/resuscitation efforts, and must include the time, amount, and route of administration of pharmaceutical agents, and the patient's response to said efforts.
- The Protocol must designate 1 or more members of the OMS team who is specifically designated to contact the emergency medical services/911 (EMS) when instructed. The time of the telephone contact must be documented in the clinical records. It is important that the OMS team member so designated is level headed and clear when imparting the requisite information to the EMS team. In addition, the OMS team designee should be instructed to remain on the telephone with EMS dispatch to maintain contact with the EMS vehicle while it is en route. An OMS team member should be designated to be stationed outside the entrance of the office to direct EMS personnel to the correct room in the most expeditious manner.
- Each member of the OMS team who has designated duties must have a specific backup personnel designated for all emergency procedures should there be a change in personnel, absences, sickness, and so forth. It is imperative that as changes in the OMS team occur the team members' duties must be redesignated accordingly. Continual education and training sessions are a must.
- The Protocol document must include details of the maintenance of all anesthesia, sedation, ventilation/resuscitation equipment, medications/pharmaceutical agents, and so

forth. It is imperative that this document is complete and up to date.

CLINICAL DOCUMENTATION

Before the initiation of sedation/anesthesia administration, a medical history must be completed, updated and reviewed by the oral and maxillofacial surgeon. The medical history form must be completed by the patient and should be witnessed by an authoritative member of the OMS team or the surgeon. There must be documentation of discussion with the patient concerning their medical history before the initiation of any administration of sedation/anesthesia including documentation of their American Society of Anesthesiologists (ASA) classification. The clinical documentation must include the fact that written preanesthesia and postanesthesia instructions were provided. If necessary, the fact that the patient was to be nil by mouth (NPO) for a requisite time period must be documented as well as the name and the relationship of the person/attendant who is responsible for the patient after the completion of the procedure.

The attendant is to bring the patient to and from the appointed procedure and is instructed that, during anesthesia recovery time, the patient should not drive or operate complicated machinery/devices, make important decisions, execute documents, and so forth.

The surgeon's treatment plan must include a specific list of the procedures that will be performed, which includes the correct Current Dental Terminology (CDT)/Current Procedural Terminology (CPT) code for the sedation/anesthesia procedure that is planned. In addition, the Ambulatory Anesthesia Report must be fully completed with all requisite information including confirmation of the correct date and the names of the personnel who are assisting in the procedure. For each sedative/anesthesia agent that is administered, the amount and time of administration must be stated and must be noted contemporaneously on the anesthesia report. All documentation for emergency and resuscitation efforts must be detailed with specificity including the time, personnel, patient response, and the time of notification of EMS/911. The vital signs monitor displays the patient's vital signs, but in some cases, the information can be lost if the monitor is turned off before the information is printed. There have been cases when vital signs monitoring equipment was turned off by EMS personnel after entering the surgical suite and none had the forethought to print the information or to document the clinical information. If the information contained within the vital signs monitor is lost, this has a significant impact on any subsequent investigation.

INFORMED CONSENT

Before any surgical procedure, the surgeon and the patient/patient's guardian must engage in the surgical procedure informed consent discussion process. In addition, a separate sedation/anesthesia informed consent discussion process must be completed. As part of the sedation/anesthesia informed consent discussion process, the patient must be provided with the requisite information to allow them to make an informed decision concerning the administration of the sedation/anesthesia that is scheduled.

The information provided to the patient during the sedation/anesthesia informed consent discussion must include an explanation of the parameters of the sedation/anesthesia procedure planned including the type of agent, the route of administration, and so forth. A discussion of all reasonable alternative sedation/anesthesia modalities available must be included; which also includes the option of having no sedation/anesthesia. The discussion must include all the material risks that may occur during the administration of sedation/anesthesia as well as the recovery phase. The informed consent process must include a discussion of the necessity of having a responsible adult attendant to transport the patient, respond to postoperative instructions including fulfillment of prescriptions, and ensure that the postanesthetic patient refrains from any analytical or complicated activity until fully competent. The adult attendant's name and contact information should be placed in the clinical documentation.

At the completion of the of the surgical procedure and sedation/anesthesia informed consent discussion processes, the discussions must be confirmed in writing, signed by the patient and/or their guardian, dated, signed by the person who is performing the surgical procedure and sedation/anesthesia, or dated and signed by an adult competent witness.

The clinical documentation must contain a statement confirming that the sedation/anesthesia informed consent discussion took place, that the patient/guardian had the opportunity to ask questions, and that all questions were responded to and understood by the patient. In the authors' experience, informed consent documents in which each paragraph of separate information is numbered with a box for the patient to initial to confirm that they have read and understood the information seem to be received better by a jury. Examples of informed consent process documentation forms are available from OMSNIC.

EMERGENCY MEDICAL SERVICES

While the EMS/911 personnel are being contacted, the surgeon and the team must continue to stabilize the patient. When the EMS/911 personnel have entered the outpatient facility/operatory and have assumed responsibility for the care/treatment/resuscitation efforts on the patient, documentation of the EMS efforts should be continued by a member of the OMS team. If the surgeon is not assisting with the resuscitation efforts, he or she should continue to document said efforts either directly in the clinical records or on a separate piece of paper to be placed in the clinical record/electronic health record at a later time.

It is important that the EMS/911 personnel are provided with all the information concerning the preoperative patient medical history, amounts, type, and route of administration of anesthesia/sedation agents, the patient reaction, description of the surgical procedure, whether completed or not, and any other relevant information. The information provided to the EMS/911 personnel should also include the patient's medical history and any salient information regarding allergies, syndromes, Mallampati score/airway issues, medication that the patient is taking, and so forth.

A specific description of the UAE should be provided to the EMS/911 personnel when transferring control of patient care and should include a description of the clinical procedure that was being performed, the specifics on the anesthesia (all drugs administered, amount, types, times, route of administration), and a specific explanation of the ventilatory resuscitative efforts performed on the patient and the patient's response. If the surgeon is assisting the EMS/911 personnel in the resuscitation of the patient, the surgeon may be requested to accompany the EMS/911 and the patient in the emergency transport vehicle. If not, another member of the OMS team may be requested to accompany the EMS/911 and the patient in the emergency vehicle.

A member of the OMS team must be assigned to provide information to the person/persons who accompanied the patient to the OMS office. Only objective information concerning the patient's condition should be provided during the stabilization process and the patient's attendant should not be allowed to witness the emergency resuscitative efforts. The OMS personnel providing this information must do so in a discreet manner so as to not generate concern in other patients present in the reception area. Be cognizant of the fact that any information that is provided to a third party can be misinterpreted/misunderstood and could be used in a subsequent Department of Health/Board of Dentistry investigation or civil litigation.

HOSPITAL EMERGENCY DEPARTMENT

The surgeon should be present at the hospital emergency department (ED) where their patient is transported to provide any information requested by emergency personnel. This may include information previously provided to EMS personnel that may require clarification. An OMS team member may be assigned to accompany the patient's family member/attendant to the ED.

While the OMS team is at the ED, they will likely be in a reception/waiting room area with the person/people who accompanied the patient to their OMS appointment. The OMS team should attempt to respond to inquiries by the patient's family/friends in a calm and objective manner. Be cognizant that any information provided by the OMS team to the patient's attendant/family may be misunderstood or misconstrued. In addition, conversations between the surgeon and members of the OMS team in the presence of third parties may be admissible in subsequent investigations/litigation. The surgeon and the OMS team should maintain a level of professionalism including empathy for the patient's condition and that of their friends and family. The OMS team discussion should not use terms of legal art including, but not limited, to negligence, liability, lawsuit, guilty, standard of care, medical error, mistake, and so forth.

REPORTING AN UAE TO THE PROFESSIONAL LIABILITY INSURANCE CARRIER

As soon as possible/practicable, the surgeon must report the UAE as an incident to their professional liability (PL) insurance carrier. The surgeon may report through an insurance agent or directly to their PL carrier. The sooner the incident is reported to the PL insurance carrier, the sooner the carrier will assign an attorney to the insured, if warranted.

The importance of timely reporting to the PL carrier is reiterated because these companies employ professionals who understand health care misadventures and can provide counsel concerning the specific mechanisms of action necessary. In addition, if the insured surgeon fails to report an incident that may provide the basis of a claim to their PL carrier within a reasonable time, this could potentially adversely affect the professional insurance coverage for that event. On balance, it is always prudent to report an incident that does not result in a claim rather than risk late reporting of an incident that does become a claim, thereby delaying the preparation of a defense strategy.

APPOINTMENT OF DEFENSE COUNSEL AND THE POST-UAE PROCEDURE

The assigned PL defense attorney (Defense Counsel) will assist with communication to the patient/family, the development of a strategy if litigation or regulatory action is forthcoming, reporting the UAE/adverse medical event to regulatory agencies, and in the drafting of narrative summary documents by the OMS team.

After Defense Counsel is appointed, they will confer with the OMS team as soon as possible to conduct interviews. A detailed narrative summary by the surgeon and each member of the OMS team is drafted using objective assessments of all facts and circumstances. The only subjective assessment should include statements made by the patient, the patient's family, and so forth. All narrative summaries should state "attorney client privilege" and "work product privilege." The narrative summaries of the OMS team members should be kept in a file separate from the clinical documentation. The file should be entitled: Litigation File "Patient Name" (Litigation File).

The clinical documentation of the patient encounter and any associated anesthesia records/report, vital signs recording data, and so forth, must be legible, complete, and correct. The documentation should be rechecked to make certain that the information included in the clinical record is comprehensive and contemporaneous. The clinical documentation and Litigation File should be sequestered from other patients' clinical documentation and placed separately in a fireproof waterproof locked safe or metal filing cabinet.

In the event of an UAE or medical misadventure, the operatory/surgical suite must remain as it was left when the EMS transported the patient to the hospital ED. Photographs of the operatory/surgical suite should be taken to ensure that no corruption of the suite has occurred. Records should not to be disposed of and any vials of anesthesia/sedation agents must be maintained in a sealed hard plastic container or in a plastic bag. Clinical operatories can be cleaned, but information must be maintained and safely stored. Equipment must be sequestered to allow inspection if there are allegations of product liability/equipment malfunction in any subsequent negligence litigation.

The surgeon and any other personnel involved with the patient's treatment must document all relevant information after the occurrence of the

UAE. The OMS team should never change or delete any existing entries in the clinical record. If needed, an amendment note should be written with careful explanation of why an amendment is necessary, particularly explaining the professional judgment involved. The team should state the facts as they are known and make no judgments concerning cause or responsibility. The same guidelines hold true for the filing of the incident report to the state regulatory agencies, which should be drafted within the requisite time period.

All discussions with the patient or family should be carefully documented in the clinical record. Although opinions may vary by jurisdiction, it is strongly suggested that the OMS team make their own set of complete personal notes, including personal opinions and observations about treatment, as soon as possible after the event. These will be extremely valuable 2 to 5 years later if necessary when preparing for testimony. It is critical that these personal notes are immediately given, as they are written, to the practitioners' attorneys, marking them "attorney client privilege"/"work product privilege" and thus preventing later discovery of the notes by anyone else.

Another potential duty of the Defense Counsel is scheduling of grief counseling for the OMS team. There is a discussion later on the effect that cataclysmic patient injuries/death resulting from a UAE can have on the OMS team, both professionally and personally.

REPORTING THE UAE TO STATE REGULATORY AGENCIES

Most states have specific requirements within their Dental Practice Act or Department of Health to report adverse anesthesia occurrences or similarly termed events to state regulatory agencies. The OMS practitioner and team must be aware of the specific requirement to report adverse anesthesia occurrences and must be familiar with the specific requirements in the states in which they practice. Some states require the initial reports to be filed within 48 hours and may require a specific delivery requirement (eg, registered mail). The Board of Dentistry/Board of Medicine governing rules outline the information that needs to be provided.

Many states also require an additional report containing more comprehensive information. Incidents that may be required to be reported are those that result in temporary, permanent, physical or mental injury requiring hospital emergency room treatment and hospitalization of a patient during, or as a result of the use of general anesthesia, deep sedation, conscious sedation, pediatric conscious sedation, oral sedation, nitrous oxide, or local anesthesia during or relating to a dental procedure. Many states require that the report includes, at a minimum, responses to the following:

- A description of the dental procedure
- A description of the preoperative physical condition of the patient
- A list of the drugs and doses administered
- A description and detail of techniques of the drugs used
- A description of adverse occurrence including not limited to
  1. Description in detail of any complication to include but not limited to the onset of any symptoms in the patient
  2. The treatment instituted on the patient
  3. Response of the patient to the treatment
- The condition of the patient and termination of any procedure undertaken[10]

In addition, if the surgeon has a double degree, DDS/DMD and MD or Doctor of Osteopathic Medicine, then they must report an adverse anesthesia occurrence to all regulatory boards under which they are presently licensed. Boards of Dentistry, Medicine, Osteopathic Medicine, and so forth may have requirements to report all outpatient medical misadventures (adverse incident reports) that do not involve the administration of local or other types of anesthesia. Again, it is imperative that the practitioner be aware of the reporting requirements in the jurisdictions within which they practice. Failure to report in a timely manner could be construed to be a violation of the Dental Practice Act or Medical Practice Act and could become probable cause for the OMS practitioner to be sanctioned by regulatory agencies, including fines, restriction of practice, mandatory continuing education, loss of anesthesia certification, suspension, or revocation of their dental/medical license.

OMS VISITATION AT THE HOSPITAL OR SERVICES

The surgeon should remain at the ED after the UAE until the patient stabilizes or a final decision is made concerning the patients' condition. The more difficult decision is whether the surgeon should visit the hospital afterward if the patient remains admitted or, in the event of death, should the surgeon attend funeral services. There is no bright line rule as to the correct decision.

The surgeon must be cognizant of the dynamics of an encounter with the family of a patient who has been admitted to a hospital as a result of a UAE. The family may not have a sufficient knowledge base to understand the reason why their family member has been hospitalized and the surgeon must realize that the environment in the hospital will be emotionally charged. Similarly, the funeral services of a patient who succumbed after a UAE could be emotionally volatile.

We advise the surgeon to contact the patient/family to inform them of their intention to visit/attend and to request their permission before their attendance at the hospital and/or services. Expressions of sympathy are appropriate as are the provision of flowers or donations to designated charities. Discussion with the patient's family/friends using terms of legal art including liability, negligence, medical error, and so forth should be avoided.

MEDIA, PROFESSIONAL, AND PATIENT INQUIRIES

The OMS team must be aware of the potential for information inquiries after a cataclysmic UAE. The OMS team should be instructed to not speak to any person except their assigned Defense Counsel concerning the facts and circumstances surrounding the UAE. This includes refraining from any discussion of the UAE with their personal family members, friends, patients, practitioners, or amongst team members themselves.

In this the era of social media, the OMS team must be cognizant that information (and misinformation) spreads quickly and may be dispersed via all types of social media platforms (Facebook, texting, Twitter, iVideo/audio from smart phones) and can be uploaded onto the World Wide Web. If the OMS office has a Facebook page, they should not respond to inquiries concerning a UAE.

During any media inquiry, the OMS team must be aware that they may be video/audio taped and should be careful when speaking with people they cannot identify on the telephone. In addition, they should be careful about speaking on cellular phones where third parties can overhear their conversation. Information maintained on computers, smart phones, and so forth, must be password protected and the password should not be shared with others.

After a UAE involving a cataclysmic outcome, the OMS office will likely receive inquiries from fellow health care practitioners concerning the specifics of the event. Some of these inquiries may come from colleagues seeking information and offering assistance, but others may be inquiries from OMS referral base practitioners. The OMS team must be aware that the provision of information involving protected health care information to a third party without the proper patient authorization would be a violation of the Healthcare Insurance Portability and Accountability Act (HIPAA).[11]

Similarly, patients may make inquiries. Again the provisions of HIPAA apply and a practitioner disclosing protected health care information without the appropriate authorizations can be subject to sanction. No specific patient information or information concerning regulatory investigation/potential litigation can be provided without the patient/family's written authorization or a subpoena from an official regulatory/judicial authority.

In the event of conventional media inquiry concerning a UAE, it is suggested that the OMS team speak with only 1 voice; preferably their Defense Counsel.

SHOULD THE ORAL MAXILLOFACIAL SURGEON RETAIN A PERSONAL COUNSEL?

As the surgeon may be aware, the Defense Attorney retained by their PL insurance carrier has a fiduciary duty to the surgeon, but their defense fees are paid by the insurance company. In cases where cataclysmic patient injuries/death occurs, there may exist potential for personal financial exposure to the surgeon above and beyond the indemnity limits of their insurance policy. Therefore, circumstances may arise when it would be prudent for the surgeon to retain a personal attorney to advise them and protect their personal interests if issues arise whereby their insured interests may not coincide with those of the PL insurance company. Each UAE would have to be assessed based on the specific facts and circumstances as to whether the retention of a personal attorney is warranted.

In some jurisdictions, the death of a patient at an ambulatory surgery facility can be investigated by the local authorities as a potential criminal event. The surgeon must be cognizant of the fact that, depending on the facts and circumstances of the specific UAE, although unlikely, they could be investigated for criminal prosecution. If that is the case, the surgeon must retain a personal criminal defense attorney to protect their interests.

WHEN IS AN APOLOGY TO A PATIENT AND/OR THEIR FAMILY APPROPRIATE?

There is much disagreement surrounding the discussion of when an apology is not an admission of liability, but rather an act of humanity. Multiple studies have demonstrated that patients clearly want errors disclosed and that they desire that clinicians apologize for their errors. However, clinicians frequently cite fear of malpractice lawsuits as a reason to avoid apologizing for an error.[12]

Many states have enacted apology statutes, which have allowed patients, next of kin, and practitioners to engage in discussions when the adverse outcome may have warranted an apology and when appropriate. Current states with apology statutes are listed in **Table 1**.

We strongly suggest that the surgeon consults their counsel/personal Defense Counsel before engaging in an apology discussion. Clearly, a poorly crafted apology can constitute an admission against the practitioner's interest. However, others have found that the act of apologizing with no admission of negligence or liability is an act of humanity that restores all parties.[13]

One health care practitioner and author has proffered that medical concepts of mistakes,

Table 1
States with apology statutes

State	Statute
Arizona	Arizona A.R.S. 12-2605 (2005)
California	California Evidence Code 1160 (2000)
Colorado	Colorado Revised Statute 13-25-135 (2003)
Connecticut	Connecticut Public Act No. 05-275 Sec.9 (2005) amended (2006) Conn. Gen. Stat. Ann. 52-184d
Delaware	Delaware Del. Code Ann. Tit. 10, 4318 (2006)
Florida	Florida Stat 90.4026 (2001)
Georgia	Georgia Title 24 code GA Annotated 24-3-37.1 (2005)
Hawaii	Hawaii HRS Sec.626-4 (2006)
Idaho	Idaho Title 9 Evidence Code Chapter 2.9-207
Illinois	Illinois Public Act 094-0677 Sec. 8-1901, 735 ILL. Comp. Stat. 5/8-1901 (2005)
Indiana	Indiana Ind. Code Ann. 34-43.5-1-1 to 34-43.5-1-5
Iowa	Iowa HF 2716 (2006)
Louisiana	Louisiana R.S. 13:3715.5 (2005)
Maine	Maine MRSA tit. 2908 (2005)
Maryland	Maryland MD Court & Judicial Proceedings Code Ann. 10-920 (2004)
Massachusetts	Massachusetts ALM GL ch. 233, 23D (1986)
Missouri	Missouri M. Ann. Stat. 538.229 (2005)
Montana	Montana Code Ann. 26-1814 (Mont. 2005)
Nebraska	Nebraska Neb. Laws L.B. 373 (2007)
New Hampshire	New Hampshire RSA 507-D:4 (2005)
North Carolina	North Carolina General Stat. 8C-1, Rule 413
North Dakota	North Dakota ND H.B. 1333 (2007)
Ohio	Ohio ORC Ann 2317.43 (2004)
Oklahoma	Oklahoma 63 OKL. St. 1-1708.1H (2004)
Oregon	Oregon Rev. Stat. 677.082 (2003)
South Carolina	South Carolina Ch.1, Title 19 Code of Laws 1976, 19-1-190 (2005)
South Dakota	South Dakota Codified Laws 19-12-14 (2005)
Tennessee	Tennessee Evid Rule 409.1 (2003)
Texas	Texas Civil Prac and Rem Code 18.061 (1999)
Utah	Utah Code Ann. 78-14-18 (2006)
Vermont	Vermont S 198 Sec. 1. 12 V.S.A. 1912 (2006)
Virginia	Virginia Code of Virginia 8.01-52.1 (2005)
Washington	Washington Rev Code
West Virginia	West Virginia 55-7-11a (2005)
Wyoming	Wyoming Wyo. Stat. Ann. 1-1-130

Data from Aon Healthcare, 2007.

errors, and bad results require medical judgments, whereas the legal concepts of fault, negligence, and culpability are defined by legal standards. Injured patients are willing to forgive if the clinician is upfront with them. Medical mistakes do not trigger most malpractice suits; they result from patient/family anger about being spurned by caregivers after something goes wrong. Most malpractice claims arise from communication breakdown and full disclosure not only improves the litigation climate but also encourages better safety practices. The acceptance of full disclosure rests primarily with health care practitioners and to a much lesser degree with lawyers and legislators.[14]

In common law, an apology that includes an admission of negligence/fault may be admissible as evidence to support the liability of the defendant health care practitioner's liability. All statements made in the course of informal settlement negotiations, including apologies, can be admitted into evidence. Statements made in the course of court ordered settlement negotiations such as at mediation are confidential and not discoverable. Therefore, an apology may be admissible as evidence at trial, and an apology that is entered into evidence is considered to be an admission by the defendant health care practitioner.

There are exceptions to the common law rule. First, apologies framed as hypothetical are not admissible; second, apologies that are preceded by exclusionary language such as "without prejudice to any of his legal rights, defendant admits..." are also inadmissible.

Based on an apology, the patient may file a complaint with the state Board of Dentistry, Board of Medicine, or Department of Health, which would result in an investigation. The apology may tempt a trial attorney to advise the patient to file a Department of Health complaint. Because the states' health care regulatory agencies are governed by consumer protection legislation, each complaint (even if anonymous) against a licensed health care practitioner must be investigated and likely will involve the subpoenaing of clinical documentation and review by an expert for the state. Therefore, if the state's investigation yields a decision of probable cause and an administrative complaint is filed against the licensee, the investigative file becomes public record. The state will have conducted an investigation with an expert opinion report that would be discoverable and admissible in subsequent medical malpractice litigation. Effectively, the state will have funded discovery of a claim and the assertion of negligent care, using tax dollars, from which the patient may file medical malpractice litigation with little or no cost to the patient or their attorney.

If the oral maxillofacial surgeon practices in 1 of the 34 states and the District of Columbia that have enacted apology statutes, the surgeon must consider several questions when investigating their apology statute.

1. Is a statement of fault admissible?
2. Whose statements are protected?
3. To whom is the apology to be made?
4. Is the apology protected if oral and written?
5. Is an offer of additional assistance to a patient discoverable? (Clearly, medical bills should be dismissed.)
6. Is there a time limit by which a health care practitioner must proffer an apology to remain protected?[15]

Several investigators have questioned whether apologies have any impact on potential medical malpractice litigation. A recent study released from the University of Michigan reported on its comprehensive program to use apologies and offer financial compensation upfront after an unanticipated outcome. According to a 2009 article in the *Journal of Health and Life Science Law*, malpractice claims against the University of Michigan Health System fell from 121 claims in 2001 to 61 claims in 2006.

Curt and dismissive comments from an oral maxillofacial surgeon or defensive posturing will not be productive. Patients and families do request an immediate unbiased investigation with complete disclosure, a nonpatronizing demeanor, practices and systems changed to prevent a similar event, standards of care mandated with regulatory systems in place and a leader in charge, and justice.

Several investigators have queried whether the health care community can characterize and address the human dimensions of medical error so that patients, families, and clinicians may reach some degree of closure and move toward forgiveness?[16] Clearly, much work remains to be performed in this area.

THE SECOND VICTIM

Mistakes and errors happen in most spheres of human life and activity, including medicine. When things go wrong during a health care encounter resulting in cataclysmic patient injury or death, there are often 2 victims; the patient who is harmed and the health care practitioner involved in the care.[17] Dr Wu coined the term "second victim" in 2000 stating that "many errors are built into existing routines and devices, setting up the unwitting physician and patient for disaster. And, although patients are the first and obvious victims of medical mistakes, doctors are wounded by the same errors: they are the second victims."[9] Second victims often feel personally responsible for the patient outcome and feel as though they failed the patient. They often second guess their clinical skills and knowledge base.[18]

The deleterious effect that a cataclysmic patient injury/death may have on the OMS team should not be diminished. Care should be taken with the decision on whether the OMS team believe they can return to administering patient care the same day as the UAE or even the next day. Grief counseling may ameliorate the immediate effect but there may be lingering consequences for months or years, evolving into to posttraumatic stress disorder.[19] Scott and colleagues[18] described the natural history of recovery for the second victim after a UAE. After interviewing 31 second victim health care providers, a predictable pattern of postevent trajectory of recovery consisting of 6 stages was identified. These are summarized in **Table 2**.

The sixth stage seemed to be the most critical in determining the ultimate fate of the heath care provider. What is of preeminent importance is that the OMS team must be secure and continue on with their professional and personal life.

A health care practitioner and a patient have developed a new program for providing trauma support services to people who have experienced unanticipated outcomes from medical care or, more particularly, the failure of medical care. Medically Induced Trauma Support Services or MITSS (http://www.mitss.org) was developed in partnership by a patient and an anesthesiologist involved in an unanticipated event that seriously harmed the patient.[20]

The emotional toll of medical error is high for both patients and clinicians, who are often unsure with whom and whether they can discuss what happened. Although institutions are increasingly adopting full disclosure policies, trainees frequently do not disclose mistakes, and faculty health care practitioners are underprepared to teach communication skills related to disclosure and apology. Several health care practitioners have developed an interactive educational program for trainees and faculty health care practitioners that assesses experiences, attitudes, and perceptions about error, explores the human impact of error through filmed patient and family narratives, develops communication skills, and offers a strategy to facilitate bedside disclosures.[21]

Between spring 2007 and fall 2008, 154 trainees (medical students/residents) and 75 medical educators completed the program. Among the learners surveyed, 62% of trainees and 88% of faculty physicians reported making medical mistakes. Of those, 62% and 78%, respectively, reported that they did not apologize. Sixty-five percent of trainees said they would turn to senior doctors for assistance after an error, but 26% were not sure where to get help. Just 20% of trainees and 21% of physicians reported adequate training to respond to error.[22]

An emotional response was reported in 82.4% of reports. Of those reports in which an emotional response was reported, a coping strategy was reported in 62.8%. The top 4 reported emotional responses were frustration (48.3%), embarrassment (31.5%), anger (12.6%), and guilt (10.1%). Physicians reported an emotional response more often than clinic staff. An emotional response was reported more often when there was a possibility of harm. Coping strategies were reported as follows: 52% talked to someone about the incident, 37.2% did nothing in response to the incident, 17.9% told the patient about the incident, and 3.6% did something else. Female physicians reported using coping strategies less often than male physicians. A coping strategy was reported more often when there was a possibility of harm.

Individuals who choose to become health care professionals are likely to be exposed to emotional turmoil repeatedly during their careers. It is normal for clinical members of health care teams to face unfortunate events with their patients. Entire health care teams can suffer when unanticipated clinical events or medical errors occur. Patient suffering from complications of treatment or consequences of medical mistakes can shake the strongest clinical foundation of seasoned health care providers, even jolting their career paths.[23]

There is a profound irony here for health care delivery systems adopting strategies of continuous quality improvement (CQI). The reality is that although the fear of legal liability/repercussions prevents open discussion concerning mistakes, it is only through disclosure and opening of attitudes that the causes of mistakes can be identified, systems can be improved, future mistakes minimized and/or prevented, and attitudes toward medical misadventures can be modified.[24]

Disclosure is 1 component of coping strategies developed for the second victim.[25] These strategies are summarized in **Table 3**.

Effective disclosure can improve doctor and patient relations, facilitate better understanding of systems, and potentially decrease medical malpractice costs. However, many health care practitioners remain wary of discussing errors with patients because of concern about litigation, the communication challenges of disclosure, and loss of self-esteem.[26]

Table 2
Research team consensus for trajectory of recovery

Stages	Stage Characteristics	Common Questions
Stage 1 Chaos and accident response	Error realized/event recognized Tell someone → get help Stabilize/treat patient May not be able to continue care of patient Distracted	How did that happen? Why did that happen?
Stage 2 Intrusive reflections	Reevaluate scenario Self isolate Haunted reenactments of event Feelings of internal inadequacy	What did I miss? Could this have been prevented?
Stage 3 Restoring personal integrity	Acceptance among work/social structure Managing gossip/grapevine Fear is prevalent	What will others think? How much trouble am I in? How come I can't concentrate?

Stage 4
Enduring the inquisition
	Realization of level of seriousness
	Reiterate case scenario
	Respond to multiple why's about
	  the event
	Interact with many different
	  event responders
	Understanding event disclosure
	  to patient/family
	Physical and psychological
	  symptoms
		How do I document?
		What happens next?
		Who can I talk to?
		Will I lose my job/license?
		How much trouble am I in?

Stage 5
Obtaining emotional first aid
	Seek personal/professional
	  support
	Getting/receiving help/support
	Litigation concerns emerge
		Why did I respond in this
		  manner?
		What is wrong with me?
		Do I need help?
		Where can I turn for help?

Stage 6
Moving on (1 of the 3
  trajectories chosen)
	Dropping out
	Transfer to a different unit or
	  facility
	Consider quitting
	Feelings of inadequacy
	Surviving
	Coping, but still have intrusive
	  thoughts
	Persistent sadness, trying to learn
	  from event
	Thriving
	Maintain life/work balance
	Gain insight/perspective
	Does not base practice/work
	  on 1 event
	Advocates for patient safety
	  initiatives
		Is this the profession I should
		  be in?
		Can I handle this kind of work?
		How could I have prevented this
		  from happening?
		Why do I still feel so badly/guilty?
		What can I do to improve our
		  patient safety?
		What can I learn from this?
		What can I do to make it better?

Adapted from Scott SD, Hirschinger LE, Cox KR. The natural history of recovery for the healthcare provider "second victim" after adverse patient events. Qual Saf Health Care 2009;18:329; with permission.

Unfortunately, providers are often reluctant to discuss these emotions with colleagues and may not seek support from others as they cope with these emotions. Recent evidence shows that health care practitioners are dissatisfied with the emotional support they receive from health care institutions after medical errors. Multiple barriers present challenges for health care leaders in designing effective support programs, including physician perceptions of efficacy, privacy, and

Table 3
Coping with mistakes and errors in judgment

1	Accept responsibility for the mistake
2	Discuss with colleagues
3	Disclose and apologize to the patient
4	Conduct an error analysis
5	Make changes in practice or practice setting designed to reduce future errors
6	Work at local and national levels to change the culture of the medical profession with regard to the management of medical mistakes

Modified from Goldberg RM, Kuhn G, Andrew LB, et al. Coping with medical mistakes and errors in judgment. Ann Emerg Med 2002;39(3):289; with permission.

availability. However, a few malpractice insurers and large medical centers have created programs that successfully provide emotional support to providers after errors through one-on-one counseling.[27]

MAINTAINING YOUR PRACTICE

As the demand for ambulatory OMS and anesthesia has increased, the incidence of UAE resulting in a cataclysmic result has also increased. The media have seized on the opportunity to increase the profile of these anesthesia misadventures in ambulatory health care.[28]

These events can and do occur in the absence of a violation of the standard of care, and their occurrence should not provide an inference that the practitioner was negligent. If an investigation of the UAE determines that the OMS team/practice requires remediation; this must be done. If an investigation involves litigation/lawsuits, those will be handled by the PL insurance carrier, the Defense Attorney, and possibly the personal attorney. The standard of care in medicine is not perfection. The most important necessity is for the OMS team to develop the ability to continue with their professional and personal lives.

REFERENCES

1. D'Eramo EM. Morbidity and mortality with outpatient anesthesia: the Massachusetts experience. J Oral Maxillofac Surg 1992;50:700.
2. D'Eramo EM. Mortality and morbidity with outpatient anesthesia: the Massachusetts experience. J Oral Maxillofac Surg 1999;61:793.
3. D'Eramo EM, Bontempi WJ, Howard JB. Anesthesia morbidity and mortality experience among Massachusetts oral and maxillofacial surgeons. J Oral Maxillofac Surg 2008;66:2421–33.
4. D'Eramo EM, Bookless SJ, Howard JB. Adverse events with outpatient anesthesia in Massachusetts. J Oral Maxillofac Surg 2003;61:793–800.
5. Hunter MJ. Morbidity and mortality with outpatient anesthesia: the experience of a residency training program. J Oral Maxillofac Surg 1997;55:684.
6. Perrott DH, Yuen JP, Andersen RV, et al. Office-based ambulatory anesthesia: outcomes of clinical practice or oral and maxillofacial surgeons. J Oral Maxillofac Surg 2003;61:983–95.
7. Rodgers SF, Rodgers MS. Safety of intravenous sedation administered by the operating oral surgeon: the second 7 years of office practice. J Oral Maxillofac Surg 2011;69:2525–9.
8. Oral and Maxillofacial Surgery National Insurance Company. Anesthesia morbidity and mortality: 2000-2011. Rosemont (IL): OMSNIC; 2012.
9. Wu AW. Medical error: the second victim. The doctor who makes the mistake needs help too. BMJ 2000;320(7237):726–7.
10. FN: Florida Administrative Code 64B-5 14.006, Formerly 21G-14.006, Amended 12-20-93, Formerly 61F5-14.006, Amended 8-8-96, Formerly 59Q-14.006, Amended 11-4-03, 12-25-06, 8-5-12.
11. Health Insurance Portability and Accountability Act of 1996 (HIPAA; Pub.L. 104–191, 110 Stat. 1936, enacted August 21, 1996).
12. Hickson GB, Clayton EW, Githens PB, et al. Factors that prompted families to file medical malpractice claims following perinatal injuries. JAMA 1992;267:1359–63.
13. McDonald WM, Gunther E. Narrative: State Laws make it necessary to say "I'm Sorry". Ann Intern Med 2008;149:811–5.
14. Sanbar SS. Medical error and disclosure and apology. In: Sanbar SS, editor. Medical malpractice survival handbook. 1st edition. Mosby/Elsevier; 2007.
15. Segal J, Sacopulos MJ. Apology laws: a variety of approaches to discussing adverse medical outcomes with patients and others. AHLA Connections 2009;13(11):26.
16. Delbanco T, Bell SK. Guilty, afraid, and alone — struggling with medical error. N Engl J Med 2007;357:17.
17. Catchpole K. Who do we blame when it all goes wrong? Qual Saf Health Care 2009;18:3–4.
18. Scott SD, Hirschinger LE, Cox KR, et al. The natural history of recovery for the healthcare provider "second victim" after adverse patient events. Qual Saf Health Care 2009;18:325–30.
19. Sakran JV, Kaafarani H, Mouawad NJ, et al. When things go wrong. Bulletin of the American College of Surgeons 2011 Aug;13–6.

20. Kenney LK, van Pelt RA. To err is human; the need for trauma support is, too – a story of the power of patient/physician partnership after a sentinel event. Patient Safety and Quality Healthcare 2005; 2(1):6–9.

21. Bell SK, Moorman DW, Delbanco T. Improving the patient, family, and clinician experience after harmful events: the "when things go wrong" curriculum. Acad Med 2010;85(6):1010–7.

22. O'Beirne M, Sterling P, Palacios-Derflingher L, et al. Emotional impact of patient safety incidents on family physicians and their office staff. J Am Board Fam Med 2012;25(2):177–83.

23. Scott SD, Hirschinger LE, Cox KR, et al. Caring for our own: deployment of a second victim rapid response system. Jt Comm J Qual Patient Saf 2010;36(5):233–40.

24. Smith ML, Forster HP. Morally managing medical mistakes. Camb Q Healthc Ethics 2000;9:38–53.

25. Goldberg RM, Kuhn G, Andrew LB, et al. Coping with medical mistakes and errors in judgment. Ann Emerg Med 2002;39(3):287–92.

26. Souter KJ, Gallagher TH. The disclosure of unanticipated outcomes of care and medical errors: what does this mean for anesthesiologists? Anesth Analg 2012;114(3):615–21.

27. White AA, Waterman A, McCotter P, et al. Supporting health care workers after medical error: considerations for healthcare leaders. J Clin Outcomes Manag 2008;15:240–7.

28. Chuchmach M, Ross B. Nightline: Death, greed at the dentist: American children at risk. ABC Nightline. New York: American Broadcasting Company; July 12, 2012.

Index

Note: Page numbers of article titles are in **boldface** type.

oralmaxsurgery.theclinics.com

Moving?

Make sure your subscription moves with you!

To notify us of your new address, find your **Clinics Account Number** (located on your mailing label above your name), and contact customer service at:

Email: journalscustomerservice-usa@elsevier.com

800-654-2452 (subscribers in the U.S. & Canada)
314-447-8871 (subscribers outside of the U.S. & Canada)

Fax number: 314-447-8029

Elsevier Health Sciences Division
Subscription Customer Service
3251 Riverport Lane
Maryland Heights, MO 63043

ELSEVIER

Moving?

Make sure your subscription moves with you!

To notify us of your new address, find your Clinics Account Number (located on your mailing label above your name), and contact customer service at:

Email: journalscustomerservice-usa@elsevier.com

800-654-2452 (subscribers in the U.S. & Canada)
314-447-8871 (subscribers outside of the U.S. & Canada)

Fax number: 314-447-8029

**Elsevier Health Sciences Division
Subscription Customer Service
3251 Riverport Lane
Maryland Heights, MO 63043**

To ensure uninterrupted delivery of your subscription, please notify us at least 4 weeks in advance of move.

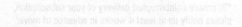

Printed and bound by CPI Group (UK) Ltd, Croydon, CR0 4YY

03/10/2024

01040370-0006